Cutaneous Oncology

Editor

DAVID E. FISHER

HEMATOLOGY/ONCOLOGY CLINICS OF NORTH AMERICA

www.hemonc.theclinics.com

Consulting Editors
GEORGE P. CANELLOS
EDWARD J. BENZ JR

October 2024 • Volume 38 • Number 5

ELSEVIER

1600 John F. Kennedy Boulevard • Suite 1800 • Philadelphia, Pennsylvania, 19103-2899

http://www.theclinics.com

HEMATOLOGY/ONCOLOGY CLINICS OF NORTH AMERICA Volume 38, Number 5
October 2024 ISSN 0889-8588, ISBN 13: 978-0-443-24652-4

Editor: Stacy Eastman
Developmental Editor: Sukirti Singh

Photocopying
Single photocopies of single articles may be made for personal use as allowed by national copyright laws. Permission of the Publisher and payment of a fee is required for all other photocopying, including multiple or systematic copying, copying for advertising or promotional purposes, resale, and all forms of document delivery. Special rates are available for educational institutions that wish to make photocopies for non-profit educational classroom use. For information on how to seek permission visit www.elsevier.com/permissions or call: (+44) 1865 843830 (UK)/(+1) 215 239 3804 (USA).

Derivative Works
Subscribers may reproduce tables of contents or prepare lists of articles including abstracts for internal circulation within their institutions. Permission of the Publisher is required for resale or distribution outside the institution. Permission of the Publisher is required for all other derivative works, including compilations and translations (please consult www.elsevier.com/permissions).

Electronic Storage or Usage
Permission of the Publisher is required to store or use electronically any material contained in this periodical, including any article or part of an article (please consult www.elsevier.com/permissions). Except as outlined above, no part of this publication may be reproduced, stored in a retrieval system or transmitted in any form or by any means, electronic, mechanical, photocopying, recording or otherwise, without prior written permission of the Publisher.

Notice
No responsibility is assumed by the Publisher for any injury and/or damage to persons or property as a matter of products liability, negligence or otherwise, or from any use or operation of any methods, products, instructions or ideas contained in the material herein. Because of rapid advances in the medical sciences, in particular, independent verification of diagnoses and drug dosages should be made.

Although all advertising material is expected to conform to ethical (medical) standards, inclusion in this publication does not constitute a guarantee or endorsement of the quality or value of such product or of the claims made of it by its manufacturer.

Hematology/Oncology Clinics (ISSN 0889-8588) is published bimonthly by Elsevier Inc., 360 Park Avenue South, New York, NY 10010-1710. Months of issue are February, April, June, August, October, and December. Business and Editorial Offices: 1600 John F. Kennedy Blvd., Ste. 1800, Philadelphia, PA 19103–2899. Customer Service Office: 3251 Riverport Lane, Maryland Heights, MO 63043. Periodicals postage paid at New York, NY and at additional mailing offices. Subscription prices are $498.00 per year (domestic individuals), $100.00 per year (domestic students/residents), $525.00 per year (Canadian individuals), $100.00 per year (Canadian students/residents), $597.00 per year (international individuals), and $255.00 per year (international students/residents). For institutional access pricing please contact Customer Service via the contact information below. International air speed delivery is included in all *Clinics* subscription prices. All prices are subject to change without notice. Orders, claims, and journal inquiries: Please visit our Support Hub page https://service.elsevier.com for assistance.

Reprints. For copies of 100 or more, of articles in this publication, please contact the Commercial Reprints Department, Elsevier Inc., 360 Park Avenue South, New York, New York 10010-1710; Tel.: 212-633-3874, Fax: 212-633-3820, E-mail: reprints@elsevier.com.

Hematology/Oncology Clinics of North America is covered in *MEDLINE/PubMed (Index Medicus), EMBASE/ Excerpta Medica, and BIOSIS.*

Contributors

CONSULTING EDITORS

GEORGE P. CANELLOS, MD
William Rosenberg Professor of Medicine, Department of Medical Oncology, Dana-Farber Cancer Institute, Boston, Massachusetts, USA

EDWARD J. BENZ Jr, MD
Professor, Pediatrics, Richard and Susan Smith Professor, Medicine, Professor, Genetics, Harvard Medical School, President and CEO Emeritus, Office of the President, Dana-Farber Cancer Institute, Boston, Massachusetts, USA

EDITOR

DAVID E. FISHER, MD, PhD
Chairman, Department of Dermatology, Cutaneous Biology Research Center, Massachusetts General Hospital, Charlestown, Massachusetts, USA; Department of Dermatology, Harvard Medical School, Massachusetts General Hospital, Boston, Massachusetts, USA

AUTHORS

YUSUF ACIKGOZ, MD
Division of Medical Oncology, Department of Internal Medicine, The Ohio State University Comprehensive Cancer Center, Columbus, Ohio, USA

DAHIANA AMARILLO, MD
Oncóloga Médica, Asistente del Servicio de Oncología Clínica, Prof Adj del, Departamento Básico de Medicina, Universidad de la República, Montevideo, Uruguay

GENEVIEVE M. BOLAND, MD, PhD
Vice Chair of Research, Department of Surgery, Massachusetts General Hospital, Boston, Massachusetts, USA

NICOLE L. BOLICK, MD, MPH, MS
Dermatology Resident Physician, Department of Dermatology, University of New Mexico School of Medicine, Albuquerque, New Mexico, USA

FABIANA BONCIMINO, PhD
Student, Research Fellow, Cutaneous Biology Research Center, Massachusetts General Hospital, Harvard Medical School, Charlestown, Massachusetts, USA

CELINE BOUTROS, MD
Oncologist, Dermatology Unit, Department of Medicine, Gustave Roussy Cancer Campus, Villejuif, France

ISAAC BROWNELL, MD, PhD
Senior Investigator, Dermatology Branch, NIAMS, NIH, Bethesda, Maryland, USA

JINA CHUNG, MD
Assistant Professor, Department of Dermatology, Perelman School of Medicine at the University of Pennsylvania, Philadelphia, Pennsylvania, USA

CAN CUI, MD, PhD
Clinical Fellow, Department of Medicine, Massachusetts General Hospital, Harvard Medical School, Boston, Massachusetts, USA

MICHAEL A. DAVIES, MD, PhD
Professor, Division of Cancer Medicine, Department of Melanoma Medical Oncology, The University of Texas MD Anderson Cancer Center, Houston, Texas, USA

SHADMEHR DEMEHRI, MD, PhD
Associate Professor, Department of Dermatology, Harvard Medical School, Massachusetts General Hospital, Principal Investigator, Center for Cancer Immunology, Center for Cancer Research, Cutaneous Biology Research Center, Boston, Massachusetts, USA

DAVID E. FISHER, MD, PhD
Chairman, Department of Dermatology, Cutaneous Biology Research Center, Massachusetts General Hospital, Charlestown, Massachusetts, USA; Department of Dermatology, Harvard Medical School, Massachusetts General Hospital, Boston, Massachusetts, USA

KEITH T. FLAHERTY, MD
Director of Clinical Research, Mass General Cancer Center, Massachusetts General Hospital, Harvard Medical School, Boston, Massachusetts, USA

JESSICA L. FLESHER, PhD
Research Fellow, Department of Dermatology, Cutaneous Biology Research Center, Massachusetts General Hospital, Harvard Medical School, Charlestown, Massachusetts, USA

ALAN C. GELLER, MPH, RN
Senior Lecturer, Department of Social and Behavioral Sciences, Harvard T.H. Chan School of Public Health, Boston, Massachusetts, USA

ANTONY HADDAD, MD
Postdoctoral Research Fellow, Department of Surgical Oncology, The University of Texas MD Anderson Cancer Center, Houston, Texas, USA

PATRICK HALLAERT, BS
Postbaccalaureate Fellow, Dermatology Branch, NIAMS, NIH, Bethesda, Maryland, USA

MERVE HASANOV, MD
Assistant Professor, Division of Medical Oncology, Department of Internal Medicine, The Ohio State University Comprehensive Cancer Center, Columbus, Ohio, USA

HUGO HERRSCHER, MD
Medical Oncologist, Oncology Unit, Saint Anne Clinic, Groupe Hospitalier Saint Vincent, Strasbourg, France

BARAA ASHRAF HIJAZ, BS
MD Candidate, Department of Dermatology, Massachusetts General Hospital, Harvard Medical School, Boston, Massachusetts, USA

ASHLEY M. HOLDER, MD
Assistant Professor, Department of Surgical Oncology, The University of Texas MD Anderson Cancer Center, Houston, Texas, USA

YANEK JIMÉNEZ-ANDRADE, PhD
Instructor, Department of Dermatology, Cutaneous Biology Research Center, Massachusetts General Hospital, Harvard Medical School, Charlestown, Massachusetts, USA

SARA YASMIN KHATTAB, BS
MD Candidate, Department of Dermatology, Massachusetts General Hospital, Boston, Massachusetts, USA

ELLEN J. KIM, MD
Professor, Department of Dermatology, Perelman School of Medicine at the University of Pennsylvania, Perelman Center for Advanced Medicine, Philadelphia, Pennsylvania, USA

TRUELIAN LEE, BA
Research Assistant, Harvard Medical School, Massachusetts General Hospital, Boston, Massachusetts, USA

ANNA MANDINOVA, MD, PhD
Associate Professor, Department of Dermatology, Cutaneous Biology Research Center, Massachusetts General Hospital, Harvard Medical School, Boston, Massachusetts, USA; Broad Institute of Harvard and MIT, 7 Cambridge Center, Harvard Stem Cell Institute, Cambridge, Massachusetts, USA

TOMONORI OKA, MD, PhD
Research Fellow, Center for Cancer Immunology, Center for Cancer Research, Department of Dermatology, Cutaneous Biology Research Center, Massachusetts General Hospital, Boston, Massachusetts, USA

STEPHEN M. OSTROWSKI, MD, PhD
Instructor, Department of Dermatology, Cutaneous Biology Research Center, Massachusetts General Hospital, Charlestown, Massachusetts, USA; Department of Dermatology, Harvard Medical School, Massachusetts General Hospital, Boston, Massachusetts, USA

PATRICK A. OTT, MD, PhD
Associate Professor of Medicine, Department of Medicine, Harvard Medical School, Department of Medical Oncology, Dana-Farber Cancer Institute, Brigham and Women's Hospital; Broad Institute of MIT and Harvard, Cambridge, Massachusetts, USA

JIN MO PARK, PhD
Associate Professor, Department of Dermatology, Cutaneous Biology Research Center, Massachusetts General Hospital, Harvard Medical School, Charlestown, Massachusetts, USA

CAROLINE ROBERT, MD, PhD
Dermatologist, Faculty of Medicine, University Paris-Saclay, Kremlin-Bicêtre, France; Co-director of the Melanoma Research Unit, INSERM Unit U981, Head of Dermatology Unit, Department of Medicine, Gustave Roussy Cancer Campus, Villejuif, France

YEVGENIY ROMANOVICH SEMENOV, MD, MA
Assistant Professor, Co-director of the Oncodermatology Program, Department of Dermatology, Massachusetts General Hospital, Harvard Medical School, Massachusetts, USA

ALAIN H. ROOK, MD
Professor, Department of Dermatology, Perelman School of Medicine, University of Pennsylvania, Philadelphia, Pennsylvania, USA

KAILAN SIERRA-DAVIDSON, MD, DPhil
Resident Physician, Department of Surgery, Massachusetts General Hospital, Boston, Massachusetts, USA

STEFANO SOL, PhD
Research Fellow, Department of Dermatology, Cutaneous Biology Research Center, Massachusetts General Hospital, Harvard Medical School, Charlestown, Massachusetts, USA

JENNIFER STRONG, BS, MRSP
Fellow, Dermatology Branch, NIAMS, NIH, Bethesda, Maryland, USA

RYAN J. SULLIVAN, MD
Physician Investigator (CI), Mass General Cancer Center, Associate Professor, Department of Medicine, Harvard Medical School, Boston, Massachusetts, USA

KRISTINA TODOROVA, PhD
Clinical Research Associate II, Department of Dermatology, Cutaneous Biology Research Center, Massachusetts General Hospital, Harvard Medical School, Charlestown, Massachusetts, USA

JENNIFER VILLASENOR-PARK, MD, PhD
Associate Professor, Department of Dermatology, Perelman School of Medicine at the University of Pennsylvania, Perelman Center for Advanced Medicine, Philadelphia, Pennsylvania, USA

DAVID M. WEINER, MD, MBE
Resident, Department of Dermatology, Johns Hopkins University School of Medicine, Baltimore, Maryland, USA

CATHERINE J. WU, MD
Professor, Department of Medicine, Harvard Medical School, Brigham and Women's Hospital, Department of Medical Oncology, Dana-Farber Cancer Institute; Broad Institute of MIT and Harvard, Cambridge, Massachusetts, USA

YIFAN ZHANG, MD, PhD
Department of Dermatology, Cutaneous Biology Research Center, Massachusetts General Hospital, Charlestown, Massachusetts, USA; Department of Dermatology, Harvard Medical School, Massachusetts General Hospital, Boston, Massachusetts, USA

Contents

Melanoma is the most commonly fatal type of skin cancer, and it is an important and growing public health problem in the United States and worldwide. Fortunately, incidence rates are decreasing in young people, stabilizing in middle-aged people, and increasing in older individuals. Herein, the authors further describe trends in melanoma incidence and mortality, review the literature on risk factors, and provide an up-to-date assessment of population-wide screening and new technology being utilized in melanoma screening.

Cutaneous imaging is a central tenant to the practice of dermatology. In this article, the authors explore various noninvasive and invasive skin imaging techniques, as well as the latest deployment of these technologies in conjunction with the use artificial intelligence and machine learning. The authors also provide insight into the benefits, limitations, and challenges around integrating these technologies into dermatologic practice.

The skin consists of several cell populations, including epithelial, immune, and stromal cells. Recently, there has been a significant increase in single-cell RNA-sequencing studies, contributing to the development of a consensus Human Skin Cell Atlas. The aim is to understand skin biology better and identify potential therapeutic targets. The present review utilized previously published single-cell RNA-sequencing datasets to explore human skin's cellular and functional heterogeneity. Additionally, it summarizes the functional significance of newly identified cell subpopulations in processes such as wound healing and aging.

Cutaneous melanoma is an aggressive form of skin cancer derived from skin melanocytes and is associated with significant morbidity and mortality. A significant fraction of melanomas are associated with precursor lesions, benign clonal proliferations of melanocytes called nevi. Nevi can be either congenital or acquired later in life. Identical oncogenic driver mutations are found in benign nevi and melanoma. While much progress has been made in our understanding of nevus formation and the molecular steps required for transformation of nevi into melanoma, the clinical diagnosis of benign versus malignant lesions remains challenging.

Kailan Sierra-Davidson and Genevieve M. Boland

Melanoma remains one of the most common cancers diagnosed in the United States, yet there have been substantial advancements in the treatment of resectable disease. Adjuvant therapy with immune checkpoint blockade (ICB) and targeted therapy with BRAF/MEK inhibitors (BRAF/MEKi) have now become standard of care for resectable stage IIIB-IV melanoma. In this article, the authors discuss recent scientific developments pertinent to the treatment of resectable melanoma including ICB, targeted therapy with BRAF/MEKi, oncolytic viruses, tumor-infiltrating lymphocyte therapy, and cancer vaccines.

Dahiana Amarillo, Keith T. Flaherty, and Ryan J. Sullivan

Melanoma, a malignant tumor of melanocytes, poses a significant clinical challenge due to its aggressive nature and high potential for metastasis. The advent of targeted therapy has revolutionized the treatment landscape of melanoma, particularly for tumors harboring specific genetic alterations such as BRAF V600E mutations. Despite the initial success of targeted agents, resistance inevitably arises, underscoring the need for novel therapeutic strategies. This review explores the latest advances in targeted therapy for melanoma, focusing on new molecular targets, combination therapies, and strategies to overcome resistance.

Celine Boutros, Hugo Herrscher, and Caroline Robert

Melanoma has seen the most remarkable therapeutic improvements among all cancers in the past decade, primarily due to the development of immune checkpoint inhibitors (ICI). Initially developed in the patients with advanced disease, ICI are now used in adjuvant and neoadjuvant settings. More recently, the development of LAG-3 blocking antibody and the combination of ICI with a personalized RNA-based vaccine have continued to lead the immunotherapeutic field. Despite these advances, primary and secondary resistances remain problematic and there is a high need for predictive biomarkers to optimize benefit/risk ratio of ICI use.

Yanek Jiménez-Andrade, Jessica L. Flesher, and Jin Mo Park

Pruritus, rash, and various other forms of dermatotoxicity are the most frequent adverse events among patients with cancer receiving targeted molecular therapy and immunotherapy. Immune checkpoint inhibitors, macrophage-targeting agents, and epidermal growth factor receptor/MEK inhibitors not only exert antitumor effects but also interfere with molecular pathways essential for skin immune homeostasis. Studying cancer therapy-induced dermatotoxicity helps us identify molecular mechanisms governing skin immunity and deepen our understanding of human biology. This review summarizes new mechanistic insights emerging from the analysis of cutaneous adverse events and discusses knowledge gaps that remain to be closed by future research.

Metastasis to the brain is a frequent complication of advanced melanoma. Historically, patients with melanoma brain metastasis (MBM) have had dismal outcomes, but outcomes have improved with the development of more effective treatments, including stereotactic radiosurgery and effective immune and targeted therapies. Despite these advances, MBM remains a leading cause of death from this disease, and many therapies show decreased efficacy against these tumors compared with extracranial metastases. This differential efficacy may be because of recently revealed unique molecular and immune features of MBMs-which may also provide rational new therapeutic strategies.

Personalized neoantigen vaccines have achieved major advancements in recent years, with studies in melanoma leading progress in the field. Early clinical trials have demonstrated their feasibility, safety, immunogenicity, and potential efficacy. Advances in sequencing technologies and neoantigen prediction algorithms have substantively improved the identification and prioritization of neoantigens. Innovative delivery platforms now support the rapid and flexible production of vaccines. Several ongoing efforts in the field are aimed at improving the integration of large datasets, refining the training of prediction models, and ensuring the functional validation of vaccine immunogenicity.

The microbiome plays a substantial role in the efficacy of immune checkpoint blockade (ICB) in patients with metastatic melanoma. While the exact gut microbiome composition and the pathways involved in this interaction are not clearly delineated, novel studies and ongoing clinical trials are likely to reveal findings applicable to the clinical setting for the prediction and optimization of response to ICB. Nevertheless, lifestyle modifications, including high fiber diet, avoidance of unnecessary antibiotic prescriptions, and careful use of probiotics may be helpful to optimize the "health" of the gut microbiome and potentially enhance response to ICB in patients with melanoma.

high-risk resectable MCC. Emerging biomarkers of tumor burden are becoming increasingly important in identifying high-risk patients and in post-treatment surveillance. Further research is needed to determine the optimal duration of anti-PD-(L)1 treatment and second-line options for patients with MCC refractory to immunotherapy. This review covers the characteristics and management of MCC including recent innovations and areas of active investigation.

HEMATOLOGY/ONCOLOGY CLINICS OF NORTH AMERICA

THE CLINICS ARE AVAILABLE ONLINE!
Access your subscription at:
www.theclinics.com

Preface

Cutaneous Oncology and Its Rapid Forward Progress

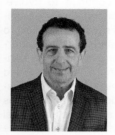

David E. Fisher, MD, PhD
Editor

Few conditions in human medicine have experienced the combination of clinical as well as conceptual advances as skin cancer in recent years. While much of this progress has stemmed from advances in melanoma, significant changes have occurred for multiple cutaneous neoplasms. This issue brings together a collection of articles that provide updated reviews on the many aspects of skin cancer that simultaneously highlight treatment advances, underlying mechanistic insights, technologic breakthroughs, and applications beyond the settings in which they were first discovered or applied.

While melanoma is one of the best characterized lethal cancers linked to an environmental carcinogen (UV), it has taken many years before decreases in incidence are starting to be observed. Roles of UV protection, early detection, and behavioral modification (such as tanning legislation) are increasingly emphasized yet remain very challenging to fully exploit. Basic immunology of the skin has proven highly relevant not only to immune surveillance of mutated premalignant neoplasms but also to the understanding of common cutaneous toxicities from immunotherapy as well as targeted therapy. The applications of systemic targeted and immune checkpoint inhibitor therapies have led to numerous FDA-approved first-line treatments for advanced highly lethal skin malignancies. Most strikingly, the clinical benefits of these treatments are frequently associated with durable regressions, likely related to combinations of broad antigen targeting, bystander-related target killing, and immunologic memory. Perhaps most dramatically, more recent studies have demonstrated significantly enhanced relapse-free survival when the same agents are applied in the adjuvant or neoadjuvant

Hematol Oncol Clin N Am 38 (2024) xiii–xv
https://doi.org/10.1016/j.hoc.2024.05.015
0889-8588/24/© 2024 Published by Elsevier Inc.

settings, thereby potentially limiting the formation of advanced disease altogether. Numerous questions arise from these extremely exciting observations of earlier disease treatments. These include the following: which drugs (or combinations) will produce optimal results for specific patient populations, how to minimize toxicity or tailor its risk, how to identify markers to recognize patients likeliest to benefit from these therapies (vs patients cured by surgery alone), and how to determine whether relapse-free survival will translate into overall/long-term survival.

Fundamental advances in modulating immune responses continue to evolve. Remarkably, the COVID-19 vaccine adoption of parenteral RNA-encoded antigen-epitopes appears to have hastened the way toward identification of significant benefit to personalized neoantigen vaccines in the adjuvant setting for melanoma. Other important advances include the adoption of these approaches to nonmelanoma skin cancers, which may similarly share high-UV mutational burden or virus-encoded (foreign) antigens. Progress in immune checkpoints applied to melanoma brain metastasis—one of the most lethal settings of melanoma—and additional approaches aiming toward combinatorial benefits with targeted radiotherapy as well as intrathecal immunotherapy for leptomeningeal disease, are pushing progress to new limits. While fundamental research in vaccines, microbiome, imaging, and targeted therapies continue to evolve at an exciting pace, it remains highly encouraging that progress has occurred on so many fronts and with such persistence in recent years. The applications of these breakthroughs to nonmelanoma cutaneous malignancies (such as Squamous Cell Carcinoma and Merkel Cell Carcinoma) are also highly encouraging, whereas distinct therapeutic approaches have been applied to other skin malignancies (like T- or B-cell Lymphomas, Basal Cell Carcinomas, and Squamous Cell Carcinomas within immunocompromised hosts).

Progress has been truly remarkable, and profound lessons in human oncology have been learned through this unprecedented period in the history of medicine. Groundbreaking technologies have been invented, in large part for applications in the diagnosis, molecular analyses, and treatment of skin cancers. And these technologies have led to key discoveries in the underlying mechanisms that drive cancer biology. Nonetheless, a painfully significant fraction of patients with these diseases does not respond adequately to the best current therapeutics. And a major fraction of patients with these life-threatening diseases might never have developed them in the first place if proper UV protection or early detection approaches had been in place. We can be proud that advances in cutaneous oncology have benefited so many skin cancer patients and begun to benefit many others with noncutaneous malignancies. But our challenge—and opportunity—remains, to push even harder toward understanding and overcoming the large pockets of treatment resistance and prevention opportunity that continue to confront us.

DISCLOSURES

David E. Fisher reports grants from the NIH (R01AR072304, R01AR043369, and P01CA163222); the Department of Defense (DoD W81XWH2220052 and DoD W81XWH2110981); and the Dr Miriam and Sheldon G. Adelson Medical Research Foundation; and a financial interest in Soltego, a company developing salt-inducible kinase inhibitors for topical skin-darkening treatments that might be used for a broad set of human applications. David E. Fisher also serves as a consultant for Coherent Medicines, Pierre Fabre, Tasca, Torqur, and Biocoz Inc. The interests of David E. Fisher were reviewed and are managed by Massachusetts General Hospital and Partners HealthCare in accordance with their conflict-of-interest policies. The author gratefully acknowledges the Lancer Family for support of the Lancer Professorship at Harvard Medical School.

David E. Fisher, MD, PhD
Department of Dermatology
Massachusetts General Hospital
Harvard Medical School
Boston, MA 02114, USA

E-mail address:
dfisher3@mgh.harvard.edu

Epidemiology and Screening for Melanoma

Nicole L. Bolick, MD, MPH, MS[a], Alan C. Geller, MPH, RN[b],*

KEYWORDS

- Epidemiology • Melanoma • Public health • Screening

KEY POINTS

- For the first time, throughout most of the world affected by melanoma, incidence rates are decreasing in young people, stabilizing in middle-aged people, and increasing in older individuals.
- Screening or other forms of early detection has saved many lives otherwise lost to melanoma and will continue to do so. However, now in the new period of advanced treatments, they are playing a very significant role in reducing the melanoma mortality burden on society.
- Attempts to reduce the disproportionate burden of melanoma in society will require a multilayered approach that concurrently focuses on the epidemiologic, behavioral, and biological roots of the disease.
- The influence of technology on melanoma screening is increasing and it is important to have all skin types represented when training artificial intelligence to reduce melanoma screening disparities and prevent decreased diagnostic accuracy for different skin types.
- There is a joint need from the dermatology and oncology communities to confront the disparities in differential immunotherapy and targeted therapy use.

INTRODUCTION

Melanoma is the most commonly fatal type of skin cancer, and it continues to be an important and growing public health problem throughout most of the developed world, especially in the United States, Australia, New Zealand, and Europe[1–11]. While incidence rates continue to rise overall throughout the world for the past 5 decades, there have been some encouraging trends among youngest populations in the United States, Australia, and New Zealand and there is new evidence of stabilizing and even decreasing rates in middle-aged populations.[11–13] Reports from the United

[a] Department of Dermatology, University of New Mexico School of Medicine, MSC08 4720 1 UNM, Albuquerque, NM 87131, USA; [b] Department of Social and Behavioral Sciences, Harvard T.H. Chan School of Public Health, Kresge Building, Room 718, 677 Huntington Avenue, Boston, MA 02115, USA
* Corresponding author.
E-mail address: ageller@hsph.harvard.edu

Hematol Oncol Clin N Am 38 (2024) 889–906
https://doi.org/10.1016/j.hoc.2024.05.003
0889-8588/24/© 2024 Elsevier Inc. All rights reserved.

States and Hungary note decreased mortality rates, likely due to the results of advanced treatments.[14,15] For example, mortality rates in the United States dropped 18% from 2013 to 2017 (most recent year provided).[14,16] Herein, the authors further describe trends in melanoma incidence and mortality, review the literature on risk factors, and provide an up-to-date assessment of population-wide screening.

MELANOMA INCIDENCE AND MORTALITY RATES
Melanoma in the United States

The number of new cases of melanoma has risen in part due to the aging of the country but as noted in the following sections, the incidence rate is beginning to stabilize. In 2016, there were 82,476 new cases of melanoma reported. In the most recent report from the American Cancer Society's (ACS's) cancer statistics report (January 17, 2024), there were 100,640 cases of which 59% were in men.[17] Via their state-by-state reporting, one can observe that 3 states—California, Florida, and Texas—reported more than 5000 cases per year and 25% of all melanomas. The ACS projects that for men ages 65 to 84 years of age, 1 in 42 will be diagnosed with melanoma during their lifetime, compared with 1 in 92 for women. By way of contrast, for men ages 65 to 84 years of age, 1 in 37 will be diagnosed with colorectal cancer during their lifetime. Melanoma is now the fifth most common cancer in men, behind only prostate, lung and bronchus, colorectal cancer, and bladder cancer. Melanoma is also the fifth most common cancer in women, following breast cancer, lung and bronchus, colon and rectum, and uterine corpus.[17]

There were reports of 8290 melanoma deaths, 5430 in men and 2860 in women, nearly a 2 to 1 difference. Melanoma deaths are disproportionately faced by non-Hispanic whites.[17.] The number of deaths and the mortality rate per 100,000 in 2020 is shown here. Non-Hispanic whites 7708 (2.62), Hispanics/Latinos 285 (0.66), blacks 121 (0.21), Asian Americans/Pacific Islanders 72 (0.33), and Alaskan Indians/American Natives 7 (1.09).[18]

Trends in melanoma incidence

Krauss-Berk and others analyzed 20 years of Surveillance, Epidemiology, and End Results incidence data (2000–2019) for individuals aged 20+ years, stratified by age and tumor thickness.[19] This was done for invasive melanoma (IM) and malignant melanoma in situ (MMIS). Notably, there was an overall increase when looking at the entire period (2000–2019) but a flattening began in 2014 to 2015 (**Fig. 1**). Similar trends were found for individuals aged 70+, historically, the population group with the largest increases in incidence. For younger age groups, individuals aged less than 40 exhibited flat or decreasing MMIS trends throughout the 20-year period and those aged less than 50 experienced a flat or decreasing IM trend. There appears to be fewer MMIS after 2015 for individuals aged 70+ and a decrease of thin T1 melanomas since 2014. However, throughout the study period, there remained a significant rate of increase in T4 (>4 mm tumors) in patients aged 70+ (**Figs. 2** and **3**).

This follows a slightly earlier study using data from 1975 to 2017 that also found recent stabilization of IM in individuals aged 15 to 44 years and males aged 45 to 54 years. This report noted an increase in MMIS, although it covered a longer period of time.[20]

Worldwide

A report from the Global Burden of Diseases (1990–2017) found that countries across the globe were found to exhibit varying levels of change in the age-standardized prevalence rates of melanoma between 1990 and 2017. Basal cell carcinoma (BCC),

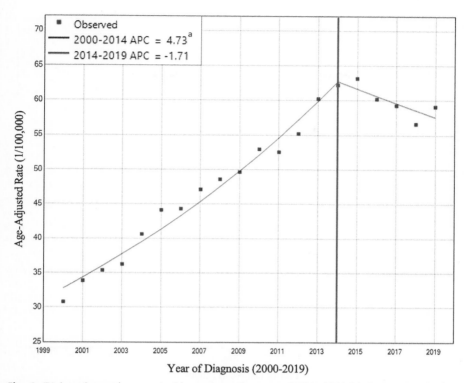

Fig. 1. T1 invasive melanoma incidence in patients aged 701, 2000-2019. T1: #1 mm thin invasive melanoma. [a]Indicates that the annual percent change is significantly different from 0 at the alpha 1⁄4 0.05 level. The red vertical line marks the year in which the annual percent change significantly changes (2014). APC, Annual percent change. *Adapted from* Berk-Krauss J, Sharma M, Polsky D, Geller AC. Cutaneous melanoma incidence-Evidence of a flattening curve. J Am Acad Dermatol. 2023 Dec 10:S0190 to 9622(23)03288-7. https:// doi.org/10.1016/j.jaad.2023.12.010. Epub ahead of print. PMID: 38086518.

squamous cell carcinoma (SCC), and melanoma were the first, fifth, and 20th leading causes of invasive neoplasms (excluding "other benign and in situ neoplasms"), respectively, in 2017. The percent changes from 1990 to 2017 were 310% for SCC, 161% for melanoma, and 77% for BCC. When the melanoma disability-adjusted life year (DALY) rates were compared between 1990 and 2017, Central Europe, Eastern Europe, Central Asia, and high-income countries consistently had more than twice and up to nearly 4 times the global average DALY rate (P<.05).[21]

In 2020, Arnold and colleagues[22], in their report on the Global Burden of Melanoma, noted that there were an estimated 325,000 persons (174,000 males and 151,000 females) worldwide who were diagnosed as having melanoma, and approximately 57,000 persons (32,000 males and 25,000 females) died of the disease. Corresponding with the most recent historical trends toward a greater proportion of deaths in middle-aged and older persons, they found that of all newly diagnosed cases in 2020, 259,000 (79.7%) were persons older than 50 years of age, and of all deaths in 2020, 50,000 persons (87.7%) were older than 50 years of age. Thus, the patterns that are seen in the United States for greater gender disparities when one looks at the effect on cases and deaths are seen here as well, for older age.

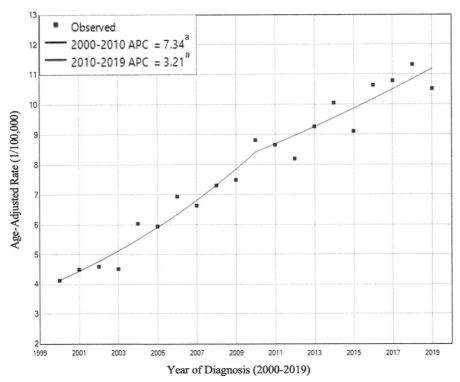

Fig. 2. Malignant melanoma in situ (MMIS). T1: ≤1 mm thin invasive melanoma. T4: greater than 4 mm thick invasive melanoma. Annual percent changes (APCs) are noted in the figure legends. [a]Indicates that the APC is significantly different from 0 at the alpha = 0.05 level. The red vertical line marks the year in which the APC significantly changes (2015 for MMIS, 2014 for T1 invasive melanoma). (*Adapted from* Berk-Krauss J, Sharma M, Polsky D, Geller AC. Cutaneous melanoma incidence-Evidence of a flattening curve. J Am Acad Dermatol. 2023 Dec 10:S0190–9622(23)03288–7. doi: Epub ahead of print. PMID: 38086518.)

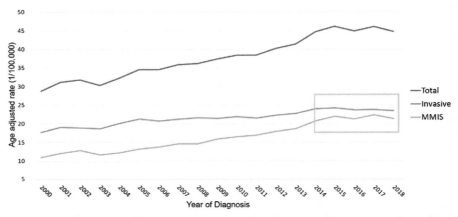

Fig. 3. Recent flattening of invasive melanoma and malignant melanoma in situ (MMIS) incidence rates, US Surveillance, Epidemiology, and End Results Program.

Sharp geographic variations existed across countries and continents, with the highest incidence rates among males (42 per 100,000 person-years) and females (31 per 100,000 person-years) noted in Australia/New Zealand, followed by Western Europe (19 per 100,000 person-years for males and females), North America (18 per 100,000 person-years for males and 14 per 100,000 person-years for females), and Northern Europe (17 per 100,000 person-years for males and 18 per 100,000 person-years for females).[22] Greater mortality to incidence ratios have been reported earlier in Eastern Europe.[11]

RISK FACTORS

Intermittent sun exposure and sunburn history are the prominent risk factors for the development of melanoma with approximately 80% of melanomas developing in locations that receive intermittent sun exposure as opposed to chronic exposure.[9] For example, an estimated 30% of all melanomas in men can be found on the back or chest, likely sites of intermittent exposure.

Over the past 25 years, additional research continues to support a correlation of melanoma risk in those who began indoor tanning at younger than 25 years of age with a 6-fold increased risk in women less than 30 years, a 3.5-fold increased risk for women 30 to 39 years, and a 2.3-fold increased risk in women 40 to 49 years.[23,24] With the addition of each primary melanoma, the odds of an individual ever having indoor tanning increase by 48%.[23,25] However, the profile is different when one tries to understand risk factors for a second melanoma. A study in Austria concluded that the development of subsequent melanomas after diagnosis of a first melanoma is most impacted by genetic variants, family history, actinic damage on the back, as well as the number of nevi.[23,26]

Although it is worth noting that ultraviolet (UV) exposure in the form of natural or artificial light is the primary culprit, lifestyle differences in melanoma risk need to be examined. Such investigations have pinpointed a moderate association between alcohol use and an increased risk of melanoma with additional research needed on this topic.[27,28] A case-control study suggested an association of vitamin D insufficiency/deficiency and melanoma as 66.2% of melanoma patients had vitamin D deficiency at the time of diagnosis and only 15.2% of non-melanoma patients were deficient.[29] Body mass may conceivably play a role in melanoma development with overweight individuals (body mass index $\geq$25) having a significantly increased melanoma risk in those less than 50 years of age (odds ratio [OR] = 1.85) although it is often difficult to distinguish the various roles of the number of moles and expanded body mass.[30] With the role that stress plays on other cancers, it is important to note one study among European populations which found that recent traumatic events such as the death of relative or personal major illness have been reported to be associated with increased melanoma risk (OR = 3.41, $P<.05$).[28] Patients receiving psoralen and UV A treatment for skin conditions such as psoriasis are at increased risk of developing melanoma after 250 treatments.[31] In a more recent study aimed at understanding the causative role of psoriasis and melanoma, researchers identified summary statistics from genome-wide association studies of psoriasis and cutaneous melanoma (CM) among 373,338 adults from predominantly European ancestry (9267 cases and 364,071 controls); genetically predicted psoriasis was identified as a significant risk factor for CM (OR, 1.69; 95% confidence interval [CI], 1.15 to 2.48; $P=.025$).[32] In postmenopausal women, aspirin use is associated with a lower risk of melanoma (21%) when compared to nonsteroidal anti-inflammatory drug nonusers with a longer duration of aspirin use providing even more protection against melanoma.[33] Most recently, a study of nationwide registries in Denmark that followed individuals aged 40 to 70 years from 1997 to 2018 (mean follow of 18.2 years) found that long-term ($\geq$5 or $\geq$ 10 years) use of aspirin was associated with $\geq$10% reductions in hazard ratios (HRs) for several cancer sites including melanoma.[34]

Socioeconomic status affects melanoma detection and disease outcome with uninsured individuals having a 67% greater risk of dying from melanoma than those with private insurance.[31] Similarly, patients with Medicaid and Medicare had worse melanoma disease outcomes than individuals with private insurance.[31]

HOST FACTORS

The risk of melanoma varies greatly by race with a lifetime risk of 0.58% for Hispanics, 0.1% for African Americans, and 2.6% for Caucasians.[31] Compared to individuals with dark skin pigmentation, Caucasians are at an approximately 10-fold risk of melanoma.[31] There is clearly controversy and difference of opinion on the relationship between the total number of moles, atypical moles, and melanoma. This is compounded further as some studies have relied on patient counts and others on physician counts. According to some, any individual with at least 1 atypical nevus should have screening from every 3 months to once a year depending on their nevi characteristics as at least 1 atypical nevus is associated with a 2-fold to 15-fold increased risk of developing melanoma.[35,36] An especially high-risk group for developing melanoma is individuals with greater than 25 nevi with 42% of melanomas being attributable to individuals with this risk factor.[35] Individuals with 11 to 25 nevi have a 1.5 times higher risk of developing melanoma with this risk doubling with each additional increase of 25 nevi.[31] In contrast to these aforementioned studies, in a survey of patients with melanoma at 2 academic sites and an affiliated Veteran Affairs medical center including physician counts of total nevi (TN) and atypical nevi (AN), most patients with melanoma had few nevi (categorized as 0–20) and no AN. In younger patients (<60 years), thick melanomas were commonly found in those with fewer TN but more AN, suggesting that physicians and patients should not rely on the total nevus count as a sole reason to perform skin examinations or to determine a patient's at-risk status.[36]

Preexisting conditions such as irritable bowel disease (IBD), Parkinson's disease (PD), and a history of childhood cancer (noted later) are associated with higher melanoma risk.[37–39] Individuals with IBD are at an increased risk of developing melanoma, with those with Crohn's disease having the greatest risk.[37] In the most recent and largest investigation of the relationship between PD and cancer, a total of 63 studies and 17,994,584 participants were included. A meta-analysis generated a pooled relative risk (RR) of 0.82 (n = 33; 95% CI 0.76–0.88; P<.001) for association between PD and total cancer, 0.76 (n = 21; 95% CI 0.67–0.85; P<.001) for PD and smoking-related cancer, and 0.92 (n = 19; 95% CI 0.84–0.99; P = .03) for non-smoking–related cancer. Notably, in contrast to other cancers, PD was associated with an increased risk of melanoma (n = 29; pooled RR = 1.75; 95% CI 1.43–2.14; P<.001) but not for other skin cancers (n = 17; pooled RR = 0.90; 95% CI 0.60–1.34; P = .60).[38] Further investigation is required to understand the mechanisms that would involve melanoma but not other skin cancers.

MULTILEVEL RISK FACTORS

Mortality to incidence ratio is an important concept used by cancer epidemiologists, biostatisticians, and cancer control planners. Recent studies have concluded that the melanoma mortality-to-incidence (MIR) can be influenced by both sociodemographic and health care differences and these factors are able to predict how MIRs vary across geographic regions within the United States.[40] After multivariable regression analysis, only the percentage of non-Hispanic whites and the number of active physicians were the 2 variables still associated with MIR.[40] One health care system–based study (Kaiser Permanente Colorado) examined incidence, recurrence, and mortality (1931 cases of IM, between January 1, 2000 and December 31, 2015). In multivariable models, the stage at initial diagnosis, gender, and age were associated with melanoma recurrence. Men were more likely to have a recurrence than women and for each decade of increasing age. Factors associated with all-cause mortality included stage (HR = 12.87, 95% CI: 6.63–24.99, for stage IV vs stage I), male gender (HR = 1.42, 95% CI: 1.12–1.79), older age at diagnosis, lower socioeconomic status, and comorbidity index.[41]

Multiple occupational exposures have been associated with melanoma development including UV radiation from both welding fumes and arc welding.[31] The UV radiation exposure in welding has been found to be associated with the development of ocular melanoma with a prior study concluding French welders were at a 7.3 increased odds of developing ocular melanoma compared to the general French population.[31]

Occupational type can also lead to differences in the risk of developing melanoma. A metanalysis concluded that individuals in the oil/petroleum industries have a slightly increased melanoma incidence.[42] and men in the oil/petroleum industries and chemical industry workers have an increased melanoma mortality rate compared to the general population.[42] This may be due to confounding factors of sun exposure habits, worse melanoma survival among males, the role of social class, and exposure to pollutants.[38] Electrical industry workers were found to have a similar melanoma incidence and mortality rates to the general population[43] Furthermore, exposure to pesticides has been shown to be significantly associated with melanoma risk with a recent meta-analysis concluding there is an increased melanoma risk after each use of a herbicide (summary RR of 1.85).[34] However, independent of the level of exposure, neither pesticides in general nor insecticides were shown to be associated with greater melanoma risk.[43] More recently, a study of astronauts found significant increases of melanoma, standardized incidence ratio 252 (95% CI 126–452), and a significant increase in mortality relative to other cancers, standardized mortality ratio 508 (95% CI 105–1485). The investigators concluded that the reported incidence of melanoma among astronauts is similar to that found among aircraft pilots, suggesting again that UV exposure may be playing a role.[44]

SCREENING FOR MELANOMA

The United States Preventive Services Task Force concludes that the current evidence is insufficient and that the balance of benefit and harms of visual skin examination by a clinician to screen for skin cancer in asymptomatic adults cannot be determined. While more formal screening programs will be discussed in the following sections, it is also worth noting that clinicians should be aware of factors related to better and worse prognosis of melanoma as they observe their patients either at the individual or population-based level. One can see that there are demographic factors to consider such as gender, age, and social class but also those related to the site of the tumor, its pathology, and biology (**Table 1**) Attempts to reduce the disproportionate burden of melanoma in society will require a multilayered, approach that concurrently focuses on the epidemiologic, behavioral, and biological roots of the disease.

When trying to tease out the effects of screening versus treatment in the recent reduction of melanoma mortality, it is important to understand that there are a number

Table 1
Demographic factors for melanoma prognosis

Better Prognosis	Worse Prognosis
Women	Men
Young	Older
Well-to-do	Low socioeconomic status
Chest	Scalp/back
Superficial spreading melanoma	Nodular melanoma
$\leq$ 1 mitosis	2+ mitoses

of factors that have made it difficult for screening to have a strong effect on the reduction of melanoma mortality. These include a cancer (a) whose incidence has historically been rising; (b) which disproportionately affects the most vulnerable populations (middle-aged and older men), (c) where access to care has not necessarily aligned with a detectable preclinical time of diagnosis; and (d) which is melanoma (particularly the case for nodular melanoma which is more fast growing and has inherent lethality attached to it). These factors and likely others converge to explain why in the absence of treatment, screening alone would not lead to a decline in mortality. Of equal importance is the argument regarding the counterfactual—how precipitously would the mortality rate have risen in the absence of physician and skin self-examination?

We reviewed relevant studies that have been conducted over the past decade as well as new screening techniques for melanoma while also discussing melanoma health disparities.

Randomized trials have not been conducted for population-wide melanoma screening, and without data from randomized trials, it is not clear that population-based screening will result in decreased mortality.[45,46] It is unlikely that one will conduct a randomized screening trial as it has been estimated that approximately 800,000 participants would be required to detect a difference in mortality because of the relatively low melanoma mortality rate.[46]

The benefits of screening for melanoma should be obvious because the prognosis of melanoma is so strongly associated with the stage and thickness but there are many challenges. Detection by screening has been associated with thinner melanomas at diagnosis, prognosis is significantly better for thinner (early-stage) compared with later-stage melanoma, CM is usually visible on the skin, visual skin examination is safe and well tolerated by patients, and risk factors for melanoma are readily identifiable.[45,46] A recent consensus on melanoma screening with a risk-stratified screening approach determined that general or lower-risk populations could be screened by a primary care physician (PCP) or regular self/partner examination, those at moderate risk could be screened by general dermatologist (GD) or a PCP, those at high risk could be screened by a pigmented lesion evaluation (PLE) expert or GD, and those at ultra-high risk should be screen by a PLE.[47] Additionally, another recent consensus report from Australia determined that there is not enough information to change to systematic melanoma screening from opportunistic screening for the Australian population and that further research is needed to determine how artificial intelligence (AI), total body imaging, and genetic information can be integrated into melanoma screening.[48]

Several limitations exist in melanoma screening. First, it is unclear how many non-dermatologist physicians are adequately trained in the skin cancer examination or have the time to perform a full body skin examination. It is estimated that 8 benign lesions must be removed by a physician with dermoscopy experience to find a single cutaneous malignant melanoma compared to more than 20 benign lesions for a primary care provider.[49] Some melanomas may not be predisposed to early detection, particularly nodular melanoma, acral lentiginous melanoma, and desmoplastic melanoma.

The most far-reaching observational trial for skin cancer screening took place first in Schleswig Holstein, a northern state in Germany. This so-called pilot study, if successful, was to lead to a nationwide screening study in Germany. The SCREEN (Skin Cancer Research to Provide Evidence for Effectiveness of Screening in Northern Germany) study started with a communications program to alert the public about the need for screening coupled with a training program of non-dermatologist physicians led by dermatologists. In all, 360,288 patients were screened (from an eligible population of 1.9 million), and 585 melanomas were detected. Mortality data from Schleswig-Holstein were compared with neighboring states and the country of Denmark and revealed a 47% mortality decline in men and 49% in women. Overall, 620 people needed to be screened to detect one melanoma. Ninety percent of melanomas detected by screening were less than 1 mm thick. Five years following the screening effort, despite a screening participation rate under 20%, mortality from melanoma among adults in the pilot program area was nearly 50% lower than in the rest of Germany and was lower than expected based on historical rates. However, the mortality decline seen at the 5-year mark was not sustained; 2 years later, mortality rates returned to the prescreening level.[50–54]

A population-based case-control study in Queensland, Australia found that when compared with unscreened patients, primary care clinician screening was associated with thinner melanoma lesions. Full skin examinations by a clinician 3 years prior to the diagnosis were associated with thinner melanomas compared with those who had not had a skin examination conferring a 14% lower risk for a melanoma greater than 0.75 mm thick. The decrease in risk was sharpest for the thickest melanomas (risk reduction 40% for lesions ≥3 mm).[55] In the Western Pennsylvania PCP-based screening intervention, clinician screening was associated with a higher rate of melanoma diagnoses, including increased diagnoses of stage T1 (≤1 mm) melanoma and melanomas in situ, but not thicker melanomas.[56] A workplace time series conducted in northern California from 1965 to 1996, involving a comprehensive initiative of pre-awareness, education, and skin screening program, led to a reduction in the incidence of thicker melanoma and a lower-than-expected death rate compared with the statewide cancer registry statistics over the time period assessed.[57]

However, when determining current screening guidelines for melanoma, it is integral that additional health disparities are not created. While white men 50 years of age and older account for 53% of melanoma deaths, it is important that other populations are still targeted for screening interventions.[58] Melanoma screening should not only focus on those at the highest risk for morbidity and death but should also target broader groups to educate them on the importance of skin screening.[58] Multiple studies support that individuals of ethnic and racial minorities often present with advanced melanoma stages and have lower survival rates.[59] A recent study determined that only 4% of non-Hispanic whites presented with distant disease compared to 14% of non-Hispanic blacks.[59] Furthermore, the 5-year melanoma specific survival for non-Hispanic blacks was only 75% compared to 93% in non-Hispanic whites.[59] It has been suggested that more emphasis should be placed on educating all individuals the signs of melanoma, including those in ethnic and racial minorities, instead of emphasizing only melanoma screening.[59]

While there is extensive melanoma research on health inequities, certain populations continue to not be represented in these studies. For example, less than 15% of studies on melanoma research regarding health inequities focused on underserved and rural populations.[60] Other less-examined melanoma health inequities include the lesbian, gay, bisexual, transgender, queer or questioning, or another diverse gender identity population and occupation status.[60]

The value of clinician training to detect melanoma has been demonstrated in several studies. Most medical professionals lack specific education in the early detection of melanoma. In a population-based screening program in the United States, the rate of melanoma diagnosis rose almost 80% among patients screened at practices with the highest proportion of providers trained using INFORMED (INternet curriculum FOR Melanoma Early Detection), an online educational system for primary care clinicians.[61–63]

Risica and colleagues[64] investigated potential psychological harms and benefits of skin examinations by conducting telephone surveys in 2015 of 187 screened participants in the western Pennsylvania study; all were ≥35 year old. Participants had their skin examined by practitioners who had completed INFORMED. Participants who were thoroughly screened did not differ on negative psychosocial measures; scored higher on measures of positive psychosocial wellbeing (Psychological Capital Questionnaire); and were more motivated to conduct monthly self-examinations and seek annual clinician skin examinations, compared to other participants ($P<.05$). Importantly, post-screening, thoroughly screened patients were more likely to report skin prevention practices (skin self-examinations to identify a concerning lesion, practitioner provided skin examination), recommend skin examinations to peers, and feel satisfied with their skin cancer education than less-thoroughly screened individuals ($P<.01$).

SCREENING OF HIGH-RISK POPULATIONS

It is vitally important to conduct randomized trials to determine the best approaches for improving screening of high-risk individuals. One such group is childhood cancer survivors who have both higher rates of skin cancer in general but also melanoma.

Working with the Childhood Cancer Survivor Study, Geller and colleagues[65] conducted a randomized controlled comparative effectiveness trial that evaluated patient activation (PAE) and provider activation (MD) (PAE + MD) **and** PAE + MD with teledermoscopy (PAE + MD + TD) compared with PAE alone, which included print materials, text messaging, and a Web site on skin cancer risk factors and screening behaviors. Seven hundred twenty-eight participants from the Childhood Cancer Survivor Study (median age at baseline 44 years), age greater than 18 years, treated with radiotherapy as children, and without previous history of skin cancer were randomly assigned (1:1:1). Primary outcomes included receiving a physician skin examination at 12 months and conducting a skin self-examination at 18 months after intervention.

Rates of physician skin examinations increased significantly from baseline to 12 months in all 3 intervention groups: PAE, 24%-39%, RR, 1.65, 95% CI, 1.32 to 2.08; PAE + MD, 24% to 39%, RR, 1.56, 95% CI, 1.25 to 1.97; PAE + MD + TD, 24% to 46%, RR, 1.89, 95% CI, 1.51 to 2.37. However, the increase in rates did not differ between groups ($P=.49$). Similarly, rates of skin self-examinations increased significantly from baseline to 18 months in all 3 groups: PAE, 29% to 50%, RR, 1.75, 95% CI, 1.42 to 2.16; PAE + MD, 31% to 58%, RR, 1.85, 95% CI, 1.52 to 2.26; PAE + MD + TD, 29% to 58%, RR, 1.95, 95% CI, 1.59 to 2.40, but the increase in rates did not differ between groups ($P=.43$).[65]

Although skin cancer screening rates increased from baseline by more than 1.5-fold in each of the intervention groups, there were no differences between groups. The investigators argued that these interventions, if implemented, could improve skin cancer prevention behaviors among childhood cancer survivors.[65]

RECENT MELANOMA SCREENING METHODS

The use of dermoscopy and reflectance confocal microscopy (RCM) can be extremely beneficial for melanoma screening. Dermoscopy greatly improves melanoma identification with a sensitivity of 90% compared to 71% with the naked eye and a specificity of 90% compared to 81% with the naked eye.[66] A risk-scoring model called the facial iDScore was developed through the use of dermoscopy by utilizing 3 objective parameters and 7 dermoscopy variables to determine a score that predicts malignant melanoma.[67] This model increased the number of lesions sent for RCM or biopsy and decreased the number of benign lesions being biopsied by 41.5%.[67] Furthermore, with the addition of RCM to dermoscopy, unnecessary biopsies decreased by 43.4%.[66] While RCM is helpful in identifying many pigmented lesions, it does not work well on deep skin lesions limiting its use on acral skin.[66] The use of paper tape and RCM for presurgical mapping procedures allows for better delineation of the subclinical margin to reduce overtreatment in cosmetically sensitive areas achieving increased tissue-sparing and preventing the need for repeat excisions.[68] A previous study determined that 92% of cases had negative margins after the first excision when using RCM with the paper tape method.[68] The use of RCM as a clinical screening tool could be utilized during dermatologic visits.[69] However, in future studies it is important that all skin types are represented in both dermoscopy and RCM research. In previous dermoscopy articles, only 5% reported ethnicity and/or race with skin phototypes I to III being the most common and no studies included participants with type VI skin phototype.[66] Representation of all skin types across both dermoscopy and RCM studies is important as melanoma presentation can differ across different skin tones.[70]

An additional exciting development in melanoma detection is the use of RNA analysis of tape strips. This is a noninvasive method to detect melanomas based on the expression levels of 2 oncogenes, KIT and PRAME.[49] The use of RNA analysis of tape strips without overlooking cutaneous malignant melanoma can reduce removal of benign lesions by one-third.[49] One limitation of this screening method is that storage time must be limited as longer storage time led to decreased ability to screen for cutaneous malignant melanomas.[49]

Deep learning convolutional neural networks (CNNs) show potential for melanoma diagnosis. Melanoma thickness at diagnosis among others depends on melanoma localization and subtype (eg, advanced thickness in acro-lentiginous or nodular melanomas). The question whether CNN may counterbalance physicians' diagnostic difficulties in these melanomas has not been addressed. The CNN showed a high-level performance in set-SSM (superficial spreading melanomas and macular nevi), set-NM (nodular melanomas and papillomatous/dermal/blue nevi), and set-LMM (lentigo maligna melanomas and facial solar lentigines/seborrhoeic keratoses/nevi) (sensitivities >93.3%, specificities >65%, receiver operating characteristics-area under the curve [ROC-AUC] >0.926).[71] In a separate study, Esteva and colleagues[72] demonstrated classification of skin lesions using a single CNN, trained end-to-end from images directly, using only pixels and disease labels as inputs. They tested its performance against 21 board-certified dermatologists on biopsy-proven clinical images with 2 critical binary classification use cases: keratinocyte carcinomas versus benign seborrheic keratoses and CMs versus benign nevi. The CNN achieved performance equal to all tested experts across both tasks, demonstrating an AI capable of classifying skin cancer with a level of competence comparable to dermatologists.

A recent systematic search determined that AI has great potential in diagnosing melanoma from dermoscopic images with AI-based algorithms achieving a greater AUC for ROC (>80%) when detecting melanomas compared to dermatologists.[73] In the future, the implementation of AI into rural clinic settings may help to not only increase melanoma screening rates but also decrease melanoma incidence and mortality in these higher risk rural communities.[73] It is important to realize that many AI models were trained on East Asian and European populations and that AI may be less accurate at diagnosing melanomas on individuals with skin of color.[73] As with dermoscopy, it is important to have all skin types represented when training AI to reduce melanoma screening disparities and prevent decreased diagnostic accuracy for different skin types.

DISPARITIES IN MELANOMA TREATMENTS

While there is much promise with the development of new melanoma treatments, there are unfortunately health disparities in who is treated with these new therapies. A prior study determined that Hispanic ethnicity was associated with a decreased likelihood of receiving immunotherapy for melanoma.[74] Furthermore, when analyzing socioeconomic factors, individuals who lived in a community with a lower household income quartile or who had Medicaid, Medicare, or no insurance were less likely to receive immunotherapy.[74] A study in North Carolina analyzing the association of systemic treatment for stage III to IV melanomas by insurance type determined that having Medicaid insurance only led to an individual being less likely to receive immunotherapy (43% lower likelihood) or systemic therapy (45% lower likelihood).[75] An additional study determined that as the percentage of minority individuals in a county increased, the delay of initiation of immune checkpoint inhibitors (ICIs) increased and the adoption of ICIs decreased.[76] A secondary analysis comparing the initiation of ICIs and race determined that the slowest initiation of ICIs in high-minority countries with the highest percentage of Hispanics.[76] This is concerning as Hispanic patients are more likely to present with melanoma at younger ages with later stages and more aggressive disease.[76] Furthermore, melanoma patients living in rural areas were less likely to receive recommended surgery for their melanomas and have indicated sentinel lymph node biopsies when compared to melanoma patients in an urban setting.[77]

There is a joint need from the dermatology and oncology communities to confront the disparities in differential immunotherapy and targeted therapy use.[78] There will be a strong and ongoing need to participate in advocacy efforts to promote support for and the implementation of policies that reduce disparities in receipt of these therapies.[78] These approaches which can be done in tandem with organizations such as The ACS and American Lung Association should include advocating for states' expansion of Medicaid coverage because patients diagnosed in states with Medicaid expansion have an increased likelihood of receiving immunotherapies and supporting expansion of oncological telemedicine availability and insurance coverage in communities with few to no oncologists.[78] Hospitals, including teaching hospitals and academic centers, need to prioritize conducting routine internal quality checks to measure disparities in the use of immunotherapies and targeted therapies.[79,80] It is important that clinicians build partnerships, engagement, and trust with patients—particularly patients from racial/ethnic minority groups and lower socioeconomic strata who have disparate access to these therapies by including these patients in focus groups to learn their perspectives on how the medical community can better address the barriers they face to receiving immunotherapy and targeted therapy.[79,80]

Gene expression profiling (GEP) in melanoma is increasing with approximately 12,000 tests being performed annually.[81] Castle Biosciences estimates that more than 8000 health care professionals have utilized DecisionDx-Melanoma into their practice with the current cost of a single test often exceeding $7000.[58] However, uninsured patients, those with limited financial means, or patients without access to a dermatologist could have limited access to a GEP test. There is potential that GEP tests may further exacerbate the aforementioned melanoma health disparities and further guidelines to prevent inequitable access to GEP are needed.[58]

The association of melanoma health disparities along insurance, race, socioeconomic status, and rural settings is concerning and future research is needed. Access to disease-oriented care by experts can decrease socioeconomic and racial melanoma health disparities.[82] Additionally, the utilization of teledermatology in rural settings could potentially mitigate melanoma health disparities.

CLINICS CARE POINTS

- When screening for melanoma lower-risk populations could be screened by a primary care physician (PCP) or regular self/partner examination, those at moderate risk could be screened by general dermatologist (GD) or a PCP, and those at high risk could be screened by a pigmented lesion evaluation (PLE) expert or GD, and those at ultra-high risk should be screen by a PLE.

- Melanoma screening should not only focus on those at highest risk for morbidity and death but should also target broader groups to educate them on the importance of skin screening.

- The use of dermoscopy and reflectance confocal microscopy (RCM) can be extremely beneficial for melanoma screening. Representation of all skin types across both dermoscopy and RCM studies is important as melanoma presentation can differ across different skin tones.

- There is a joint need from the dermatology and oncology communities to confront the disparities in differential immunotherapy and targeted therapy use among different patient populations.

- There is potential that Gene expression profiling (GEP) tests may further exacerbate melanoma health disparities and further guidelines to prevent inequitable access to GEP is needed.

DISCLOSURE

The authors have nothing to disclosure.

REFERENCES

1. Koh HK, U.S. Department of Health and Human Services. The Surgeon General's Call to Action to Prevent Skin Cancer. Washington, DC: U.S. Dept of Health and Human Services, Office of the Surgeon General; 2014. p. 112.
2. Whiteman DC, Green AC, Olsen CM. The growing burden of invasive melanoma: projections of incidence rates and numbers of new cases in six susceptible populations through 2031. J Invest Dermatol 2016;136(6):1161–71.

3. Guy GP Jr, Thomas CC, Thompson T, et al. Vital signs: melanoma incidence and mortality trends and projections - United States, 1982-2030. MMWR Morb Mortal Wkly Rep 2015;64(21):591–6.

4. Karimkhani C, Green AC, Nijsten T, et al. The global burden of melanoma: results from the Global Burden of Disease Study 2015. Br J Dermatol 2017;177(1):134–40.

5. Dimitriou F, Krattinger R, Ramelyte E, et al. The World of Melanoma: epidemiologic, genetic, and anatomic differences of melanoma across the globe. Curr Oncol Rep 2018;20(11):87.

6. Fitzmaurice C. Global Burden of Disease Cancer Collaboration. Global, regional, and national cancer incidence, mortality, years of life lost, years lived with disability, and disability-adjusted life-years for 29 cancer groups, 2006 to 2016: A systematic analysis for the Global Burden of Disease study. J Clin Oncol 2018;36(15_suppl):1568.

7. Aitken JF, Youlden DR, Baade PD, et al. Generational shift in melanoma incidence and mortality in Queensland, Australia, 1995-2014: Generational shift in melanoma. Int J Cancer 2018;142(8):1528–35.

8. Forsea AM, del Marmol V, de Vries E, et al. Melanoma incidence and mortality in Europe: new estimates, persistent disparities: Melanoma incidence and mortality disparities in Europe. Br J Dermatol 2012;167(5):1124–30.

9. Garbe C, Leiter U. Melanoma epidemiology and trends. Clin Dermatol 2009;27(1):3–9.

10. Forsea AM, del Marmol V, Stratigos A, et al. Melanoma prognosis in Europe: far from equal. Br J Dermatol 2014;171(1):179–82.

11. Thrift AP, Gudenkauf FJ. Melanoma incidence among non-hispanic whites in All 50 US States From 2001 Through 2015. JNCI J Natl Cancer Inst 2019;djz153.

12. Blazek K, Furestad E, Ryan D, et al. The impact of skin cancer prevention efforts in New South Wales, Australia: Generational trends in melanoma incidence and mortality. Cancer Epidemiol 2022 Dec;81:102263. Epub 2022 Sep 26. PMID: 36174452.

13. Leiter U, Keim U, Garbe C. Epidemiology of skin cancer: Update 2019. Adv Exp Med Biol 2020;1268:123–39. PMID: 32918216.

14. Berk-Krauss J, Stein JA, Weber J, et al. New systematic therapies and trends in cutaneous melanoma deaths among US Whites, 1986-2016. Am J Public Health 2020;110(5):731–3. Epub 2020 Mar 19. PMID: 32191523; PMCID: PMC7144422.

15. Liszkay G, Benedek A, Polgár C, et al. Significant improvement in melanoma survival over the last decade: A Hungarian nationwide study between 2011 and 2019. J Eur Acad Dermatol Venereol 2023 May;37(5):932–40. Epub 2023 Mar 18. PMID: 36785988.

16. Kahlon N, Doddi S, Yousif R, et al. Melanoma treatments and mortality rate trends in the US, 1975 to 2019. JAMA Netw Open 2022 Dec 1;5(12):e2245269. PMID: 36472871; PMCID: PMC9856246.

17. Siegel RL, Giaquinto AN, Jemal A. Cancer statistics, 2024. CA Cancer J Clin 2024 Jan-Feb;74(1):12–49. Epub 2024 Jan 17. PMID: 38230766.

18. U.S. Cancer Statistics Working Group. U.S. Cancer Statistics Data Visualizations Tool, based on 2022 submission data (1999–2020): U.S. Department of Health and Human Services, Centers for Disease Control and Prevention and National Cancer Institute. 2023. Available at: https://www.cdc.gov/cancer/dataviz. [Accessed 25 January 2024].

19. Berk-Krauss J, Sharma M, Polsky D, et al. Cutaneous melanoma incidence-Evidence of a flattening curve. J Am Acad Dermatol 2023;10. S0190-S9622(23) 03288-3297.

20. Kurtansky NR, Dusza SW, Halpern AC, et al. An epidemiologic analysis of melanoma overdiagnosis in the United States, 1975-2017. J Invest Dermatol 2022 Jul; 142(7):1804–11.e6. Epub 2021 Dec 11. PMID: 34902365; PMCID: PMC9187775.

21. Urban K, Mehrmal S, Uppal P, et al. The global burden of skin cancer: A longitudinal analysis from the Global Burden of Disease Study, 1990-2017. JAAD Int 2021 Jan 4;2:98–108. PMID: 34409358; PMCID: PMC8362234.

22. Arnold M, Singh D, Laversanne M, et al. Global burden of cutaneous melanoma in 2020 and projections to 2040. JAMA Dermatol 2022;158:495.

23. Suppa M, Gandini S. Sunbeds and melanoma risk: time to close the debate. Curr Opinion Oncol 2019;31:65–71.

24. Lazovich D, Isaksson Vogel R, Weinstock MA, et al. Association between indoor tanning and melanoma in younger men and women. JAMA Dermatol 2016; 152(3):268.

25. Li Y, Kulkarni M, Trinkaus K, et al. Second primary melanomas: Increased risk and decreased time to presentation in patients exposed to tanning beds. J Am Acad Dermatol 2018;79(6):1101–8.

26. Müller C, Wendt J, Rauscher S, et al. Risk factors of subsequent primary melanomas in Austria. JAMA Dermatol 2019;155(2):188.

27. Gandini S, Masala G, Palli D, et al. Alcohol, alcoholic beverages, and melanoma risk: a systematic literature review and dose–response meta-analysis. Eur J Nutr 2018;57(7):2323–32.

28. de Vries E, Trakatelli M, Kalabalikis D, et al. Known and potential new risk factors for skin cancer in European populations: a multicentre case-control study: Risk factors for skin cancer in European populations. Br J Dermatol 2012;167:1–13.

29. Cattaruzza MS, Pisani D, Fidanza L, et al. 25-Hydroxyvitamin D serum levels and melanoma risk: a case–control study and evidence synthesis of clinical epidemiological studies. Eur J Cancer Prev 2019;28(3):203–11.

30. De Giorgi V, Gori A, Savarese I, et al. Role of BMI and hormone therapy in melanoma risk: a case–control study. J Cancer Res Clin Oncol 2017;143(7):1191–7.

31. Carr S, Smith C, Wernberg J. Epidemiology and Risk Factors of Melanoma. Surg Clin North Am 2020;100(1):1–12.

32. Zhao N, Guo P, Tang M, et al. Evidence for a causal relationship between psoriasis and cutaneous melanoma: A bidirectional two-sample Mendelian randomized study. Front Immunol 2023;14:1201167.

33. Gamba CA, Swetter SM, Stefanick ML, et al. Aspirin is associated with lower melanoma risk among postmenopausal Caucasian women: The Women's Health Initiative. Cancer 2013;119(8):1562–9.

34. Skriver C, Maltesen T, Dehlendorff C, et al. Long-Term Aspirin Use and Cancer Risk: a 20-Year Cohort Study. J Natl Cancer Inst 2023;djad231. Epub ahead of print. PMID: 37966913.

35. Mayer JE, Swetter SM, Fu T, et al. Screening, early detection, education, and trends for melanoma: Current status (2007-2013) and future directions. J Am Acad Dermatol 2014;71(4):611.e1–10.

36. Geller AC, Mayer JE, Sober AJ, et al. Total Nevi, Atypical Nevi, and Melanoma Thickness: An Analysis of 566 Patients at 2 US Centers. JAMA Dermatol 2016; 152(4):413–8. PMID: 26934430.

37. Long MD, Martin CF, Pipkin CA, et al. Risk of Melanoma and Nonmelanoma Skin Cancer Among Patients With Inflammatory Bowel Disease. Gastroenterology 2012;143(2):390–9.e1.

38. Pappo AS, Armstrong GT, Liu W, et al. Melanoma as a subsequent neoplasm in adult survivors of childhood cancer: A report from the childhood cancer survivor study. Pediatr Blood Cancer 2013;60(3):461–6.

39. Zhang X, Guarin D, Mohammadzadehhonarvar N, et al. Parkinson's disease and cancer: a systematic review and meta-analysis of over 17 million participants. BMJ Open 2021 Jul 2;11(7):e046329. Erratum in: BMJ Open. 2021 Sep 22;11(9): e046329corr1. PMID: 34215604; PMCID: PMC8256737.

40. Hopkins ZH, Moreno C, Carlisle R, et al. Melanoma prognosis in the United States: Identifying barriers for improved care. J Am Acad Dermatol 2019;80(5): 1256–62.

41. Feigelson HS, Powers JD, Kumar M, et al. Melanoma incidence, recurrence, and mortality in an integrated healthcare system: A retrospective cohort study. Cancer Med 2019 Aug;8(9):4508–16. Epub 2019 Jun 19. PMID: 31215776; PMCID: PMC6675720.

42. Vujic I, Gandini S, Stanganelli I, et al. A meta-analysis of melanoma risk in industrial workers. Melanoma Res 2018;1. https://doi.org/10.1097/CMR.0000000000000531.

43. Stanganelli I, De Felici MB, Mandel VD, et al. The association between pesticide use and cutaneous melanoma: a systematic review and meta-analysis. J Eur Acad Dermatol Venereol 2020;34(4):691–708.

44. Reynolds R, Little MP, Day S, et al. Cancer incidence and mortality in the USA Astronaut Corps, 1959-2017. Occup Environ Med 2021;78(12):869–75. Epub 2021 May 26. PMID: 34039755.

45. US Preventive Services Task Force, Bibbins-Domingo K, Grossman DC, et al. Screening for Skin Cancer: US Preventive Services Task Force Recommendation Statement. JAMA 2016;316(4):429.

46. Wolff T. Screening for Skin Cancer: An Update of the Evidence for the U.S. Preventive Services Task Force. Ann Intern Med 2009;150(3):194.

47. Kashani-Sabet M, Leachman SA, Stein JA, et al. Early detection and prognostic assessment of cutaneous melanoma: consensus on optimal practice and the role of gene expression profile testing. JAMA Dermatol 2023;159(5):545.

48. Janda M, Cust AE, Neale RE, et al. Early detection of melanoma: a consensus report from the Australian Skin and Skin Cancer Research Centre Melanoma Screening Summit. Aust N Z J Public Health 2020;44(2):111–5. Epub 2020 Mar 19. PMID: 32190955.

49. Heerfordt IM, Philipsen PA, Andersen JD, et al. RNA analysis of tape strips to rule out melanoma in lesions clinically assessed as cutaneous malignant melanoma: A diagnostic study. J Am Acad Dermatol 2023;89(3):537–43.

50. Breitbart EW, Waldmann A, Nolte S, et al. Systematic skin cancer screening in Northern Germany. J Am Acad Dermatol 2012;66(2):201–11.

51. Waldmann A, Nolte S, Geller AC, et al. Frequency of excisions and yields of malignant skin tumors in a population-based screening intervention of 360 288 whole-body examinations. Arch Dermatol 2012;148(8).

52. Boniol M, Autier P, Gandini S. Melanoma mortality following skin cancer screening in Germany. BMJ Open 2015;5(9):e008158.

53. Katalinic A, Waldmann A, Weinstock MA, et al. Does skin cancer screening save lives?: An observational study comparing trends in melanoma mortality in regions with and without screening. Cancer 2012;118(21):5395–402.

54. Stang A, Jöckel K. Does skin cancer screening save lives? A detailed analysis of mortality time trends in Schleswig-Holstein and Germany. Cancer 2016;122(3): 432–7.

55. Aitken JF, Elwood M, Baade PD, et al. Clinical whole-body skin examination reduces the incidence of thick melanomas. Int J Cancer 2010;126(2):450–8.

56. Ferris LK, Saul MI, Lin Y, et al. A large skin cancer screening quality initiative: description and first-year outcomes. JAMA Oncol 2017;3(8):1112.

57. Schneider JS, Moore DH, Mendelsohn ML. Screening program reduced melanoma mortality at the Lawrence Livermore National Laboratory, 1984 to 1996. J Am Acad Dermatol 2008;58(5):741–9.

58. Geller AC, Weinstock MA. Public health and diagnostic approaches to risk stratification for melanoma. JAMA Dermatol. 2023;159(5):475.

59. Kolla AM, Berwick M, Polsky D. Differentiating Between Lead-Time Bias and True Survival Benefits When Discussing Racial and Ethnic Disparities in Melanoma. JAMA Dermatol 2022;158(6):701.

60. Clark P, Howard H, Garrett E, et al. Health inequities in melanoma: A scoping review. J Am Acad Dermatol 2023. https://doi.org/10.1016/j.jaad.2023.09.068. S019096222302892X.

61. Eide MJ, Asgari MM, Fletcher SW, et al. Effects on Skills and Practice from a Web-Based Skin Cancer Course for Primary Care Providers. J Am Board Fam Med 2013;26(6):648–57.

62. INFORMED. Melanoma and skin cancer early detection. Available at: http://Www. Skinsight.Com/Info/For_professionals/Skin-Cancer-Detection-Informed/Skin-Cancer-Education. [Accessed 6 July 2012].

63. Shaikh WR, Geller A, Alexander G, et al. Developing an interactive web-based learning program on skin cancer: the learning experiences of clinical educators. J Cancer Educ 2012;27(4):709–16.

64. Risica PM, Matthews NH, Dionne L, et al. Psychosocial consequences of skin cancer screening. Prev Med Rep 2018;10:310–6.

65. Geller AC, Coroiu A, Keske RR, et al. Advancing Survivors Knowledge (ASK Study) of Skin Cancer Surveillance After Childhood Cancer: A Randomized Controlled Trial in the Childhood Cancer Survivor Study. J Clin Oncol 2023; 41(12):2269–80. Epub 2023 Jan 9. PMID: 36623247; PMCID: PMC10448942.

66. Faldetta C, Kaleci S, Chester J, et al. Melanoma clinicopathological groups characterized and compared with dermoscopy and reflectance confocal microscopy. J Am Acad Dermatol 2023. S0190962223030141.

67. Tognetti L, Cartocci A, Żychowska M, et al. A risk-scoring model for the differential diagnosis of lentigo maligna and other atypical pigmented facial lesions of the face: The *facial iDScore*. J Eur Acad Dermatol Venereol 2023;37(11):2301–10.

68. Cabrioli C, Maione V, Arisi M, et al. Surgical margin mapping for lentigo maligna and lentigo maligna melanoma: traditional technique (visual inspection with dermoscopy) versus combined paper tape and reflectance confocal microscopy technique. Int J Dermatol 2023;62(6):805–11.

69. Longo C, Sticchi A, Curti A, et al. Lentigo maligna and lentigo maligna melanoma in patients younger than 50 years: a multicentre international clinical–dermoscopic study. Clin Exp Dermatol 2023;llad325.

70. Fahmy LM, Karantza IM, Schreidah CM, et al. Skin of color representation in dermoscopy studies distinguishing benign from malignant skin lesions: A scoping review. JAAD Int 2023;13:179–80.

71. Winkler JK, Sies K, Fink C, et al. Melanoma recognition by a deep learning convolutional neural network—Performance in different melanoma subtypes and localisations. Eur J Cancer 2020;127:21–9.
72. Esteva A, Kuprel B, Novoa RA, et al. Dermatologist-level classification of skin cancer with deep neural networks. Nature 2017;542(7639):115–8.
73. Patel RH, Foltz EA, Witkowski A, et al. Analysis of artificial intelligence-based approaches applied to non-invasive imaging for early detection of melanoma: a systematic review. Cancers 2023;15(19):4694.
74. Ermer T, Canavan ME, Maduka RC, et al. Association between food and drug administration approval and disparities in immunotherapy use among patients with cancer in the US. JAMA Netw Open 2022;5(6):e2219535.
75. Adamson AS, Jackson BE, Baggett CD, et al. Association of Receipt of Systemic Treatment for Melanoma With Insurance Type in North Carolina. Med Care 2023; 61(12):829–35.
76. Li M, Liao K, Nowakowska M, et al. Disparity in initiation of checkpoint inhibitors among commercially insured and Medicare Advantage patients with metastatic melanoma. J Manag Care Spec Pharm 2023;29(11):1232–41.
77. Hernandez AE, Benck KN, Huerta CT, et al. Rural Melanoma Patients Have Less Surgery and Higher Melanoma-Specific Mortality. Am Surg 2023. 00031348231216485.
78. Ashrafzadeh S, Asgari MM, Geller AC. The Need for Critical Examination of Disparities in Immunotherapy and Targeted Therapy Use Among Patients With Cancer. JAMA Oncol 2021;7(8):1115–6. PMID: 34042941.
79. Charlton M, Schlichting J, Chioreso C, et al. Challenges of Rural Cancer Care in the United States. Oncology (Williston Park) 2015 Sep;29(9):633–40. PMID: 26384798.
80. Moyers JT, Patel A, Shih W, et al. Association of Sociodemographic Factors With Immunotherapy Receipt for Metastatic Melanoma in the US. JAMA Netw Open 2020;3(9):e2015656. PMID: 32876684; PMCID: PMC7489862.
81. Chan WH, Tsao H. Consensus, controversy, and conversations about gene expression profiling in melanoma. JAMA Dermatol. 2020;156(9):949.
82. Mirsky MM, Mitchell C, Hong A, et al. Outcomes of Antineoplastic Immunotherapy at a Large Healthcare Organization: Impact of Provider, Race and Socioeconomic Status. Cancer Manag Res 2023;15:913–27.

Cutaneous Imaging Techniques

Sara Yasmin Khattab, BS[a], Baraa Ashraf Hijaz, BS[a,b],
Yevgeniy Romanovich Semenov, MD, MA[a,b],*

KEYWORDS

- Cutaneous • Imaging • Dermoscopy • TBP • RCM • OCT • Dermatopathology

KEY POINTS

- Skin imaging provides dermatologists with an objective means to capture information about individual lesions and track changes in these lesions over time.
- Skin imaging can be divided into invasive and noninvasive approaches, with several modalities available in both categories.
- Skin imaging techniques can be combined with one another and analyzed using emerging machine learning computational approaches to extract additional diagnostic and prognostic information.

INTRODUCTION

Capturing images of the skin has become a central component of modern dermatology. Shortly after the invention of photography in 1865, Dr Alexander John Balmanno Squire first used photography to document cutaneous disease.[1] Since then, the field has come to rely increasingly on the use of technology in capturing visual documentation of the skin for clinical, research, and teaching purposes.[1] Furthermore, the advent of artificial intelligence (AI) and machine learning (ML) have begun to play a central role in integrating new technologies and advancing existing capabilities in skin imaging. Dermatology, which is predicated on large volumes of imaging data, has naturally become an ideal candidate for these types of tools. However, in comparison to other medical fields, the use of novel clinical imaging techniques in dermatology remains underutilized.[2] In this article, we provide an overview of various noninvasive skin imaging modalities, followed by cutaneous histopathologic imaging technologies, and the growing role of AI and ML approaches in the field of skin imaging. This list includes commonly used imaging techniques in clinical and research settings but will not be an exhaustive review of all skin imaging techniques available. We discuss the uses, benefits, and limitations of these technologies as well as the broader implications and challenges surrounding the implementation of these tools.

---

[a] Department of Dermatology, Massachusetts General Hospital, 40 Blossom Street, Bartlett Hall 6R, Room 626, Boston, MA 02114, USA; [b] Harvard Medical School, Boston, MA 02115, USA
* Corresponding author. 40 Blossom Street, Bartlett Hall 6R, Room 626, Boston, MA 02114.
E-mail address: ysemenov@mgh.harvard.edu

Hematol Oncol Clin N Am 38 (2024) 907–919
https://doi.org/10.1016/j.hoc.2024.05.011
0889-8588/24/© 2024 Elsevier Inc. All rights reserved, including those for text and data mining, AI training, and similar technologies.
hemonc.theclinics.com

NONINVASIVE TECHNIQUES
Dermoscopy

Dermoscopy was first used in 1971 by Dr Ronald Mackie for the detection of melanoma.[3] A dermatoscope, which has become a handheld staple among practicing dermatologists and trainees, allows for real-time visualization of the skin using magnification and illumination to visualize multiple layers of the skin simultaneously.[4]

Benefits

One of the primary benefits of dermoscopy is the ability to examine structures within the reticular dermis, providing a greater level of detail than is visible with the naked eye.[5] It is primarily used by dermatologists to differentiate malignant versus nonmalignant lesions in the melanocytic domain.[6] Beyond its uses to examine suspicious lesions, dermoscopy also has applications in trichology (examination of hair follicles), onychology (examination of nail units), examination of inflammatory lesions, and examination of skin infections.[5] In addition to its diagnostic versatility, the utility of dermoscopy can be expanded when combined with photography to allow for tracking of magnified lesions across time, known as serial digital dermoscopy.[7] This modality also enables expansion of access to dermatologic care via teledermoscopy.[8] By using dermoscopic lenses that can be attached to smartphone cameras, general practitioners and other nondermatology providers can consult their dermatology colleagues with high-resolution images to facilitate more accurate diagnosis.[9] High-quality, high-resolution images acquired by dermoscopy can also be analyzed using ML algorithms to aid and supplant diagnostics.[10] Indeed, multiple studies have demonstrated enhanced diagnostic accuracy when deploying ML to classify images with known diagnoses.[11] Further, when combining dermoscopic image information with patient demographic and historical medical information, higher level of diagnostic accuracy can be achieved.[12]

Limitations

As described in a meta-analysis of 27 studies by Kittler and colleagues, the diagnostic accuracy of dermoscopy is dependent on user experience.[13] For inexperienced users, dermoscopy does not provide benefits beyond examination with the naked eye.[14] This is due, at least in part, to inconsistent and nonformalized training in dermoscopy across the country.[15] Therefore, the utility of dermoscopy is highly dependent on the level of familiarity with interpreting dermatoscopic findings and can be a source of subjectivity.[16] This is particularly true when leveraging ML techniques for dermoscopic image classification and analysis. Variable lighting conditions, the angle of the photo, and noise within the image, such as the presence of hair or a ruler, can reduce the effectiveness of these tools.[17] Teledermoscopy (remote evaluation of dermoscopic images by an experienced reviewer) can be used as a means of mitigating the issue of user experience.[18] On the ML front, systems have been built that the use millions of images in their training sets so that photographic variability can be mitigated.[19] Public databases, such as the International Skin Imaging Collaboration (ISIC), have been developed to aggregate large volumes of dermoscopic images to aid in the development of ML approaches for the diagnosis of malignant skin lesions. As of this writing, ISIC has amassed over 80,000 high-quality and standardized dermoscopic images.[20] Finally, the nature of dermoscopy requires each lesion to be evaluated individually, which can be time-consuming, particularly for new or inexperienced users.[21]

Total Body Photography

Total body digital photography (TBP) has been used clinically as an objective means of longitudinally capturing comprehensive information on the whole body using a standardized approach.[22] There are 2 types of TBP: 2 dimensional (2D) and 3 dimensional (3D).[23] In 2D TBP, patients are placed in predetermined standardized positions against a typically blue-colored background with a standardized and fixed lighting source. High-resolution digital photographs are then taken and can be used for tracking of large areas of the skin and individual lesions over time.[24–26] A 3D TBP, a more recent innovation in skin imaging, reconstructs a 3D map of the skin surface using a combination of digital photography and dermoscopy.[27] This allows for tracking suspicious lesions over time in more detail.[28] Although there are no broadly accepted clinical guidelines in the United States regarding which patients should receive TBP, a recent survey-based study of a group of dermatologists recommended TBP for patients meeting any of the criteria listed in **Table 1**.[29]

Benefits

Advantages of using TBP include the ability to establish a baseline for pre-existing lesions, accurately track the evolution of these lesions, and identify new lesions in an objective manner.[22,30] This helps prevent biopsies of benign lesions, saving the patient from discomfort and unnecessary additional costs to the health care system.[31] This also helps provide more comprehensive and robust documentation of skin lesions.[32] Hornung and colleagues found that 12,082 patients who received TBP had lower melanoma Breslow depth and were more likely to have melanoma in situ rather than invasive melanoma by comparison to patients who were followed using conventional skin examination.[32] Another advantage of TBP includes expanding access to health care, whereby local clinics can offer these services to patients living in locations with limited access to dermatology, and the images can be interpreted by a dermatologist remotely via telehealth.[27] Furthermore, the objective, standardized, high-resolution images captured using TBP are an ideal foundation for AI-enabled precision medicine.[33,34] For example, most TBP vendors incorporate AI into their software, providing real-time analysis of lesion evolution that may not be as easily detected by the human eye.[35]

Limitations

Limitations to TBP include large setup requiring consistent availability of space and high upfront cost to establish.[24,36] For 3D TBP specifically, imaging of skin folds, genitals, scalp, and acral regions is not possible which may lead to missed cancers and a false sense of security.[27] Additionally, despite its potential applications, most health insurance companies do not provide coverage for TBP, forcing the patient to absorb this additional cost.[9] Furthermore, no prospective studies have been conducted to assess

Table 1	
Waldman et al dermatologist survey results for total body digital photography recommendations	
Condition	
Family history of atypical multiple mole melanoma syndrome OR	
>50 nevi AND	Personal history of multiple melanomas
	Personal history of amelanotic melanoma
	Multiple atypical nevi
	Multiple pink nevi
	Genetic predisposition to melanoma

From Waldman RA, Grant-Kels JM, Curiel CN, et al. Consensus recommendations for the use of noninvasive melanoma detection techniques based on results of an international Delphi process. *J Am Acad Dermatol.* 2021;85(3):745-749.

the clinical utility of TBP, and systematic review and meta-analysis comprising greater than 40,000 patients demonstrated high levels of heterogeneity in its diagnostic accuracy.[37] Nevertheless, it remains an important and frequently used imaging modality for clinical monitoring of high-risk patient populations (**Table 2**).

High-frequency Ultrasound

High-frequency ultrasound (HFUS) and ultra-HFUS with adjunct use of Doppler are relatively inexpensive imaging techniques that use greater than 10 MHz sound waves to assess the skin from the stratum corneum to the deep fascia.[2,38] The layers of the epidermis, dermis, and subcutis are distinguishable from one another on ultrasound due to their varying echogenicity.[39] The higher frequency waves are unable to penetrate the deeper tissues beyond the fascia, but in exchange are able to produce high-resolution details superficially.[4,38]

Benefits

HFUS has very broad dermatologic applications that can provide important clinical information ranging from diagnosis, monitoring disease progression, tracking response to therapy, guiding treatment location, and cosmetics.[38] HFUS has been valuable in the diagnosis of melanoma, where it has been able to accurately predict histologic Breslow thickness (although thickness tends to be overestimated by comparison to histologic evaluation due to tissue shrinkage during histologic processing).[40,41] ML tools that combine digital photography with HFUS have been developed to achieve diagnostic accuracy that is on par and often more accurate than expert diagnostics alone.[42] Although there are many applications for HFUS in dermatology, it has not yet become a widely used tool.[43]

Limitations

One drawback of HFUS, as with all ultrasound imaging, is that acoustic shadowing from hyper and hypoechogenic regions may limit diagnostic accuracy. This becomes especially relevant in dermatologic applications of HFUS when interrogating hyperkeratotic lesions such as cutaneous squamous cell carcinomas.[38,44] Another drawback of HFUS is the nontrivial expertise required to acquire and interpret the images, with

Table 2
Comparison of noninvasive skin imaging techniques

	Depth	Resolution	Space Requirement	User Experience
Total body photography	Naked eye	++	++++	+
Dermoscopy	10x magnification	+++	+	+++
High-frequency ultrasound	Variable[a,45]	+	+++	++++
Optical coherence tomography	1–2 mm	+++	+++[b]	++++
Reflective confocal microscopy	350 μm	++++	+++[b]	++++
Infrared thermography	2-3 mm	+	+	++

"+" ranges from "+" to "++++". For resolution, which describes the level of granular detail the image produces, higher "+" corresponds to higher resolution. For space requirement, higher "+" corresponds to the requirement of a greater amount of physical space. For user experience, higher "+" corresponds to increased user friendliness and usability.

[a] Will vary depending on the probe frequency selected; for instance, 8–9 mm can be achieved at 50 MHz.
[b] New, handheld devices have been developed, reducing the space requirement.

most practicing dermatologists having had no training in HFUS.[46] Finally, although much progress has been achieved in the quality of detail produced by HFUS of the skin, other noninvasive techniques are able to provide greater resolution.[46]

Reflectance Confocal Microscopy

Reflectance confocal microscopy (RCM) is a noninvasive, in vivo, skin imaging technique that produces horizontal cross sections of tissue at cellular-level resolution.[47] Thus, it allows for the real-time observation of skin under the microscope.[48] In RCM, a microscope emits a laser, which passes through the skin, and is reflected at different areas of the skin composition with different refractive indices.[49] This allows for the construction of a visual representation of specific planes beneath the surface of the skin.[50] The reflected light is used to compose a 2D image providing cellular-level detail with visualization down to the dermal–epidermal junction.[51]

Benefits

RCM provides the greatest resolution of the available noninvasive skin imaging technologies and is the closest modality to the current diagnostic gold standard of histopathologic evaluation.[48] For this reason, its primary use has been in imaging lesions that a dermatologist may otherwise be reluctant to biopsy.[52] RCM has many applications across dermatology, including in diagnosing cutaneous malignancies, inflammatory disease, and in the evaluation of mucosal, nail, and follicular pathologies.[53] Other uses of RCM include confirming surgical margins and longitudinally tracking changes in individual lesions.[54] This imaging modality has also been reported to have increased specificity in the diagnosis of melanoma compared to dermoscopy alone.[55] Furthermore, it has been shown to be even more effective in combination with dermoscopy, resulting in a 50% reduction in unnecessary biopsies.[52,56] These images can also be integrated into ML pipelines for lesion classification, with studies demonstrating accuracy levels leveraging ML tools that are on par with experts in RCM.[57,58]

Limitations

The maximum depth of penetration from RCM is 350 μm.[59] As a result, due to its thickness, acral skin is difficult to evaluate by RCM.[60] Additionally, given its reliance on reflectance, highly heterogeneous or deep lesions (eg, highly keratotic, ulcerated, deep, and nodular lesions, as well as lesions in densely hair-bearing regions) are difficult to penetrate using RCM.[53] As with all noninvasive skin imaging techniques, RCM carries the risk of misclassifying otherwise benign lesions, leading to unnecessary sampling, discomfort, and cost.[61] RCM requires extensive expertise and substantial time for image interpretation, which further limits the feasibility of widespread application of this technique.[52] Another limitation of RCM includes its high initial cost to set up. Unlike optical coherence tomography (OCT), however, category I current procedural terminology (CPT) codes have been issued for skin imaging using RCM, mitigating some barriers to implementation.[62]

Optical Coherence Tomography

Cutaneous OCT is a noninvasive skin imaging technique that utilizes 1300 nm focused laser beams to measure the scattering properties of light.[63] Upon entering the skin, these beams interact with a reference beam to construct a vertically oriented image of the simultaneous layers of the skin based on their differing light scattering properties.[64,65] Ultimately, a real-time, high-resolution cross-sectional image of tissues and underlying vascular structures can be constructed using this noninvasive technique.[66]

Benefits

OCT provides images that are more detailed than HFUS, with resolutions of 4–10 μm, and with deeper visibility than RCM, up to 1 to 2 mm.[67,68] It has capabilities of imaging up to the upper layers of the dermis and has been shown to prevent the need for biopsy in one-third of basal cell cancers.[65,67] Sahu and colleagues suggest that the combination of OCT and RCM in a single probe may be used not only to diagnose new basal cell carcinomas and determine their depth, but also to identify residual cancer in previously biopsied basal cell carcinomas (BCC).[69] In addition to aiding in cancer diagnostics, OCT can also be used to track vascular changes in inflammatory pathologies, ranging from psoriasis to a number of connective tissue diseases.[66] There have also been advances in the use of ML to enhance care using OCT devices. A recent study leveraged ML to classify and detect abnormal features extracted from OCT images to enhance tissue excision accuracy in Mohs micrographic surgery.[70]

Limitations

OCT is limited in its inability to gain adequate depth for some advanced tumors as well as with the discernment of pigmented lesions.[71] In addition, it does not allow for the visualization of cellular-level detail.[62] Further, these images can be difficult to interpret and are reliant on high levels of technical expertise to both acquire and interpret them.[66] Studies have demonstrated that even among highly trained users, common benign cutaneous processes can be misclassified as malignant.[65] Furthermore, formal and structured curricular integration in graduate medical education as well as among trained dermatologists is limited.[66] Other barriers to implementation include difficulties in reimbursement and device cost. In 2017, the American Medical Association granted 2 category III CPT codes for the usage of OCT: 0470T as indicated for the imaging and interpretation of skin morphology and microarchitecture and 0471T for subsequent images acquired.[72] While beneficial in paving the way for reimbursement, category III CPT codes are investigational and therefore limit the ability to reimburse for many insurance carriers. In addition, traditional OCT device costs can range between $50,000 and $120,000 while weighing up to 60 pounds. Although newer, handheld OCT devices have been developed, their cost of approximately $15,000 remains too prohibitive for most clinical dermatology settings.[73]

Infrared Thermography

A wealth of important clinical information can be extracted based on temperature changes experienced on the skin, particularly within the context of inflammatory or infectious dermatoses.

Infrared thermography takes advantage of this property and leverages the electromagnetic/infrared radiation emitted as temperatures exceeding absolute zero to map out temperature changes on the skin.[74] Conventional color gradients are then often used to map warm (red) or cool (blue) areas on the skin.[75] Two types of infrared thermography exist: passive and active. In passive thermography, temperature information is obtained from the skin in its natural state, whereas in active thermography, an external cooling source is applied to the skin after which rewarming is measured.[76] ML models have already been deployed to aid in diagnostics and disease classification based on the gradients produced using this image technology, ranging from improved diagnostics for cutaneous malignancies to aid in the recognition of allergic reactions.[77,78]

Benefits

Infrared thermography is able to provide information 2–3 mm in depth.[79] Hypothesizing that the increased heat generation within cutaneous malignancies results in detectable increases in skin temperature, Godoy and colleagues showed that infrared imaging could be used to accurately distinguish malignant lesions from nonmalignant lesions with 83% specificity and 95% sensitivity.[80] Thermography can also be used to more accurately estimate the depth of burn wounds and in diagnosing and monitoring response to treatment in cellulitis patients.[79,81]

Limitations

Thermography can be influenced by room temperature and humidity.[82] Additionally, the depth of thermography may be limited by skin surface texture, such as the presence of crusting.[79] The cost of cameras used for infrared thermography ranges from $200 to $600.[76] As indications for its uses continue to expand, so too will the cost savings of using this tool. Lower cost, attachable cameras have also been developed and have demonstrated comparable performance.[83]

ADVANCED HISTOLOGIC EVALUATION

While the abovementioned techniques can be leveraged to reduce the need for biopsies in arriving at an accurate diagnosis, histopathologic evaluation remains the gold standard for diagnosis of cutaneous pathology.[84] The standard clinical staining technique used is hematoxylin and eosin (H&E) staining, however, when necessary other staining modalities are employed to capture additional information.[85,86] Histopathologic evaluation techniques can provide a lot of information, including information that has not yet been clinically leveraged. For instance, in addition to diagnosis, we can leverage the wealth of information provided by histopathologic evaluation in prognostication. To this end, several advanced histopathologic imaging techniques have been developed. Additionally, there has been a growing effort to shift toward incorporating digital histopathology in clinical and research settings,[87] providing the pathologist with an ability to read slides from a remote setting, transmit information more seamlessly to the referring clinician, and leverage these images in research settings.[88]

Multiplex Immunofluorescence

Multiplex immunofluorescence is a staining technique where antibodies are used to bind antigens of interest in the tissue.[89] Subsequently, a secondary antibody with an associated fluorophore is linked to the primary antibody to provide a signal.[89] Typically 3 to 4 stains are applied to the slide, though some recent approaches have enabled the visualization of up to 60 stains.[90] Once the slides are scanned, the information from all the rounds of staining can be superimposed and displayed concurrently. This technique has allowed scientists to learn more about the tumor microenvironment (TME) and how cells within the TME interact with one another using visual inspection and automated analyses using ML.[91] For example, Wan and colleagues leveraged ML to characterize molecular, cellular, and spatial features within TMEs from these images,[92] including detailed investigations of region-based cell composition and development of indices to measure tumor proliferation, immune cell infiltration, and tumor immune cell engagement.

Orion

Orion is an emerging staining technique where slides first undergo multiplex staining followed by one round of H&E on the same tissue section.[93] This approach allows for the superimposition of the data from both types of imaging modalities, enabling more seamless integration into existing ML pipelines.[93]

SUMMARY

In conclusion, in this article, we demonstrated that there are many imaging modalities, both noninvasive and invasive, that can be leveraged by dermatologists and pathologists to accurately diagnose and track concerning lesions. These methods can be combined with emerging ML and AI approaches to increase specificity and manage increasingly high volumes of clinical and imaging data.

CLINICS CARE POINTS

Pearls
- Dermoscopy has become a prime target for innovation in skin imaging, with applications expanding beyond illuminated magnification into domains of ML and teledermoscopy.
- Reflectance coherence microscopy provides the greatest known resolution of the available noninvasive skin imaging techniques, boasting a 50% reduction in unnecessary biopsies when coupled with dermoscopy.[52,56]
- The advent of digital pathology has opened avenues for innovation in the gold standard for dermatologic imaging, ranging from using ML to elucidate the TME to the integration of multiple staining techniques.

Pitfalls
- There exists a lack of structured and formal education around the proper use of dermoscopy, which may propagate into the efficacy of emerging ML algorithms that rely on this technique.
- The inability to reimburse for advanced and emerging techniques, namely OCT, will continue to pose a barrier to implementation, despite favorable evidence demonstrating improved care for patients (eg, a reduction in the need for biopsy when using OCT).
- While imaging in dermatology ripe for innovation, the cost to purchase these technologies remains a key barrier to implementation for many dermatology practices.

DISCLOSURE

Dr Y.R. Semenov is an advisory board member/consultant and has received honoraria from Incyte Corporation, Castle Biosciences, Galderma, and Sanofi outside of the submitted work. Dr Y.R. Semenov is supported in part by the Melanoma Research Alliance Young Investigator Award.

REFERENCES

1. Ferreira IG, Weber MB, Bonamigo RR. History of dermatology: the study of skin diseases over the centuries. An Bras Dermatol 2021;96(3):332–45.
2. Aspres N, Egerton IB, Lim AC, Shumack SP. Imaging the skin. Australas J Dermatol 2003;44(1):19–27.
3. Buch J, Criton S. Dermoscopy saga - a tale of 5 centuries. Indian J Dermatol 2021;66(2):174–8.
4. Campos-do-Carmo G, Ramos-e-Silva M. Dermoscopy: basic concepts. Int J Dermatol 2008;47(7):712–9.
5. Sonthalia S, Yumeen S, Kaliyadan F. Dermoscopy overview and Extradiagnostic applications. Treasure Island, FL: StatPearls Publishing; 2023.
6. Crotty KA, Menzies SW. Dermoscopy and its role in diagnosing melanocytic lesions: a guide for pathologists. Pathology 2004;36(5):470–7.
7. Tschandl P. Sequential digital dermatoscopic imaging of patients with multiple atypical nevi. Dermatol Pract Concept 2018;8(3):231.

8. Uppal SK, Beer J, Hadeler E, et al. The clinical utility of teledermoscopy in the era of telemedicine. Dermatol Ther 2021;34(2):e14766.

9. Lee KJ, Soyer HP. Future developments in teledermoscopy and total body photography. Int J Dermatol Venereol 2019;2(1):15.

10. García AJL, García ZB. Detection of pigment network in dermoscopy images using supervised machine learning and structural analysis. Comput Biol Med 2014; 44:144–57.

11. Chan S, Reddy V, Myers B, et al. Machine Learning in Dermatology: Current Applications, Opportunities, and Limitations. Dermatol Ther (Heidelb) 2020;10(3): 365–86.

12. Haenssle HA, Fink C, Schneiderbauer R, et al. Man against machine: diagnostic performance of a deep learning convolutional neural network for dermoscopic melanoma recognition in comparison to 58 dermatologists. Ann Oncol 2018; 29(8):1836–42.

13. Kittler H, Pehamberger H, Wolff K, Binder M. Diagnostic accuracy of dermoscopy. Lancet Oncol 2002;3(3):159–65.

14. Hoorens I, Vossaert K, Lanssens S, et al. Value of Dermoscopy in a Population-Based Screening Sample by Dermatologists. Dermatol Pract Concept 2019; 9(3):200–6.

15. Wu TP, Newlove T, Smith L, et al. The importance of dedicated dermoscopy training during residency: a survey of US dermatology chief residents. J Am Acad Dermatol 2013;68(6):1000–5.

16. Celebi ME, Kingravi HA, Uddin B, et al. A methodological approach to the classification of dermoscopy images. Comput Med Imaging Graph 2007;31(6):362–73.

17. Avanaki ARN, Espig K, Xthona A, et al. Perceptual image quality in digital dermoscopy. In: Samuelson FW, Taylor-Phillips S, editors. Medical imaging 2020: image perception, observer performance, and technology assessment11316. Houston, TX: SPIE; 2020. p. 235–41.

18. Lee KJ, Finnane A, Peter Soyer H. Recent trends in teledermatology and teledermoscopy. Dermatol Pract Concept 2018;8(3):214.

19. Esteva A, Kuprel B, Novoa RA, et al. Dermatologist-level classification of skin cancer with deep neural networks. Nature 2017;542(7639):115–8.

20. ISIC. ISIC. Available at: https://www.isic-archive.com/. [Accessed 31 January 2024].

21. Zalaudek I, Kittler H, Marghoob AA, et al. Time required for a complete skin examination with and without dermoscopy. Arch Dermatol 2008;144(4). https://doi.org/10.1001/archderm.144.4.509.

22. Salerni G, Carrera C, Lovatto L, et al. Benefits of total body photography and digital dermatoscopy ("two-step method of digital follow-up") in the early diagnosis of melanoma in patients at high risk for melanoma. J Am Acad Dermatol 2012; 67(1):e17–27.

23. Grochulska K, Betz-Stablein B, Rutjes C, et al. The additive value of 3D total body imaging for sequential monitoring of skin lesions: a case series. Dermatology 2022;238(1):12–7.

24. Dengel LT, Petroni GR, Judge J, et al. Total body photography for skin cancer screening. Int J Dermatol 2015;54(11):1250–4.

25. Korotkov K, Quintana J, Campos R, et al. An improved skin lesion matching scheme in total body photography. IEEE J Biomed Health Inform 2019;23(2):586–98.

26. Halpern AC, Marghoob AA, Bialoglow TW, et al. Standardized positioning of patients (poses) for whole body cutaneous photography. J Am Acad Dermatol 2003; 49(4):593–8.

27. Rayner JE, Laino AM, Nufer KL, et al. Clinical perspective of 3D total body photography for early detection and screening of melanoma. Front Med (Lausanne) 2018;5. https://doi.org/10.3389/fmed.2018.00152.

28. Huang WL, Tashayyod D, Kang J, et al. Skin lesion correspondence localization in total body photography. In: Lecture notes in computer science. Lecture notes in computer science. Switzerland: Springer Nature; 2023. p. 260–9.

29. Waldman RA, Grant-Kels JM, Curiel CN, et al. Consensus recommendations for the use of noninvasive melanoma detection techniques based on results of an international Delphi process. J Am Acad Dermatol 2021;85(3):745–9.

30. Risser J, Pressley Z, Veledar E, et al. The impact of total body photography on biopsy rate in patients from a pigmented lesion clinic. J Am Acad Dermatol 2007;57(3):428–34.

31. Truong A, Strazzulla L, March J, et al. Reduction in nevus biopsies in patients monitored by total body photography. J Am Acad Dermatol 2016;75(1):135–43.e5.

32. Hornung A, Steeb T, Wessely A, et al. The value of total body photography for the early detection of melanoma: a systematic review. Int J Environ Res Publ Health 2021;18(4):1726.

33. Cerminara SE, Cheng P, Kostner L, et al. Diagnostic performance of augmented intelligence with 2D and 3D total body photography and convolutional neural networks in a high-risk population for melanoma under real-world conditions: A new era of skin cancer screening? Eur J Cancer 2023;190(112954):112954.

34. Primiero CA, Rezze GG, Caffery LJ, et al. A narrative review: opportunities and challenges in artificial intelligence skin image analyses using total body photography. J Invest Dermatol 2024;16. https://doi.org/10.1016/j.jid.2023.11.007.

35. Brancaccio G, Balato A, Malvehy J, et al. Artificial intelligence in skin cancer diagnosis: a reality check. J Invest Dermatol 2024;144(3):492–9.

36. Hona TWPT, Horsham C, Silva CV, et al. Consumer views of melanoma early detection using 3D total-body photography: cross-sectional survey. Int J Dermatol 2023;62(4):524–33.

37. Ji-Xu A, Dinnes J, Matin RN. Total body photography for the diagnosis of cutaneous melanoma in adults: a systematic review and meta-analysis. Br J Dermatol 2021;185(2):302–12.

38. Levy J, Barrett DL, Harris N, et al. High-frequency ultrasound in clinical dermatology: a review. Ultrasound J 2021;13(1):24.

39. Almuhanna N, Wortsman X, Wohlmuth-Wieser I, et al. Overview of ultrasound imaging applications in dermatology [Formula: see text]. J Cutan Med Surg 2021;25(5):521–9.

40. Reginelli A, Belfiore MP, Russo A, et al. A preliminary study for quantitative assessment with HFUS (high- frequency ultrasound) of nodular skin melanoma Breslow thickness in adults before surgery: Interdisciplinary team experience. Curr Radiopharm 2020;13(1):48–55.

41. Piłat P, Borzęcki A, Jazienicki M, et al. Evaluation of the clinical usefulness of high-frequency ultrasonography in pre-operative evaluation of cutaneous melanoma - a prospective study. Postepy Dermatol Alergol 2020;37(2):207–13.

42. Zhu AQ, Wang Q, Shi YL, et al. A deep learning fusion network trained with clinical and high-frequency ultrasound images in the multi-classification of skin diseases in comparison with dermatologists: a prospective and multicenter study. EClinicalMedicine 2024;67(102391):102391.

43. Schmid-Wendtner MH, Dill-Müller D. Ultrasound technology in dermatology. Semin Cutan Med Surg 2008;27(1):44–51.

44. Polańska A, Dańczak-Pazdrowska A, Jałowska M, et al. Current applications of high-frequency ultrasonography in dermatology. Postepy Dermatol Alergol 2017;34(6):535–42.

45. Shung KK. High frequency ultrasonic imaging. J Med Ultrasound 2009;17(1): 25–30.

46. Polańska A, Jenerowicz D, Paszyńska E, et al. High-frequency ultrasonography-possibilities and perspectives of the use of 20 MHz in teledermatology. Front Med (Lausanne) 2021;8:619965.

47. Kang HY, Bahadoran P, Suzuki I, et al. *In vivo* reflectance confocal microscopy detects pigmentary changes in melasma at a cellular level resolution. Exp Dermatol 2010;19(8). https://doi.org/10.1111/j.1600-0625.2009.01057.x.

48. Waddell A, Star P, Guitera P. Advances in the use of reflectance confocal microscopy in melanoma. Melanoma Manag 2018;5(1):MMT04.

49. Calzavara-Pinton P, Longo C, Venturini M, et al. Reflectance confocal microscopy for in vivo skin imaging. Photochem Photobiol 2008;84(6):1421–30.

50. Braghiroli NF, Sugerik S, Freitas LAR, et al. The skin through reflectance confocal microscopy - Historical background, technical principles, and its correlation with histopathology. An Bras Dermatol 2022;97(6):697–703.

51. Wielowieyska-Szybińska D, Białek-Galas K, Podolec K, Wojas-Pelc A. The use of reflectance confocal microscopy for examination of benign and malignant skin tumors. Postepy Dermatol Alergol 2014;6(6):380–7.

52. Levine A, Markowitz O. In vivo reflectance confocal microscopy. Cutis 2017; 99(6). Available at: https://pubmed.ncbi.nlm.nih.gov/28686758/. [Accessed 31 January 2024].

53. Franceschini C, Persechino F, Ardigò M. In vivo reflectance confocal microscopy in general dermatology: How to choose the right indication. Dermatol Pract Concept 2020;10(2):e2020032.

54. Lupu M, Voiculescu VM, Caruntu A, et al. Preoperative Evaluation through Dermoscopy and Reflectance Confocal Microscopy of the Lateral Excision Margins for Primary Basal Cell Carcinoma. Diagnostics (Basel) 2021;11(1):120.

55. Stanganelli I, Longo C, Mazzoni L, et al. Integration of reflectance confocal microscopy in sequential dermoscopy follow-up improves melanoma detection accuracy. Br J Dermatol 2015;172(2):365–71.

56. Muzumdar S, Wu R, Rothe MJ, Grant-Kels JM. Reflectance confocal microscopy decreases the cost of skin lesion diagnosis: a single institution retrospective chart review. J Am Acad Dermatol 2022;86(1):209–11.

57. Campanella G, Navarrete-Dechent C, Liopyris K, et al. Deep learning for basal cell carcinoma detection for reflectance confocal microscopy. J Invest Dermatol 2022;142(1):97–103.

58. Li J, Garfinkel J, Zhang X, et al. Biopsy-free in vivo virtual histology of skin using deep learning. Light Sci Appl 2021;10(1):1–22.

59. Hofmann-Wellenhof R, Wurm EMT, Ahlgrimm-Siess V, et al. Reflectance confocal microscopy—state-of-art and research overview. Semin Cutan Med Surg 2009; 28(3):172–9.

60. Puig S, Carrera C, Lovato L, Hanke-Martinez M. Acral volar skin, facial skin and mucous membrane. In: Reflectance confocal microscopy for skin diseases. Berlin, Heidelberg: Springer; 2012. p. 33–8.

61. Menge TD, Hibler BP, Cordova MA, et al. Concordance of handheld reflectance confocal microscopy (RCM) with histopathology in the diagnosis of lentigo maligna (LM): A prospective study. J Am Acad Dermatol 2016;74(6):1114–20.

62. Rajadhyaksha M, Marghoob A, Rossi A, et al. Reflectance confocal microscopy of skin in vivo: From bench to bedside. Lasers Surg Med 2017;49(1):7–19.

63. Xu J, Song S, Men S, Wang RK. Long ranging swept-source optical coherence tomography- based angiography outperforms its spectral-domain counterpart in imaging human skin microcirculations. J Biomed Opt 2017;22(11):1.

64. Babalola O, Mamalis A, Lev-Tov H, Jagdeo J. Optical coherence tomography (OCT) of collagen in normal skin and skin fibrosis. Arch Derm Res 2014;306(1):1–9.

65. Olsen J, Holmes J, Jemec GBE. Advances in optical coherence tomography in dermatology—a review. J Biomed Opt 2018;23(04):1.

66. Wan B, Ganier C, Du-Harpur X, et al. Applications and future directions for optical coherence tomography in dermatology. Br J Dermatol 2021;184(6):1014–22.

67. Steiner R, Kunzi-Rapp K, Scharffetter-Kochanek K. Optical coherence tomography: Clinical applications in dermatology. Med Laser Appl 2003;18(3):249–59.

68. Mamalis A, Ho D, Jagdeo J. Optical coherence tomography imaging of normal, chronologically aged, photoaged and photodamaged skin. Dermatol Surg 2015;41(9):993–1005.

69. Sahu A, Yélamos O, Iftimia N, et al. Evaluation of a combined reflectance confocal microscopy–optical coherence tomography device for detection and depth assessment of basal cell carcinoma. JAMA Dermatol 2018;154(10):1175.

70. Liu X, Ouellette S, Jamgochian M, et al. One-class machine learning classification of skin tissue based on manually scanned optical coherence tomography imaging. Sci Rep 2023;13(1):1–9.

71. Michelle Schwartz BA, Levine A, Markowitz O. Optical coherence tomography in dermatology. 2017. Available at: https://www.mdedge.com/dermatology/article/146053/melanoma/optical-coherence-tomography-dermatology. [Accessed 31 January 2024].

72. Ba MS, Levine A, Markowitz O. Optical coherence tomography in dermatology. Available at: https://cdn.mdedge.com/files/s3fs-public/Document/August-2017/CT100003163.PDF. [Accessed 31 January 2024].

73. Thompson C. Low-cost retinal scanner could help prevent blindness worldwide. Duke Pratt School of Engineering 2019. Available at: https://pratt.duke.edu/news/low-cost-oct/. [Accessed 31 January 2024].

74. Vergilio MM, Gomes G, Aiello LM, et al. Evaluation of skin using infrared thermal imaging for dermatology and aesthetic applications. J Cosmet Dermatol 2022;21(3):895–904.

75. Sarawade AA, Charniya NN. Infrared Thermography and its Applications: A Review. In: 2018 3rd international conference on communication and electronics systems (ICCES). Coimbatore, India: IEEE; 2018. p. 280–5.

76. Speeckaert R, Hoorens I, Lambert J, et al. Beyond visual inspection: The value of infrared thermography in skin diseases, a scoping review. J Eur Acad Dermatol Venereol 2024. https://doi.org/10.1111/jdv.19796.

77. Magalhaes C, Tavares JMRS, Mendes J, Vardasca R. Comparison of machine learning strategies for infrared thermography of skin cancer. Biomed Signal Process Control 2021;69(102872):102872.

78. Neumann Ł, Nowak R, Stępień J, et al. Thermography based skin allergic reaction recognition by convolutional neural networks. Sci Rep 2022;12(1):1–10.

79. Gurjarpadhye AA, Parekh MB, Dubnika A, et al. Infrared imaging tools for diagnostic applications in dermatology. SM J Clin Med Imaging 2015;1(1):1–5.

80. Godoy SE, Ramirez DA, Myers SA, et al. Dynamic infrared imaging for skin cancer screening. Infrared Phys Technol 2015;70:147–52.

81. Amendola JA, Segre AM, Miller AC, et al. Using thermal imaging to track cellulitis. Open Forum Infect Dis 2023;10(5):ofad214.
82. Verstockt J, Verspeek S, Thiessen F, et al. Skin cancer detection using infrared thermography: Measurement setup, procedure and equipment. Sensors (Basel) 2022;22(9):3327.
83. Villa E, Arteaga-Marrero N, Ruiz-Alzola J. Performance assessment of low-cost thermal cameras for medical applications. Sensors (Basel) 2020;20(5):1321.
84. Ahmadi O, Das M, Hajarizadeh B, Mathy JA. Impact of shave biopsy on diagnosis and management of cutaneous melanoma: A systematic review and meta-analysis. Ann Surg Oncol 2021;28(11):6168–76.
85. Peters N, Schubert M, Metzler G, et al. Diagnostic accuracy of a new *ex vivo* confocal laser scanning microscope compared to H&E-stained paraffin slides for micrographic surgery of basal cell carcinoma. J Eur Acad Dermatol Venereol 2019;33(2):298–304.
86. Van Herck Y, Antoranz A, Andhari MD, et al. Multiplexed immunohistochemistry and digital pathology as the foundation for next-generation pathology in melanoma: Methodological comparison and future clinical applications. Front Oncol 2021;11. https://doi.org/10.3389/fonc.2021.636681.
87. Glines KR, Haidari W, Ramani L, et al. Digital future of dermatology. Dermatol Online J 2020;26(10). https://doi.org/10.5070/d32610050455.
88. Vodovnik A, Aghdam MRF. Complete routine remote digital pathology services. J Pathol Inform 2018;9(1):36.
89. Magaki S, Hojat SA, Wei B, et al. An introduction to the performance of immunohistochemistry. In: Methods in molecular biology. Vol 1897. Methods in molecular biology (clifton, N.J). New York: Springer; 2019. p. 289–98.
90. Shah AA, Frierson HF Jr, Cathro HP. Analysis of immunohistochemical stain usage in different pathology practice settings. Am J Clin Pathol 2012;138(6):831–6.
91. Harms PW, Frankel TL, Moutafi M, et al. Multiplex immunohistochemistry and immunofluorescence: A practical update for pathologists. Mod Pathol 2023; 36(7):100197.
92. Wan G, Maliga Z, Yan B, et al. SpatialCells: Automated profiling of tumor microenvironments with spatially resolved multiplexed single-cell data. bioRxiv 2023. https://doi.org/10.1101/2023.11.10.566378.
93. Lin JR, Chen YA, Campton D, et al. High-plex immunofluorescence imaging and traditional histology of the same tissue section for discovering image-based biomarkers. Nat Cancer 2023;4(7):1036–52.

Unraveling the Functional Heterogeneity of Human Skin at Single-Cell Resolution

Stefano Sol, PhD[a], Fabiana Boncimino, PhD[a],
Kristina Todorova, PhD[a], Anna Mandinova, MD, PhD[a,b,c],*

KEYWORDS

• Keratinocytes • Stem cells • Epidermis • Dermis • Single-cell sequencing

KEY POINTS

• Human skin represents our interface with the environment and comprises 3 different functional layers: the epidermis, dermis, and hypodermis.

• The epidermal basal layer's keratinocytes undergo a terminal differentiation while migrating to the skin surface. Based on morphologic and proliferation studies, it has been suggested that there are distinct differentiation trajectories for the interfollicular epidermis.

• Several single-cell and spatial transcriptomic studies of the skin have provided essential insights into the heterogeneity of the epidermis and dermis cell subpopulations.

• The Human Cell Atlas is developing a consensus Human Skin Cell Atlas of diverse skin cell types across several conditions, such as age, gender, ancestral group, and body site.

• Aging and wound healing single-cell analysis highlighted the dysregulation of cell-type-specific transcriptional networks, providing help in the identification of novel therapeutic targets or compounds.

INTRODUCTION

Human skin, the body's largest organ, is a multilayered interface between the internal and external environment, representing the first line of defense against trauma, ultraviolet radiation, and chemical and pathogenic insults.[1,2] The skin protects internal tissues and organs, provides sensory innervation, prevents moisture loss to avoid dehydration, and regulates temperature homeostasis via control of peripheral vascular resistance.

[a] Cutaneous Biology Research Center, Massachusetts General Hospital and Harvard Medical School, Charlestown, MA 02129, USA; [b] Broad Institute of Harvard and MIT, 7 Cambridge Center, MA 02142, USA; [c] Harvard Stem Cell Institute, 7 Divinity Avenue Cambridge, MA 02138, USA
* Corresponding author. Cutaneous Biology Research Center, Massachusetts General Hospital, Harvard Medical School, 149 13th Street, Boston, MA 02129.
E-mail address: amandinova@mgh.harvard.edu

Hematol Oncol Clin N Am 38 (2024) 921–938
https://doi.org/10.1016/j.hoc.2024.05.001
hemonc.theclinics.com
0889-8588/24/© 2024 Elsevier Inc. All rights reserved.

The 3 layers of the skin, the epidermis, dermis, and hypodermis, vary significantly in their anatomy and function. Differentiation between layers of human skin has long been a focal point for research and is critical for refining treatment methods. Furthermore, recent research has revealed molecular diversity within these layers as well. Understanding the precise molecular processes orchestrating cell distribution and renewal across and between the skin's layers is crucial for developing practical therapeutic approaches. High-resolution single-cell transcriptomic techniques have emerged as precious tools for further investigating molecular heterogeneity. This new technology made it possible to identify disease-specific drivers and therapeutic targets, supporting the development of personalized therapies.[3] Despite the extensive data produced in mouse studies that initially helped to characterize cellular and functional heterogeneity of the skin, murine and human skin display significant histologic differences.[4–6] Therefore, in the present review, the authors focused on summarizing exclusively the latest findings on the transcriptomic profiling of human skin, analyzed from human biopsy, focusing on physiologic context, wound healing, and aging.

EPIDERMIS

The barrier function is mediated by the epidermis,[7] a stratified squamous epithelium divided into several differentiated layers and the basal stem cell (SC) layer anchored to the basement membrane (BM). In detail, from inside to outside there are stratum basale (the deepest portion of the epidermis), stratum spinosum, stratum granulosum, stratum lucidum, and stratum corneum (the most superficial portion of the epidermis).

Epidermal Stem Cell and Differentiation

The human epidermis is one of the tissues with the highest turnover in the human body. Basal SCs, attached to the BM, undergo self-renewal throughout adulthood, giving rise to the differentiating cells of the spinous and granular layers. These cells successively lose their nucleus and cytoplasmic organelles to form cornified cells.[2] The layers of cornified cells are a significant physical barrier against environmental stresses, keeping out invading pathogens and preventing dehydration of the underlying tissues. Basal SCs continuously generate terminally differentiated cells to replace lost ones and to maintain tissue homeostasis.[8] Nonetheless, the process of transitioning from undifferentiated SCs into differentiated cells, which are both molecularly unique and spatially distinct after cell division, remains unclear (**Fig. 1**).

Research has indicated functional heterogeneity within the interfollicular epidermis (IFE), leading to several theories about its formation. First, the Epidermal Proliferative Unit (EPU) Model comes from studies on morphology and cell proliferation, which have suggested that the IFE is structured in EPUs. In each EPU, a slow-cycling SC population produces transit-amplifying cell (TA) progeny. These TAs have a limited proliferation capacity and are predestined to undergo terminal differentiation.[9–11]

In contrast, evidence from lineage tracing of randomly labeled basal cells and label dilution experiments has led to the Single Progenitor Model. This model supports the presence of a single committed progenitor (CP) cell population responsible for both cell division and differentiation.[12–15]

Other models involving a SC population include the Stem Cell and Committed Progenitor Model, in which the SC population gives rise to CP cells that directly differentiate,[16,17] and the 2 stem cell model, in which there are 2 independent SC populations, each with distinct proliferation and differentiation patterns[18] (**Fig. 2**).

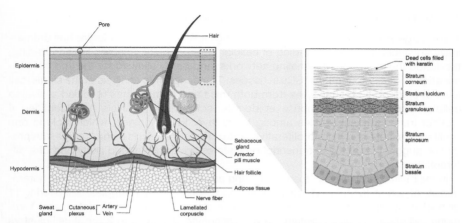

Fig. 1. Structure of human skin. Representation of the 3 layers of the skin, the epidermis, dermis, and hypodermis, with associated adnexal structures such as hair follicles, sweat glands, and sebaceous glands. The epidermis is a stratified squamous epithelium composed of the stratum basale, stratum spinosum, stratum granulosum, stratum lucidum, and stratum corneum. (Created with BioRender.com.)

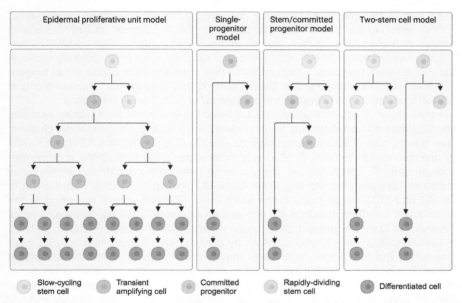

Fig. 2. Models for self-renewal and differentiation. The EPU model suggests that quiescent slow-cycling stem cells generate transit-amplifying cells, which undergo 3 rounds of symmetric division before terminal differentiation. The single-progenitor model says that, on division, a single population of committed progenitors (CP) generates other proliferative committed progenitors or differentiated cells through stochastic fate. The stem/committed progenitor model argues that slow-cycling stem cells within the basal layer generate rapidly cycling committed progenitors. In this model, the differentiated cells arise only from committed progenitors. The 2 stem cell model suggests the presence of 2 independent stem cell populations with different proliferation and differentiation rates. (Created with BioRender.com.)

Cellular Composition at Single-cell RNA-sequencing Level

The emergence of single-cell RNA-sequencing (scRNA-seq) technologies has dramatically advanced our understanding of cellular heterogeneity, enabled lineage tracing, facilitated the inference of signaling networks, and partly allowed for the spatial identification of distinct functional SCs in tissues. Transcriptomic analysis at the single-cell level of epidermal keratinocytes from both mice and humans has revealed a diverse cellular landscape.[5,19] In mouse epidermis, scRNA-seq analysis has identified 4 distinct transcriptional profiles among basal layer keratinocytes, which include one proliferative state and 3 nonproliferative states. Further analysis using lineage fate prediction suggests that these transcriptional states are transient and likely part of a differentiation hierarchy.[5]

In their initial scRNA-seq research, Cheng and colleagues examined cellular heterogeneity of human keratinocytes in 9 healthy and 3 inflamed skin samples, discovering 11 distinct transcriptional clusters: 8 keratinocyte states, 2 melanocyte states, and 1 immune cell state.[20] They classified the 8 keratinocyte clusters into 2 basal cell clusters with high expression of KRT5 and KRT14, termed "basal1" and "basal2," respectively, one "spinous" cluster with peak levels of KRT1 and KRT10 expression, and one "granular" cluster characterized by markers of advanced differentiation, including LOR, FLG, and SPINK5. The other 4 keratinocyte clusters were classified into one "mitotic" cluster with high expression of cell cycle markers such as PCNA and KI67, one "channel" cluster defined by ion channel and cell–cell communication transcripts including ATP1A1, GJB2, and GJB6, one "WNT1" cluster distinguished by expression of genes related to WNT signaling such as SFRP1, FRZB, DKK3, and 1 "follicular" cluster expressing markers of human follicular root sheaths and sebaceous gland, such as MGST1 and S100A2. Remarkably, "WNT1" and "follicular" clusters were predominantly found in skin derived from the scalp, which confirms their involvement in follicular hair biogenesis. The authors identified a third basal cluster called "basal3" that is present only in foreskin biopsies and is based on the expression of AREG, an EGFR ligand.

In their study, Wang and colleagues analyzed the epidermis from human neonatal foreskin obtained from 5 healthy donors, identifying 7 distinct transcriptional clusters: 4 basal keratinocyte states (comprising about 23%, BAS-I, BAS-II, BAS-III, and BAS-IV), one spinous (about 54%, SPN), one granular state (about 16%, GRN), and one melanocyte state.[19] These findings imply a linear differentiation pathway within basal epidermal keratinocytes, starting at the basal SC population (BAS-I), transitioning to the SC and ITGB1-high populations (BAS-II and BAS-III), and culminating in the commitment to differentiation in the progenitor population (BAS-IV). While all 4 basal keratinocyte states express typical basal keratinocyte markers, including KRT14, KRT5, and CDH3, each is characterized by distinct gene markers and specific locations within the rete ridges, which are projections of epidermis into the underlying dermis. The BAS-I and BAS-II basal clusters are enriched with cell cycle marker genes (akin to the basal3 cluster from Cheng and colleagues[20]) but are distinguished by different gene expressions: PTTG1 and CDC20 for BAS-I, and RRM2, HELLS, UHRF1, and PLAF for BAS-II.[20] ASS1, COL17A1, and POSTN expression define the BAS-III cluster. GJB2, KRT6A, and KRT16 expression define the BAS-IV basal cluster. The spinous cluster, SPN, represented more than half of the entire population pool and exhibited increased expression of KRT1, KRT10, DSG1, and CDH1—genes whose expression persists in granular keratinocytes. DSC1, KRT2, IVL, and TGM3 differentiation gene markers distinguish differentiated granular keratinocytes (GRN).

In another study by Negri and colleagues, researchers identified 13 distinct keratinocyte subpopulations.[21] Consistent with scRNA-seq findings from neonatal foreskin keratinocytes, they confirmed heterogeneity within the basal epidermal layer. They identified 3 nondividing cell subpopulations—"Basal I," "Basal II," and "Basal III"—based on the expression of basal layer markers such as KRT5 and KRT14, alongside one proliferative cell subpopulation named "Proliferation." The Proliferation cluster was characterized by high levels of cyclin-dependent kinase 1 (CDK1) and the proliferation marker Ki-67 (MKI67).[19] The distribution of integrin subunits varies across the basal clusters, with ITGA3 and ITGA6 being the most abundant in Basal II and ITGA2 and ITGB1 predominating in Basal III. Basal II cells were identified as the most stem-like state, indicated by several SC markers, such as COL17A1, POSTN, DLL1, and CD46. Two clusters were recognized as transition states due to the expression of pro-commitment genes such as DUSP6 and DUSP10, with DUSP6 mainly upregulated in "Transition I" and DUSP10 in both "Transition I" and "Transition II" Fields.[22] Five clusters corresponded to the first spinous cell layers, indicated by the expression of KRT1 and KRT10, while a higher FLG expression defined a small cluster of granular cells. Additionally, they found a population of keratinocytes classified as immune-related, identified by the coexpression of basal (KRT5, KRT14) and suprabasal (KRT10) markers, along with high levels of CD74, which is the receptor for macrophage migration inhibitory factor.

The study by Ganier and colleagues provides a more comprehensive analysis of various keratinocyte subpopulations in adnexal structures, such as hair follicles, sweat glands, and sebaceous glands. The research examines healthy human skin from multiple body sites, including the ear, nose, cheek, forehead, temple, and basal cell carcinoma (BCC).[23] More specifically, they showed the presence of 6 distinct transcriptomic profiles, 3 for the hair follicle—"upper hair follicle," "inner" and "outer bulb K"; one for the sweat gland—"gland secretory luminal cell"; and one for sebaceous gland—"Sebocytes." The upper hair follicle K cluster was characterized by the highest expression of KRT6a and KRT6B, whereas inner and outer bulb K clusters were defined based on KRT17 and SFRP1/WIF1 expression, respectively. KRT7, KRT19, and DCD mark gland secretory luminal cells, while MGST1 characterizes the Sebocytes cluster. The authors identified 4 different transcriptionally keratinocyte clusters specific to the IFE, comprising 1 undifferentiated ("IFE Basal K," KRT14$^+$/POSTN$^+$/DLL1$^+$) and 2 differentiated ("IFE Spinous K," KRT1$^+$/KRT10$^+$, and "IFE Granular K," LYPD3$^+$/SPPINK3$^+$), 1 "Dividing K" (CDK1$^+$/PCNA$^+$), and 1 "Transitional K" (JUN$^+$/JUNB$^+$/FOS$^+$) clusters.

DERMIS
Dermis Structure: Upper Versus Lower Dermis

The dermis is a connective tissue composed of collagen and elastic fibers that provide flexibility and support the overlying epidermis.[24,25] Histologically, 2 distinct layers are identified in the human skin dermis: (1) the upper papillary dermis, which is the layer adjacent to the epidermis that has a higher cell density with less extracellular matrix (ECM), and (2) the lower reticular dermis, which is a thicker layer that contains fewer fibroblasts and more ECM.[26,27] The reticular dermis overlies the hypodermis, or the dermal and subcutaneous white adipose tissue.[28,29] The dermis accommodates other extracellular components, including vessels, nerves, hair follicles, and glands.[30] The principal resident cell type of the dermis is fibroblast, which produces the connective tissue components but also exerts roles in skin inflammatory response, wound healing, and skin aging.[31] Besides the fibroblast, the dermis comprises other cell types such as pericytes, closely associated with blood vessels and mast cells, involved in the immune and inflammatory responses, melanocytes, and adipocytes.[32] Several published studies individualized two main fibroblast populations, papillary and reticular fibroblasts, with distinct morphology and function by their localization in the dermis.[26,33,34] RNA extracted from microdissected papillary (upper 100 µm dermis) and reticular dermis (lower 200–500 µm dermis) was subjected to RNA sequencing analysis, and it showed that cells in papillary and reticular dermis had distinct gene expression profile.[35] Expression of COL6A5 and components of the Wnt pathway was highly enriched in the papillary dermis, while CD36 was upregulated in the lower reticular dermis and hypodermis. Although most of the studies recognized these two fibroblast subpopulations, univocal markers to distinguish them have yet to be determined, and subsequent studies elucidated a newly functional heterogeneity that remained hidden until then.

Cellular Composition at Single-Cell RNA-Sequencing Level

The progress in scRNA seq analysis has provided a new insight into fibroblast heterogeneity. Multiple research groups attempted to explain the transcriptomic heterogeneity of the human skin dermis, taking advantage of scRNA-seq and identifying distinct functional fibroblast subpopulations. However, the results of these studies could be more precise. Foremost, Tabib and colleagues revealed two central fibroblast populations characterized by SFRP2/DPP4 and FMO1/LSP1 markers.[36] SFRP2/DPP4 fibroblasts expressed higher levels of ECM genes, including type I collagen, fibrillin, and fibronectin. The other population of fibroblasts strongly agreed with CXCL12, suggesting a role in immune surveillance. Besides these two main populations, different marker genes definite five minor cell populations characterized by the expression of CRABP1, COL11A1, PRG4, ANGPTL7, and SFRP4, respectively, with just CRABP1 cells actual in their function of dermal papilla cells as described previously.[37,38] Recently, Wiedemann and colleagues discerned three subpopulations, with two of those matching with the previous study of Tabib and colleagues, with a first group defined by FMO1/LSP1 expression implicated in immune surveillance and a second group defined by SFRP2 and DPP4 involved in ECM homeostasis.[39] These 2 major fibroblast subtypes were not associated with papillary and reticular fibroblasts. Instead, Philippeos and colleagues have identified at least 4 fibroblast populations with distinct functions related to their localization in the dermis.[35] The upper dermal fibroblasts are defined by lin−CD90+CD39+CD26− cell surface markers and are characterized by the expression of COL6A5 and upregulation of Wnt signaling. Lin- CD90+CD36+ are markers of the lower dermal fibroblasts, including preadipocytes. Also localized in the reticular dermis are lin- CD90+CD39-RGS5+, that correspond to pericytes[40], lin- CD90+CD39+CD26+ and lin- CD90+CD39-RGS5− that are not yet characterized fibroblasts. Likewise, Solè-Boldo and colleagues classified 4 main young fibroblast subpopulations, 2 of these described as secretory-reticular fibroblasts and secretory-papillary fibroblasts correlated with the production of collagen and ECM organization; meanwhile, the other 2 subpopulations both have a more prominent reticular localization but one with a mesenchymal potential and the other with proinflammatory functions.[41] In comparison with the previous studies, Sole-Boldo and colleagues found that the expression of FMO1 was deficient in all dermal fibroblasts, and SFRP2 was expressed in almost every fibroblast subpopulation, while most of the genes used to define the 5 subpopulations by Philippeos and colleagues did not have a significant expression level in their dataset. Afterward, Vorstandlechner and colleagues described 6 fibroblast clusters.[42] The larger fibroblast subpopulation was discernible by DPP4/CD26 markers, and the overexpression of collagen I, ECM proteins, and metalloproteases characterized it. The other 2 groups, expressing WIF1, CXCL1, and THY1, were functionally related to immune response and leukocyte migration. Of the other subpopulation, the first correlated to cartilage development and leptin signaling, the second was associated with growth factors response, and the last subpopulation was connected to interferon-gamma response and p38 and NF-κB signaling. Also, this study found no expression of FMO1 in any cell subtypes, and SFRP2 expression was distributed homogenously along the different fibroblast subsets. Ascensión and colleagues reanalyzed all published datasets and revealed a remarkable agreement between them, considering that the skin was sampled from diverse body areas and heterogenous donors of dissimilar age and sex and with a different experimental approach.[43] Overall, they showed that it is possible to classify the fibroblast into three populations: (1) the primary group is defined by the expression of ELN, MMP2, QPCT, and SFRP2 and it appears to be involved in ECM homeostasis; (2) fibroblasts defined by APOE, C7, CYGB, and IGFBP7 expression have a role in immune response and inflammation; (3) the last group of fibroblasts is instead defined by DKK3, TNMD, TNN, and SFRP1 expression and it includes dermal papilla cells and dermo-hypodermal junction fibroblasts. Based on these studies, the traditional classification of fibroblasts in reticular and papillary subpopulations is not robust due to their anatomic location. Fibroblast subsets with similar functions are most probably disseminated throughout the dermal layers.

The previously cited study of Ganier and colleagues has shed light on spatial transcriptomic information of the dermis through the integration of scRNA-seq, spatial global transcriptional profiling (ST), and in situ sequencing (ISS).[23] Integrating the already published dataset from body sites with their scRNAseq data from facial skin samples, they identified 4 central populations of fibroblasts, which were characterized by high expression of APOD, SFRP2, PTGDS, and POSTN, respectively.[36,41] The abundance and distribution of fibroblast clusters differed between body and face samples. APOD + fibroblasts, more abundant in facial skin than body skin, highly expressed APOE and are implicated in immune responses. Global ST data and ISS data showed an association between APOD + fibroblasts and blood vessels, and this explains the increased prevalence of APOD + fibroblasts in facial skin because of the increased vascular density compared to body skin. SFRP2 + fibroblasts coexpressed WISP2, a Wnt inhibitor, and GO terms are correlated to ECM organization and negative regulation of BMP signaling, which is essential in regulating hair follicle (HF) growth. SFRP2 + fibroblasts were overrepresented in body skin compared to facial skin, and they are distributed throughout the dermis with a higher concentration in the reticular dermis. PTGDS + fibroblasts, present in a similar amount in the face and body skin, are also related to ECM remodeling, collagen fibril organization, and TGF-ß response. PTGDS + fibroblasts were primarily localized in the papillary dermis and in proximity to the upper HF. Lastly, POSTN + fibroblasts are involved in ECM deposition and collagen fibril organization, similar to PTGDS + fibroblasts, which colocalize around HFs. This study shows how a combination of scRNA-seq and spatial techniques can contribute to creating a spatial atlas of different cell populations of various human skin body sites that can be used by skin research and dermatology communities. Besides the steps forward in understanding fibroblast heterogeneity, many aspects must be further investigated to build a consistent resource for skin research.

Extracellular Matrix

The ECM is the most significant component of the dermal skin layer. The ECM primarily comprises water, proteins, and polysaccharides, and its composition can dynamically remodel in response to environmental stimuli. It provides physical support for cells through its complex chemical composition and organization.[44] The ECM primarily comprises 2 main classes of macromolecules: fibrous proteins, including elastin and collagens (mainly types I and III), and glycoproteins, including fibronectin, proteoglycans, and laminin. In contrast to the predominantly fibrillar structure of collagens, proteoglycans' intrinsic characteristic to bind water provides hydration and resistance.[45] Dermal ECM composition differs between the papillary layer with thin collagen fibers and the reticular dermis with dense collagen fibers. Collagen I is mainly deposited into the deeper reticular dermis. In contrast, collagen VII is mainly deposited by the papillary fibroblast to the BM that separates the epidermis from the dermis.[46]

BASEMENT MEMBRANE

The epidermis and the underlying dermis are connected at the dermal–epidermal junction (DEJ) by the BM, a thin layer composed of extracellular matrix.[47,48] The BM provides structural support to keratinocytes and is essential in maintaining skin processes, such as barrier function, cell differentiation, proliferation, and polarization.[49] More specifically, the BM constituents preserve the SC pool of keratinocytes due to the release of signals essential to establish cell polarity, thus allowing asymmetric cell divisions of keratinocytes, which undergo a terminal differentiation while transiting from the basal to the suprabasal cell layers. Furthermore, the BM could regulate the interaction between ligand and cell surface receptors by binding and retaining growth factors, thereby modulating signaling processes such as tissue growth, cell migration, and cell survival.[50,51] The BM has 2 bifunctional sides: the epithelial face is enriched in laminins and is stiffer than the stromal side, which is enriched in collagen proteins.[52] The extracellular matrix proteins within the BM belong to 4 categories: collagen IV, the glycoproteins laminin, nidogen, and the heparan sulfate proteoglycan perlecan.[53] Glycosaminoglycans and proteoglycans are in the form of hydrogels, which are a pool of growth factors and permit resistance to the mechanical stress to which the skin is constantly exposed. Collagen proteins have a triple-helical structure, and cross-linking provides stiffness and flexibility. Collagen IV is the most abundant structural component of the BM, and it is essential to stabilizing its structure.[54] The optimal stiffness and the other peculiar characteristics of this layer are due to the precise molecular organization and the specific interactions between the structural domains of each constituent, some of which are synthesized by either fibroblasts or keratinocytes. In contrast, others are produced by both cell types.[55] The well-defined architecture and the characteristic anchoring complexes assured the attachment of the dermis to the epidermis layers. The anchoring complexes link the stroma to the intermediate filament of the basal keratinocytes' cytoskeleton, consisting of hemidesmosome and anchoring fibril.[56] Hemidesmosomes are highly organized adhesion structures, while the anchoring fibrils are composed of a6b4 integrin, laminin isoform 332 (LM-332), and collagens VII and XVII.[57] LM-332 is associated with basal epidermal keratinocytes, and the binding of LM-332 to collagen VII is critical for the initial assembly of hemidesmosomes at the basolateral surface of cells. Then collagen VII interacts with b4 integrin and plectin, which in turn binds intermediate filaments in the cytoplasm.[58] Collagen XVIII is also involved in many connections in this network, thus having a vital role in the keratinocyte anchorage.[59]

HUMAN SKIN CELL ATLAS

The rapidly advancing technological development in scRNA seq opened new scenarios, enabling the definition of new cell types, disease-specific drivers, and new therapeutic targets. To allow wider distribution of these data within the scientific community, a new program called The Human Cell Atlas (HCA; humancellatlas.org) was launched in 2016.[60] The HCA aims to map all cell types in the body to achieve a higher knowledge level of normal human physiology and disease. In this context, the ambition of the Skin Biological Network is to develop a consensus Human Skin Cell Atlas (HSCA), as part of the HCA, of diverse skin cell types across several scales. At the same time, to create a comprehensive map of cell populations at single-cell resolution, different research groups are integrating scRNA-seq data with several complementary approaches to localize cells within human skin.[23,61] A new public web interface (https://spatial-skin-atlas.cellgeni.sanger.ac.uk/) was created to facilitate the use of this spatial skin atlas.

Indeed, massive work must be done to represent skin's full anatomic and functional diversity at a single-cell level. The HSCA should include several body sites that differ in dominant features (epidermis thickness and hair follicle size, density, and growth cycle),[62] skin microbiome profile,[63] prominent age-dependent changes of many skin sites,[64,65] wound healing scale,[66–69] difference between genders,[70] and the ancestral groups that show different cutaneous anatomic features, such as skin pigmentation, sweat gland, and hair follicle differences and are underrepresented in biomedical research[71,72] (Fig. 3).

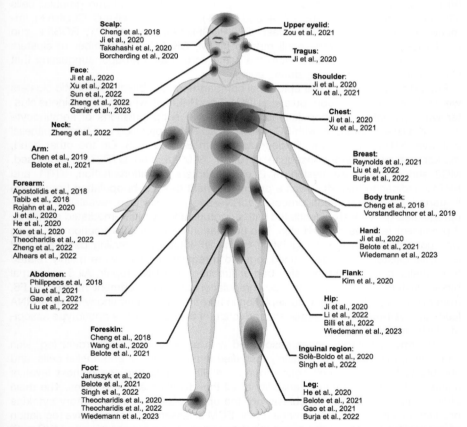

Fig. 3. Summary of skin scRNA-seq studies subdivided on the base of biopsy excision sites. Representation of the different body areas from which skin specimens were collected and analyzed with single-cell techniques. (Created with BioRender.com.).

References to the papers that generated the scRNA-seq dataset are listed chronologically for each location: scalp[20,73–75]; upper eyelid[76]; face[23,73,77–79]; tragus[73]; neck[79]; shoulder[73,77]; chest[73,77]; breast[80–82]; body trunk[20,42]; arm[83,84]; forearm[36,73,79,85–90]; hand[39,73,84]; abdomen[35,81,91,92]; flank[93]; hip[39,67,73,94]; foreskin[19,20,84]; inguinal region[41,68]; leg[82,84,87,92]; foot.[66,68,69,82,84,89]

Created with BioRender.com.

Aging

Zou and colleagues were the first to apply scRNA-seq technologies to whole-skin aging in humans, using eyelid skin samples from a group of healthy female donors of different ages, dividing into young (Y, 18–28 year old), middle-aged (M, 35–48 year old), and old (O, 70–76 year old) groups.[76] Indeed, human facial skin is predisposed to aging-related changes not only for the intrinsic chronologic effect but also because of the influence of UV exposure.[95,96] Overall, the main morphologic changes during skin aging are the decrease of epidermal thickness and dermal collagen density with accumulation of p16INK4a-positive cells as hallmarks of increased senescence in both epidermis and dermis.[97] The authors identified 11 clusters based on specific markers, including basal (BC, KRT14+), mitotic (MC, MKI67+); vellus hair follicles (VHF, SOX9+, KRT6B+, and SFRP1+), spinous (SC, KRT10+) and granular cells (GC, FLG+), melanocyte (ME, TYR+ and DCT+), endothelial cell (EC, CLDN5+), immune cell (IC, PTPRC+), fibroblast (FB, PDGFRA+), pericyte (PT, RGS5+ and PDGFRB+), and orbicularis oculi muscle (OOM, CKM+). The number of clusters and the cell-type distributions were the same across all 3 groups, suggesting that skin maintains its cell identity during aging.

Regarding the interfollicular epidermal compartment, the basal and mitotic clusters were subdivided into 3 subpopulations (BC1-3 and MC1-3), whereas the spinous cluster was split into 2 subpopulations (SC1-2). All 9 subpopulations of keratinocyte showed a linear hierarchy, with SC marker COL17A1 expression and basal epithelial cell layer KRT14 that gradually decreased from BC1 to BC3. On the other hand, markers of inflammatory response (S100A9, S100A8, and CYP27A1) increased. MC2 showed high expression of 2 early markers of differentiation, KRT1 and KRT10, indicating that MC2 was a procommitment basal subpopulation from which it started the differentiation process. scRNA-seq analysis also revealed that age-upregulated genes were associated with apoptotic and cytokine-mediated signaling, 2 prominent features of aged skin. The correlation between inflammation and aging was consistent with the upregulation of the NF-kappa B signaling pathway in all epithelial clusters with age. Indeed, age-downregulated genes were mainly related to epithelial cell proliferation, skin barrier function, and DNA repair. All 3 epidermal basal clusters showed a strong downregulation of a development marker, KLF6, from middle age. In contrast, its depletion in human primary keratinocytes via shRNA leads to a self-renewal decrease and induction of the senescence phenotype associated with inflammation.

Furthermore, hotspot genes associated with aging and skin disorders (eg, skin carcinoma, melanoma) were mainly identified in melanocytes, endothelial cells, and fibroblasts.[98] Zou and colleagues found that fibroblasts had the highest level of aging-related transcriptional variability of all the identified skin cell types. The main changes in aged dermal fibroblasts are the up-regulation of inflammatory cytokine production pathways, DNA damage repair, ECM disassembly, and negative regulation of cell proliferation. In contrast, genes related to ribosome biogenesis and MYC activation pathways were downregulated. These findings are in accordance with the already documented tendency of a lower proliferation rate of aged dermal fibroblasts and with alteration in ECM deposition linked to the thinning of the dermis.[65,99] Moreover, Zou and colleagues found that among the top downregulated genes, the transcription factor HES1 is a critical downstream target of the Notch signaling.[100] It was shown that its downregulation promotes cellular senescence and may drive physiologic fibroblast aging.

Solè-Boldo and colleagues also investigated the effect of aging at the transcriptional level in dermal fibroblasts, showing a reduced proliferative capacity of old fibroblasts in the proinflammatory, secretory-papillary and slightly secretory-reticular cell subpopulations.[41] Moreover, the aged fibroblast showed a loss of the functional annotations for each cluster, with a less prominent reticular gene expression signature for the reticular fibroblasts. In contrast, the old papillary fibroblasts displayed a higher reticular instead of the papillary gene expression signatures. Thus, this study suggested an age-related loss of fibroblast priming. More recent scRNA-seq study by Ahlers and colleagues confirmed the previous observations of age-related changes across fibroblast populations, such as the loss of fibroblast priming and a neuroprotective effect of HES1.[90] These acknowledgments may help identify novel therapeutic targets or compounds against human skin aging and related diseases.

Wound Healing

Wound healing is a complex and highly coordinated process that involves interactions between the different cell types. Chronic wounds are a significant public health challenge and scRNA-seq data generated from acute and chronic wounds would represent a successful tool for diagnosis and therapy.[101] Li and colleagues performed a scRNA-seq analysis in pressure ulcer (PU), a type of chronic nonhealing wound in which there is a dysregulation of inflammation that inhibits the regeneration process.[67,102] They identified 6 clusters: melanocyte, immune cell, and 4 keratinocytes (KC). KC_1 (K10+ cells) and KC_3 (S100A7 + cells) represented spinous and granular KCs, respectively, whereas KC_2 (IFITM1 + cells) and KC_4 (IGFBP3 + cells) were both basal layer KCs. Both KC_2 and KC_4 cells were associated with focal adhesion and extracellular matrix organization; KC_1 subpopulation was correlated to lipid metabolism, Ras signal transduction, and Notch signaling pathway; KC_3 is implicated in immune response and epidermis/hair follicle development. They found differences in cell composition and gene expression in PU samples compared to healthy skin. Granular KC_3 and epidermal immune cells were more abundant in PU than in skin or acute wound AW, while fewer spinous KC_1 and basal layer KC_4 cells were detected. PU KCs highly expressed genes involved in neutrophil-mediated immunity (eg, S100A7) and apoptosis (eg, DUSP1 and RHOB). Immunostaining in the PU samples confirmed increased cleaved caspase-3-positive cells. PU KCs also showed dysregulation in the differentiation program, with a lower proportion of proliferating cells. However, in AW healing, there was an increased frequency of spinous KC_1 and granular KC_3 cells with a higher proportion of proliferating KCs expressing the early differentiation markers K1 and K10. This finding is based on previous studies in which humans' significant proliferative and tissue-regenerative capacity early differentiates KCs.[103]

Another study published by Singh and colleagues focused on human unwounded (UW) skin and chronic wound edge (WE) at a single-cell resolution.[68] They identified 11 clusters corresponding to 10 cell types: fibroblasts, endothelial cells, smooth muscle cells, NK cells, myeloid cells, mast cells, B cells, lymphatic endothelial cells, melanocytes, and 2 different clusters of keratinocytes defined as Kera1 (KRT14+KRT1+) and Kera2 (KRT19+KRT7+). Kera1 was detected in both WE and UW skin samples. WE samples showed significant downregulation of genes associated with TP53–FOXO-mediated regulation of transcription while upregulation of genes related to ECM degradation and keratinization. In contrast, Kera2 was characterized by a higher expression of genes implied in cellular metabolism and glycolysis. Still, this subpopulation was substantially loss in the chronic WE tissue compared to UW skin. Thus, this likely suggested a contribution to wound chronicity. Reanalyzing the data of Li and colleagues, they found that unlikely from WE sample depletion of Kera2 subpopulation was not observed.[67] Moreover, Kera1 of AW did not present a downregulation of TP53, NOTCH1, and TWIST1. Still, it displayed a downregulated iron uptake and transport pathways, upregulation of keratinization, and formation of the cornified envelope, denoting an active re-epithelialization process.

Meanwhile, scRNA-seq performed by Januszyk and colleagues on wound tissue from human diabetic and nondiabetic plantar foot ulcers identified the altered distribution of fibroblast subpopulations with differing fibrotic potentials.[66] Of the 3 subclusters recognized, subcluster 1 (sc1) corresponded to traditionally defined PDGFRA + fibroblasts, the second subcluster (sc2) may represent a basal population of collagen-producing fibroblasts, and subcluster 3 (sc3) as a pro-fibrotic population. The collagen-producing sc2 and profibrotic sc3 populations were more prominent in diabetic foot ulcer (DFU) cells. Diabetic wound fibroblasts are characterized by a higher expression of COL1A1, COL3A1, and COL6A1, associated with ECM deposition and fibrosis, overexpression of profibrotic and myofibroblast markers such as FOS, POSTN, and ACTA2, and elevated inflammatory state defined by CXCL8 and CD44 expression. Among the downregulated genes, there were FGF2 and APOD associated with fibroblast survival and regeneration. Theocharidis and colleagues also investigated differences between DFU and nonulcerated tissue.[69] Ulcer samples showed a distinct cellular composition, with the identification of 3 clusters instead of the 5 individualized in healthy skin, with an upregulation of genes related to blood vessel development and ECM organization, suggesting a role in promoting neo-angiogenesis. Moreover, the papillary fibroblast cluster was enriched for COL7A1 (collagen Type VII), which plays a vital role in the DEJ's structure and wound healing. Further single-cell analysis of wound specimens is needed to improve the knowledge regarding the complex wound-compartmentalized microenvironment in human skin.

SUMMARY

In conclusion, the present review underscores the ever-growing knowledge of skin's complexity as a multifunctional organ, highlighting the pivotal role of cellular diversity and communication in maintaining skin integrity and function. Advances in scRNA seq have revealed intricate details about skin cell heterogeneity, offering new insights into the aging process, skin diseases, and wound healing mechanisms. This knowledge opens up promising avenues for developing targeted therapies and personalized medical approaches. However, it also emphasizes the need for further research to fully understand the molecular underpinnings of skin health and translate these findings into clinical applications.

CLINICS CARE POINTS

- The skin is the largest and one of the most complex and heterogeneous organs in the human body. It comprises diverse cell types, each strategically positioned to provide structure and perform specialized functions.

- The primary function of the skin is to protect the body from the external environment. It serves as the first line of defense against physical trauma, ultraviolet radiation, and chemical and pathogenic assaults.

- The human epidermis is one of the tissues with the highest turnover rate in the body. Basal stem cells, attached to the basement membrane, undergo self-renewal throughout adulthood. They give rise to the differentiating cells of the spinous and granular layers, which eventually lose their nucleus and cytoplasmic organelles to form cornified cells.

- The dermis is a connective tissue composed of collagen and elastic fibers, providing flexibility and support to the overlying epidermis. Histologically, the dermis has two distinct layers: (i) the upper papillary dermis, adjacent to the epidermis, which has a higher cell density and less extracellular matrix (ECM), and (ii) the lower reticular dermis, a thicker layer with fewer fibroblasts and more ECM.

- Gaining a deeper understanding of the molecular mechanisms and pathways that maintain skin homeostasis is crucial for developing effective therapeutic strategies.

- Advances in single-cell RNA sequencing (scRNA-seq) have provided detailed insights into skin cell heterogeneity, revealing new information about aging, skin diseases, and wound healing mechanisms. This knowledge paves the way for developing targeted therapies and personalized medical approaches.

ACKNOWLEDGMENTS

The authors thank Sarah Waszyn for editing the article.

DISCLOSURE

A. Mandinova is a co-founder (with equity) of New Frontier Bio, a consumer health company developing skincare and anti-aging products, and has equity in DermBiont, a private company advancing targeted topical therapeutics for dermatologic indications. K. Todorova has a financial interest in New Frontier Bio.

REFERENCES

1. Fuchs E. Scratching the surface of skin development. Nature 2007;445(7130): 834–42.
2. Watt FM. Mammalian skin cell biology: at the interface between laboratory and clinic. Science 2014;346(6212):937–40.
3. Dubois A, Gopee N, Olabi B, et al. Defining the skin cellular community using single-cell genomics to advance precision medicine. J Invest Dermatol 2021; 141(2):255–64.
4. Blanpain C, Fuchs E. Epidermal homeostasis: a balancing act of stem cells in the skin. Nat Rev Mol Cell Biol 2009;10(3):207–17.
5. Haensel D, Jin S, Sun P, et al. Defining epidermal basal cell states during skin homeostasis and wound healing using single-cell transcriptomics. Cell Rep 2020;30(11):3932–3947 e6.
6. Joost S, Annusver K, Jacob T, et al. The molecular anatomy of mouse skin during hair growth and rest. Cell Stem Cell 2020;26(3):441–457 e7.
7. Fuchs E. Finding one's niche in the skin. Cell Stem Cell 2009;4(6):499–502.
8. Cockburn K, Annusver K, Gonzalez DG, et al. Gradual differentiation uncoupled from cell cycle exit generates heterogeneity in the epidermal stem cell layer. Nat Cell Biol 2022;24(12):1692–700.

9. Mackenzie IC. Retroviral transduction of murine epidermal stem cells demonstrates clonal units of epidermal structure. J Invest Dermatol 1997;109(3): 377–83.

10. Potten CS. The epidermal proliferative unit: the possible role of the central basal cell. Cell Tissue Kinet 1974;7(1):77–88.

11. Potten CS, Saffhill R, Maibach HI. Measurement of the transit time for cells through the epidermis and stratum corneum of the mouse and guinea-pig. Cell Tissue Kinet 1987;20(5):461–72.

12. Clayton E, Doupé DP, Klein AM, et al. A single type of progenitor cell maintains normal epidermis. Nature 2007;446(7132):185–9.

13. Doupe DP, Klein AM, Simons BD, et al. The ordered architecture of murine ear epidermis is maintained by progenitor cells with random fate. Dev Cell 2010; 18(2):317–23.

14. Rompolas P, Mesa KR, Kawaguchi K, et al. Spatiotemporal coordination of stem cell commitment during epidermal homeostasis. Science 2016;352(6292): 1471–4.

15. Piedrafita G, Kostiou V, Wabik A, et al. A single-progenitor model as the unifying paradigm of epidermal and esophageal epithelial maintenance in mice. Nat Commun 2020;11(1):1429.

16. Mascre G, Dekoninck S, Drogat B, et al. Distinct contribution of stem and progenitor cells to epidermal maintenance. Nature 2012;489(7415):257–62.

17. Sanchez-Danes A, Hannezo E, Larsimont JC, et al. Defining the clonal dynamics leading to mouse skin tumour initiation. Nature 2016;536(7616):298–303.

18. Sada A, Jacob F, Leung E, et al. Defining the cellular lineage hierarchy in the interfollicular epidermis of adult skin. Nat Cell Biol 2016;18(6):619–31.

19. Wang S, Drummond ML, Guerrero-Juarez CF, et al. Single cell transcriptomics of human epidermis identifies basal stem cell transition states. Nat Commun 2020; 11(1):4239.

20. Cheng JB, Sedgewick AJ, Finnegan AI, et al. Transcriptional Programming of Normal and Inflamed Human Epidermis at Single-Cell Resolution. Cell Rep 2018;25(4):871–83.

21. Negri VA, Louis B, Zijl S, et al. Single-cell RNA sequencing of human epidermis identifies Lunatic fringe as a novel regulator of the stem cell compartment. Stem Cell Rep 2023;18(11):2047–55.

22. Mishra A, Oulès B, Pisco AO, et al. A protein phosphatase network controls the temporal and spatial dynamics of differentiation commitment in human epidermis. Elife 2017;6.

23. Ganier C, Mazin P, Herrera-Oropeza G, et al. Multiscale spatial mapping of cell populations across anatomical sites in healthy human skin and basal cell carcinoma. Proc Natl Acad Sci U S A 2024;121(2). e2313326120.

24. Parsonage G, Filer AD, Haworth O, et al. A stromal address code defined by fibroblasts. Trends Immunol 2005;26(3):150–6.

25. Watt FM, Fujiwara H. Cell-extracellular matrix interactions in normal and diseased skin. Cold Spring Harb Perspect Biol 2011;3(4).

26. Harper RA, Grove G. Human skin fibroblasts derived from papillary and reticular dermis: differences in growth potential in vitro. Science 1979;204(4392):526–7.

27. Korosec A, Frech S, Gesslbauer B, et al. Lineage identity and location within the dermis determine the function of papillary and reticular fibroblasts in human skin. J Invest Dermatol 2019;139(2):342–51.

28. Driskell RR, Jahoda CAB, Chuong CM, et al. Defining dermal adipose tissue. Exp Dermatol 2014;23(9):629–31.

29. Festa E, Fretz J, Berry R, et al. Adipocyte lineage cells contribute to the skin stem cell niche to drive hair cycling. Cell 2011;146(5):761–71.
30. Brown TM, Krishnamurthy K. Histology, Dermis, *StatPearls*. Treasure Island, FL: StatPearls Publishing; 2022.
31. Plikus MV, Wang X, Sinha S, et al. Fibroblasts: Origins, definitions, and functions in health and disease. Cell 2021;184(15):3852–72.
32. Paquet-Fifield S, Schlüter H, Li A, et al. A role for pericytes as microenvironmental regulators of human skin tissue regeneration. J Clin Invest 2009; 119(9):2795–806.
33. Hiraoka C, Toki F, Shiraishi K, et al. Two clonal types of human skin fibroblasts with different potentials for proliferation and tissue remodeling ability. J Dermatol Sci 2016;82(2):84–94.
34. Janson DG, Saintigny G, van Adrichem A, et al. Different gene expression patterns in human papillary and reticular fibroblasts. J Invest Dermatol 2012; 132(11):2565–72.
35. Philippeos C, Telerman SB, Oulès B, et al. Spatial and single-cell transcriptional profiling identifies functionally distinct human dermal fibroblast subpopulations. J Invest Dermatol 2018;138(4):811–25.
36. Tabib T, Morse C, Wang T, et al. SFRP2/DPP4 and FMO1/LSP1 Define Major Fibroblast Populations in Human Skin. J Invest Dermatol 2018;138(4):802–10.
37. Driskell RR, Lichtenberger BM, Hoste E, et al. Distinct fibroblast lineages determine dermal architecture in skin development and repair. Nature 2013; 504(7479):277–81.
38. Driskell RR, Watt FM. Understanding fibroblast heterogeneity in the skin. Trends Cell Biol 2015;25(2):92–9.
39. Wiedemann J, Billi AC, Bocci F, et al. Differential cell composition and split epidermal differentiation in human palm, sole, and hip skin. Cell Rep 2023; 42(1):111994.
40. Bondjers C, Kalén M, Hellström M, et al. Transcription profiling of platelet-derived growth factor-B-deficient mouse embryos identifies RGS5 as a novel marker for pericytes and vascular smooth muscle cells. Am J Pathol 2003; 162(3):721–9.
41. Sole-Boldo L, Raddatz G, Schütz S, et al. Single-cell transcriptomes of the human skin reveal age-related loss of fibroblast priming. Commun Biol 2020; 3(1):188.
42. Vorstandlechner V, Laggner M, Kalinina P, et al. Deciphering the functional heterogeneity of skin fibroblasts using single-cell RNA sequencing. FASEB J 2020; 34(3):3677–92.
43. Ascension AM, Fuertes-Álvarez S, Ibañez-Solé O, et al. Human dermal fibroblast subpopulations are conserved across single-cell RNA sequencing studies. J Invest Dermatol 2021;141(7):1735–1744 e35.
44. Mouw JK, Ou G, Weaver VM. Extracellular matrix assembly: a multiscale deconstruction. Nat Rev Mol Cell Biol 2014;15(12):771–85.
45. Watt FM, Huck WT. Role of the extracellular matrix in regulating stem cell fate. Nat Rev Mol Cell Biol 2013;14(8):467–73.
46. Huang J, Heng S, Zhang W, et al. Dermal extracellular matrix molecules in skin development, homeostasis, wound regeneration and diseases. Semin Cell Dev Biol 2022;128:137–44.
47. McMillan JR, Akiyama M, Shimizu H. Epidermal basement membrane zone components: ultrastructural distribution and molecular interactions. J Dermatol Sci 2003;31(3):169–77.

48. Merker HJ. Morphology of the basement membrane. Microsc Res Tech 1994; 28(2):95–124.

49. Candiello J, Balasubramani M, Schreiber EM, et al. Biomechanical properties of native basement membranes. FEBS J 2007;274(11):2897–908.

50. Breitkreutz D, Koxholt I, Thiemann K, et al. Skin basement membrane: the foundation of epidermal integrity–BM functions and diverse roles of bridging molecules nidogen and perlecan. BioMed Res Int 2013;2013:179784.

51. Yurchenco PD. Basement membranes: cell scaffoldings and signaling platforms. Cold Spring Harb Perspect Biol 2011;3(2).

52. Halfter W, Oertle P, Monnier CA, et al. New concepts in basement membrane biology. FEBS J 2015;282(23):4466–79.

53. Pozzi A, Yurchenco PD, Iozzo RV. The nature and biology of basement membranes. Matrix Biol 2017;57-58:1–11.

54. Crouch E, Sage H, Bornstein P. Structural basis for apparent heterogeneity of collagens in human basement membranes: type IV procollagen contains two distinct chains. Proc Natl Acad Sci U S A 1980;77(2):745–9.

55. Aumailley M. Laminins and interaction partners in the architecture of the basement membrane at the dermal-epidermal junction. Exp Dermatol 2021;30(1): 17–24.

56. Rousselle P, Laigle C, Rousselet G. The basement membrane in epidermal polarity, stemness, and regeneration. Am J Physiol Cell Physiol 2022;323(6): C1807–22.

57. Roig-Rosello E, Rousselle P. The human epidermal basement membrane: a shaped and cell instructive platform that aging slowly alters. Biomolecules 2020;10(12).

58. Winograd-Katz SE, Fässler R, Geiger B, et al. The integrin adhesome: from genes and proteins to human disease. Nat Rev Mol Cell Biol 2014;15(4):273–88.

59. Heljasvaara R, Aikio M, Ruotsalainen H, et al. Collagen XVIII in tissue homeostasis and dysregulation - Lessons learned from model organisms and human patients. Matrix Biol 2017;57-58:55–75.

60. Regev A, Teichmann SA, Lander ES, et al. The human cell atlas. Elife 2017;6.

61. Thrane K, Winge MCG, Wang H, et al. Single-cell and spatial transcriptomic analysis of human skin delineates intercellular communication and pathogenic cells. J Invest Dermatol 2023;143(11):2177–2192 e13.

62. Sandby-Moller J, Poulsen T, Wulf HC. Epidermal thickness at different body sites: relationship to age, gender, pigmentation, blood content, skin type and smoking habits. Acta Derm Venereol 2003;83(6):410–3.

63. Byrd AL, Belkaid Y, Segre JA. The human skin microbiome. Nat Rev Microbiol 2018;16(3):143–55.

64. Farage MA, Miller KW, Elsner P, et al. Characteristics of the aging skin. Adv Wound Care 2013;2(1):5–10.

65. Haydont V, Bernard BA, Fortunel NO. Age-related evolutions of the dermis: Clinical signs, fibroblast and extracellular matrix dynamics. Mech Ageing Dev 2019; 177:150–6.

66. Januszyk M, Chen K, Henn D, et al. Characterization of diabetic and non-diabetic foot ulcers using single-cell RNA-sequencing. Micromachines 2020;11(9).

67. Li D, Cheng S, Pei Y, et al. Single-cell analysis reveals major histocompatibility complex II–expressing keratinocytes in pressure ulcers with worse healing outcomes. J Invest Dermatol 2022;142(3 Pt A):705–16.

68. Singh K, Rustagi Y, Abouhashem AS, et al. Genome-wide DNA hypermethylation opposes healing in patients with chronic wounds by impairing epithelial-mesenchymal transition. J Clin Invest 2022;132(17).
69. Theocharidis G, Baltzis D, Roustit M, et al. Integrated skin transcriptomics and serum multiplex assays reveal novel mechanisms of wound healing in diabetic foot ulcers. Diabetes 2020;69(10):2157–69.
70. Dao H Jr, Kazin RA. Gender differences in skin: a review of the literature. Gend Med 2007;4(4):308–28.
71. Hirano SA, Murray SB, Harvey VM. Reporting, representation, and subgroup analysis of race and ethnicity in published clinical trials of atopic dermatitis in the United States between 2000 and 2009. Pediatr Dermatol 2012;29(6):749–55.
72. Ma MA, Gutiérrez DE, Frausto JM, et al. Minority representation in clinical trials in the United States: Trends Over the Past 25 Years. Mayo Clin Proc 2021;96(1):264–6.
73. Ji AL, Rubin AJ, Thrane K, et al. Multimodal analysis of composition and spatial architecture in human squamous cell carcinoma. Cell 2020;182(2):497–514 e22.
74. Takahashi R, Grzenda A, Allison TF, et al. Defining transcriptional signatures of human hair follicle cell states. J Invest Dermatol 2020;140(4):764–773 e4.
75. Borcherding N, Crotts SB, Ortolan LS, et al. A transcriptomic map of murine and human alopecia areata. JCI Insight 2020;5(13).
76. Zou Z, Long X, Zhao Q, et al. A single-cell transcriptomic atlas of human skin aging. Dev Cell 2021;56(3):383–397 e8.
77. Xu Z, Chen D, Hu Y, et al. Anatomically distinct fibroblast subsets determine skin autoimmune patterns. Nature 2022;601(7891):118–24.
78. Sun Y, Xu L, Li Y, et al. Single-cell transcriptomics uncover key regulators of skin regeneration in human long-term mechanical stretch-mediated expansion therapy. Front Cell Dev Biol 2022;10:865983.
79. Zheng M, Hu Z, Mei X, et al. Single-cell sequencing shows cellular heterogeneity of cutaneous lesions in lupus erythematosus. Nat Commun 2022;13(1):7489.
80. Reynolds G, Vegh P, Fletcher J, et al. Developmental cell programs are co-opted in inflammatory skin disease. Science 2021;371(6527).
81. Liu Y, Wang H, Taylor M, et al. Classification of human chronic inflammatory skin disease based on single-cell immune profiling. Sci Immunol 2022;7(70):eabl9165.
82. Burja B, Paul D, Tastanova A, et al. An optimized tissue dissociation protocol for single-Cell RNA sequencing analysis of fresh and cultured human skin biopsies. Front Cell Dev Biol 2022;10:872688.
83. Chen YL, Gomes T, Hardman CS, et al. Re-evaluation of human BDCA-2+ DC during acute sterile skin inflammation. J Exp Med 2020;217(3).
84. Belote RL, Le D, Maynard A, et al. Human melanocyte development and melanoma dedifferentiation at single-cell resolution. Nat Cell Biol 2021;23(9):1035–47.
85. Apostolidis SA, Stifano G, Tabib T, et al. Single Cell RNA Sequencing Identifies HSPG2 and APLNR as Markers of Endothelial Cell Injury in Systemic Sclerosis Skin. Front Immunol 2018;9:2191.
86. Rojahn TB, Vorstandlechner V, Krausgruber T, et al. Single-cell transcriptomics combined with interstitial fluid proteomics defines cell type-specific immune regulation in atopic dermatitis. J Allergy Clin Immunol 2020;146(5):1056–69.
87. He H, Suryawanshi H, Morozov P, et al. Single-cell transcriptome analysis of human skin identifies novel fibroblast subpopulation and enrichment of immune subsets in atopic dermatitis. J Allergy Clin Immunol 2020;145(6):1615–28.

88. Xue D, Tabib T, Morse C, et al. Transcriptome landscape of myeloid cells in human skin reveals diversity, rare populations and putative DC progenitors. J Dermatol Sci 2020;97(1):41–9.

89. Theocharidis G, Thomas BE, Sarkar D, et al. Single cell transcriptomic landscape of diabetic foot ulcers. Nat Commun 2022;13(1):181.

90. Ahlers JMD, Falckenhayn C, Holzscheck N, et al. Single-Cell RNA profiling of human skin reveals age-related loss of dermal sheath cells and their contribution to a juvenile phenotype. Front Genet 2021;12:797747.

91. Liu J, Chang HW, Huang ZM, et al. Single-cell RNA sequencing of psoriatic skin identifies pathogenic Tc17 cell subsets and reveals distinctions between CD8(+) T cells in autoimmunity and cancer. J Allergy Clin Immunol 2021; 147(6):2370–80.

92. Gao Y, Yao X, Zhai Y, et al. Single cell transcriptional zonation of human psoriasis skin identifies an alternative immunoregulatory axis conducted by skin resident cells. Cell Death Dis 2021;12(5):450.

93. Kim D, Kobayashi T, Voisin B, et al. Targeted therapy guided by single-cell transcriptomic analysis in drug-induced hypersensitivity syndrome: a case report. Nat Med 2020;26(2):236–43.

94. Billi AC, Ma F, Plazyo O, et al. Nonlesional lupus skin contributes to inflammatory education of myeloid cells and primes for cutaneous inflammation. Sci Transl Med 2022;14(642):eabn2263.

95. Flament F, Bazin R, Laquieze S, et al. Effect of the sun on visible clinical signs of aging in Caucasian skin. Clin Cosmet Investig Dermatol 2013;6:221–32.

96. Abyzov A, Mariani J, Palejev D, et al. Somatic copy number mosaicism in human skin revealed by induced pluripotent stem cells. Nature 2012;492(7429): 438–42.

97. Lorencini M, Brohem CA, Dieamant GC, et al. Active ingredients against human epidermal aging. Ageing Res Rev 2014;15:100–15.

98. Tacutu R, Thornton D, Johnson E, et al. Human Ageing Genomic Resources: new and updated databases. Nucleic Acids Res 2018;46(D1):D1083–90.

99. Mahmoudi S, Mancini E, Xu L, et al. Heterogeneity in old fibroblasts is linked to variability in reprogramming and wound healing. Nature 2019;574(7779):553–8.

100. Dhanesh SB, Subashini C, James J. Hes1: the maestro in neurogenesis. Cell Mol Life Sci 2016;73(21):4019–42.

101. Martinengo L, Olsson M, Bajpai R, et al. Prevalence of chronic wounds in the general population: systematic review and meta-analysis of observational studies. Ann Epidemiol 2019;29:8–15.

102. Martin P, Nunan R. Cellular and molecular mechanisms of repair in acute and chronic wound healing. Br J Dermatol 2015;173(2):370–8.

103. Li A, Pouliot N, Redvers R, et al. Extensive tissue-regenerative capacity of neonatal human keratinocyte stem cells and their progeny. J Clin Invest 2004; 113(3):390–400.

Nevi and Melanoma

Yifan Zhang, MD, PhD[a,b], Stephen M. Ostrowski, MD, PhD[a,b],
David E. Fisher, MD, PhD[a,b],*

KEYWORDS

- Nevus • Atypical nevus • Dysplastic nevus • Melanoma • Senescence

KEY POINTS

- Nevi are benign lesions, but some, at low frequency, can progress to melanoma.
- Approximately 30% of primary melanomas have an identifiable nevus precursor.
- Identical oncogenic mutations in BRAF and NRAS are found in both nevi and melanoma.
- The mechanisms that allow nevus senescence after BRAF and NRAS mutation are unclear.
- Many benign nevi have clinically and histologically atypical features, making clinical diagnosis difficult.

INTRODUCTION

Cutaneous melanoma is an aggressive form of skin cancer derived from skin melanocytes and is associated with significant morbidity and mortality. A significant fraction of melanomas is associated with precursor lesions, benign clonal proliferations of melanocytes called nevi. Nevi can be either congenital or acquired later in life. Though generally considered benign, nevus cells are histologically distinct from ordinary melanocytes and have a wide spectrum of histologic presentations. Identical oncogenic driver mutations are found in benign nevi and melanoma. While much progress has been made in our understanding of nevus formation and the molecular steps required for transformation of nevus into melanoma, the clinical diagnosis of benign versus malignant lesions remains challenging.

ACQUIRED MELANOCYTIC NEVI

Acquired melanocytic nevi appear after birth; nevus number increases during early childhood and adolescence and peaks during the third and fourth decades of life.[1] Acquired melanocytic nevi are the most common type of nevi and are most common in fair-skinned individuals[2] (**Fig. 1**A). Nevus formation is regulated both by genetic

[a] Department of Dermatology, Cutaneous Biology Research Center, Massachusetts General Hospital, 149 13th Street, Charlestown, MA 02129, USA; [b] Department of Dermatology, Harvard Medical School, Massachusetts General Hospital, Boston, MA 02114, USA
* Corresponding author.
E-mail address: dfisher3@mgh.harvard.edu

Hematol Oncol Clin N Am 38 (2024) 939–952
https://doi.org/10.1016/j.hoc.2024.05.005
0889-8588/24/© 2024 Elsevier Inc. All rights reserved.

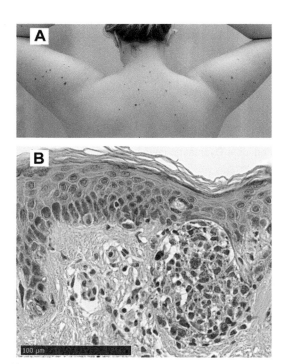

Fig. 1. Clinical and histologic appearance of nevi. (*A*) A patient with high density of nevi, including nevi with clinical atypia. (*B*) Histologic appearance of a junctional nevus, showing nested proliferation of melanocytes. (*From* Drozdowski et al. Dysplastic nevus part I: Historical perspective, classification, and epidemiology. J Am Acad Dermatol 88(1):1-10 (Elsevier).[75](A).)

factors and environmental ultraviolet (UV) radiation exposure.[3,4] Most acquired nevi are typically stable or slowly regress over time; however, a small fraction of these lesions gain further mutations required for transformation into melanoma, estimated at 1:3000 to 1:10,000 lifetime transformation risk for any particular nevus.[5]

Histologically Categorization of Acquired Melanocytic Nevi

Junctional nevi
Junctional nevi are characterized histologically by increased number of melanocytes at the dermoepidermal junction (DEJ) with or without the presence of melanocytic nests (see **Fig. 1**B), without dermal involvement. Clinically, they manifest as uniformly pigmented macules under 6 mm with slight accentuation of skin markings.

Intradermal nevi
Located mostly in the dermis, these nevi clinically appear as skin-colored, dome-shaped papules or nodules, are common in adults, and are less prone to melanoma transformation. Histologically, they are identified by melanocyte nests or cords in the dermis, often with notable fibrosis and no junctional activity. They display various morphologies, including cellular, mixed, and spindle forms.

Compound nevi
Compound nevi have melanocytes at the DEJ and within the dermis. They have variable elevation, with a darker central area and a lighter halo. Histologically, they show melanocyte nests in both epidermis and dermis.

Nevi have traditionally been thought to arise from proliferations of epidermal melanocytes at the DEJ, which then migrate deep to form compound and intradermal nevi (Paul Gerson Unna's theory of Abtropfung, "dropping off"); however, longitudinal dermoscopic and reflectance confocal microscopic imaging studies have shown nevi to have minimal change in superficial or deep movement even with changes in nevi size.[1,6,7] Junctional nevi are typically associated with multiple classic melanocytic markers (tyrosinase related protein 1 [TYRP1], premelanosome protein [PMEL]) while deeper nevi tend to have fewer markers, suggesting some level of dedifferentiation with depth.[8,9] In addition, reticular dermoscopic pattern has been associated with junctional differentiation and decreased likelihood of B-raf proto-oncogene, serine/threonine kinase (BRAF)^{V600E} mutation, while globular dermoscopic pattern has been associated with intradermal differentiation and almost always associated with BRAF^{V600E} mutation.[10–12] Overall, this suggests that histologic subtypes of nevi are stable lesions that have distinct developmental trajectories.

GENETIC MUTATIONS AND MOLECULAR PATHOLOGY

The defining genetic characteristic of acquired melanocytic nevi is the presence of oncogenic driver mutation in the BRAF or NRAS proto-oncogene, GTPase (NRAS) gene.[13] While these mutations are not canonical "UV signature" mutations, there is evidence UVB irradiation is capable of inducing this spectrum of mutations.[14] It is thought that oncogenic mutation is a rare event that leads to early nevus proliferation, followed by senescence, though there is debate if nevus senescence is caused either by oncogene-induced senescence or by other mechanisms.[15,16]

BRAF Mutations

The BRAF^{V600E} mutation is the most prevalent in acquired melanocytic nevi, present in up to 80% of cases.[17] This mutation leads to the activation of the mitogen-activated protein kinases (MAPK)/extracellular signal-regulated kinase signaling pathway, driving the proliferation of melanocytes and is sufficient to induce nevogenesis in an animal model.[18]

NRAS Mutations

NRAS^{Q61} mutations, though less common than BRAF mutations, are found in about 15% to 20% of acquired melanocytic nevi and also stimulate the MAPK pathway.[19]

Genetic Diversity and Mutational Load

Whole exome and whole genome sequencing of nevi have shown that in addition to BRAF/NRAS driver mutations, nevi exhibit a significant number of predominantly "UV signature" of mutations, with a mutation burden from 0 to 12 single nucleotide variants per megabase (SNV/Mb). These findings support the role of UVB-induced mutations in nevogenesis.[20–22] Importantly, in a given nevus, most mutations occurred at similar allele fraction as that of the BRAF or NRAS driver mutation, supporting nevi as clonal proliferations and suggesting that UV-induced mutations occurred before or concurrently with BRAF or NRAS mutation.[21] An unanswered question is if the presence of a high mutational burden or specific genomic or genetic alterations in a nevus is associated with a higher risk of melanoma transformation. Interestingly, normal melanocytes from sun-exposed skin exhibit a high mutational burden, suggesting that many UV-induced mutations may represent passenger mutations that do not contribute to disease pathogenesis.[23]

NEVUS DEVELOPMENT AND RISK FACTORS

The development of acquired melanocytic nevi is influenced by various factors:

- *Skin type*: Individuals with lighter skin are more prone to develop a higher number of nevi, with the exception of fair-skinned, red-haired individuals who have the lowest nevus counts.[24,25]
- *UV radiation*: Exposure to UV light, especially acute intermittent exposures during childhood, is a significant risk factor for nevus development; sun protection has been shown to decrease risk of nevus formation.[26,27]
- *Immunosuppression*: Immunosuppressed individuals, such as organ transplant recipients or those with HIV infection, show an increased tendency for nevus formation.[28,29]

NEVI AND MELANOMA

Acquired melanocytic nevi are important in the context of melanoma for several reasons:

Nevus Count and Melanoma Risk

A higher nevus count is associated with an increased risk of melanoma.[30] Interestingly, there seems to be only a slight increase in the ratio of nevus-associated to de novo melanoma in patients with high nevus counts as compared to patients with low nevus counts.[31,32] In addition, several genetic variants (detailed in later discussion) have been shown to increase the risk of development of nevi and melanoma. This suggests that nevus formation and melanoma formation are regulated by the same factors.

Genetic Links

Nevi are growth arrested proliferations of melanocytes driven by mutations in key melanoma oncogenes such as BRAF or NRAS. Other genetic factors have been found to modulate nevus counts, suggesting that BRAF/NRAS oncogene mutation may not be entirely sufficient for nevus formation and may be modulated by host genetic factors. For example, genome-wide association studies have implicated variations in several genes, including cyclin dependent kinase inhibitor 2A (CDKN2A), interferon regulatory factor 4 (IRF4), and phospholipase A2 group VI (PLA2G6), in nevus formation.[33–35]

Melanoma Formation Trajectories

Melanomas can arise de novo or from pre-existing nevi. Whiteman and colleagues first proposed the divergent pathway hypothesis, suggesting divergent mechanisms for melanoma formation on chronically sun-exposed and chronic non-sun-exposed sites.[36] This hypothesis has been extensively validated, and it has been demonstrated that melanomas on chronic sun-exposed sites are associated with host factors such as increased age, cumulative sun exposure, and inability to tan, while melanomas that occur on nonexposed sites are associated with younger age, association with nevus precursor, and BRAF[V600E] positivity.[37,38] At the molecular level, CSD melanomas have increased mutational burden, and increased incidence of non-BRAF[V600E] mutations such as NRAS and c-KIT.[39]

OTHER TYPES OF NEVI

In addition to acquired melanocytic nevi, several other classes of benign nevi exist. These share common factors that include being composed of melanocytic cells, exhibiting a similar oncogene-induced growth phase followed by senescence, and a low risk of transformation of melanoma. However, the histopathological features and the nature of the oncogenic mutation differ between these subtypes, and it is thought that this might reflect differing cells of origin.[40]

Congenital Melanocytic Nevus

Congenital melanocytic nevi, CMNs, are present from birth or within the first few months of life, and can appear on any part of the body in varying sizes. CMNs are rare, estimated to occur in approximately 1% to 3% of newborns.[41] They can have irregular borders and variations in color within a single lesion.[42] Tardive congenital nevi appear after birth and share clinical and dermoscopic feature with CMNs.[43]

CMNs are categorized by the size the lesion is expected to attain by adulthood.[44] Small (<1.5 cm) and medium (1.5–20 cm) lesions are most frequently associated with BRAF^{V600E} mutation and have a low risk of transformation. Large (20–40 cm) and giant (>40 cm) CMNs are almost exclusively associated with mutations in NRAS; the risk of melanoma development within large and giant CMNs in these lesions is a significant concern and may exceed 10% lifetime risk.[45,46] The management of CMNs involves regular monitoring and, in some cases, surgical intervention.[42] It is crucial to balance the risk of melanoma with the potential morbidity of surgical procedures. Medical management using topical therapies is also being explored.[47] Early detection and appropriate management strategies are key in reducing the risk of melanoma associated with CMNs.

Spitz Nevus

Spitz nevi are distinctive melanocytic lesions that often present a diagnostic challenge due to their atypical features, which can resemble melanoma. Clinically, they manifest as raised, classically pink/red but also brown papules (**Fig. 2**A). Seventy percentage of cases occur in children and adolescents, but Spitz nevi can also appear in adults.[48,49] Histologically, Spitz nevi are characterized by large spindle or epithelioid melanocytes,

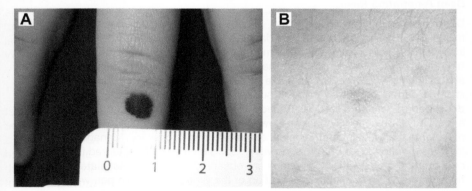

Fig. 2. Classes of melanocytic nevi. In addition to common acquired nevi, several distinct types of nevi have been identified (*A*) Blue nevus. Note that this lesion is macular and that the blue/gray color is due to deep dermal infiltration of nevus melanocytes. (*B*) Spitz nevus on the finger of a 5 year old child. These lesions often present a diagnostic and therapeutic challenge.(*From* Baykal et al. The spectrum of benign dermal dendritic melanocytic proliferations. J Eur Acad Dermatol Venereol, 3(6):1029-1041 (A) Cheng TW, Ahern MC and Giubellino A (2022) The Spectrum of Spitz Melanocytic Lesions: From Morphologic Diagnosis to Molecular Classification. Front. Oncol. 12:889223. https://doi.org/10.3389/fonc.2022. 889223. (B).)

which are arranged in a vertical pattern and may show Kamino bodies—periodic acid–schiff stain (PAS)+ eosinophilic hyaline globules that are helpful in diagnosis.[48,49]

It is often challenging to definitively distinguish Spitz nevi and spitzoid melanomas. Molecularly, Spitz nevi frequently have genetic alterations distinct from those seen in spitzoid melanomas, such as HRAS mutations, receptor tyrosine kinase fusions, or fusions of MAPK pathway members, which can aid in their classification and management.[40,50] Due to their ambiguous nature, Spitz nevi require careful clinical and histologic evaluation to differentiate them from melanoma. Management typically involves close observation with consideration for excision, depending on the features and behavior of the lesion.

Blue Nevus

Blue nevi are typically isolated melanocytic lesions that derive their name from the distinctive blue coloration visible on the skin (see **Fig. 2**B). This coloration is due to the melanin being deeper in the dermis, which causes a light scattering effect known as the Tyndall effect. Blue nevi are typically acquired but can be associated with syndromes such as LAMB (lentigines, atrial myxomas, and blue nevi) and NAME (nevi, atrial myxoma, myxoid neurofibromas, and ephelides) where they are diffusely distributed. Histologically, blue nevi are composed of densely packed spindle-shaped melanocytes and melanophages. They are often located on the dorsal hands, feet, face, and buttocks. While blue nevi are usually stable, any changes in size, shape, or color warrant evaluation to rule out malignancy. Histologic features such as atypia, vascular invasion, or necrosis may be suggestive of blue nevus-like melanoma. Management of blue nevi is conservative, with surgical excision being reserved for atypical cases or for diagnostic clarification. Genetically, blue nevi are most frequently associated with hotspot mutations in G protein subunit alpha Q (GNAQ) or G protein subunit alpha 11 (GNA11) and, less commonly, mutations in cysteinyl leukotriene receptor 2 (CYSLTR2) or fusions of protein kinase C isoforms.[40]

Deep Penetrating Nevus

Deep penetrating nevi (DPNs) are uncommon melanocytic lesions that can be mistaken for melanoma due to their dark coloration and deep dermal infiltration. Clinically, DPNs typically appear as pigmented papules or nodules with a blue-black or blue-gray color, often located on the face, arms, or shoulders. Histologically, they are distinguished by nests of spindle or epithelioid melanocytes that extend deeply into the dermis and often into the subcutaneous fat, with a pattern that has been described as "inverted wedge-shaped." Despite their concerning depth and appearance, DPNs are generally benign. However, due to their potential to be confused with melanoma, careful histopathological examination is necessary. Management usually involves monitoring for changes; however, excision may be considered for diagnostic confirmation or if significant changes are observed. DPNs are associated with mutations that result in constitutive activation of the Wnt/beta-catenin pathway.[40]

TRANSFORMATION TO MELANOMA
Nevus Formation and Nevus Senescence

Acquired nevi undergo a period of rapid proliferation after BRAF or NRAS gene mutation. After the proliferative phase, the lesion enters senescence, a form of stable cell cycle arrest, to form a nevus[51] (**Fig. 3**A–B). This process has been best studied in the BRAF context, where the activation BRAF^{V600E} causes unphysiologically high downstream MAPK signaling leading to cell stress and CDKN2A-mediated G1 cell cycle arrest.[52]

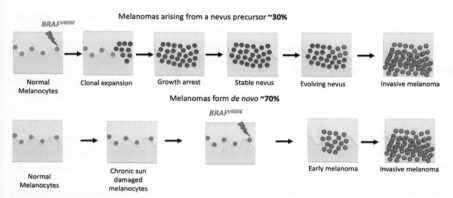

Fig. 3. Melanoma may be derived either from nevus precursor or from de novo. (*A*) BRAF^V600E mutation leads for melanocyte proliferation followed by oncogene-induced senescence, resulting in formation of a benign nevus. At low frequency, nevi transform to melanoma. (*B*) A significant fraction of melanomas form in the absence of a nevus precursor. It has been hypothesized that highly mutated epidermal melanocytes are at high risk for melanoma transformation following BRAF^V600E mutation.

These nevus cells do not reenter the cell cycle even in the presence of mitogenic stimuli and are positive for senescence associated markers CDKN2A and beta-galactosidase.[51,53] A recent study demonstrates that in a mouse model, BRAF-mutated melanocytes do not exhibit transcriptional signatures of senescence, leading to the hypothesis that nevus growth arrest is not due to oncogene-induced senescence.[15]

Genomic and Genetic Progression from Nevus to Melanoma

At low frequency, nevi can transform to melanoma; nevus to melanoma transition has been extensively characterized at the molecular level.[54–58] In a study of melanomas and adjacent precursor nevi, the earliest genomic changes were telomerase reverse transcriptase (TERT) promoter mutations, which occurred at the melanoma-in-situ stage. Biallelic inactivation of *CDKN2A*, MAPK pathway amplification, and mutation of epigenetic modifiers such as ARID2 occurred at the stage of early invasive melanoma stage, while mutation of the tumor suppressors phosphatase and tensin homolog (PTEN) and P53 occurred only in advance melanomas. The point-mutation burden increased from benign through intermediate lesions to melanoma, with a strong signature of the effects of ultraviolet radiation detectable at all evolutionary stages. Copy-number alterations became prevalent only in invasive melanomas.

Clinical Differences in Nevus-associated versus Nonnevus-associated Melanoma

While there are clear differences in the clinical risk factors, histopathologic features, and molecular features between nevus associated and de novo melanomas, almost all studies suggest that there is identical prognosis after correcting for factors such as Breslow depth and ulceration.[37,38,59–62] To date, no studies have examined therapy response in patients with metastatic melanoma whose primary melanoma was de novo versus nevus-associated, though this would be a question with important clinical implications.

CLINICAL MONITORING AND MANAGEMENT OF NEVI AND DYSPLASTIC NEVI
Surveillance/Monitoring of Benign and Atypical Nevi

While an increased number of nevi is a strong melanoma risk factor, each individual nevus has a low risk of melanoma transformation, and most melanomas are nonnevus associated. Thus, prophylactic removal of nevi is recognized as an inappropriate approach. Instead, patients are monitored closely either for the development of new lesions or changes in existing nevi that have a high concern for malignant transformation.

Methods for nevus monitoring

The cornerstone of early melanoma diagnosis is expert clinical examination to discriminate benign pigmented lesions from early melanoma. The clinical features that discriminate melanoma from benign lesions have been summarized by the mnemonic "ABCDE" (asymmetry, border irregularity, color variegation, diameter >6 mm, and evolution over time).[63] Patient education on ABCDE is coupled with guidance for self-examination, and there is evidence that self-examination improves the detection of early melanomas.[64] One disadvantage of the ABCDE rule is that these features can be present in benign lesions (seborrheic keratosis, lentigo, congenital nevus, and dysplastic nevus) and absent in nodular and amelanotic melanomas. It is also important to note that some melanomas may not exhibit every ABCDE feature; an increasing number of features are likely to be seen in melanomas diagnosed by nondermatologists.[65]

A dermoscope, a skin surface microscope, is used by dermatologists for a more detailed examination of pigmented lesions enhancing the visualization of subsurface structures that are not visible to the naked eye. One key feature of dermoscopy is that it can allow the identification of a lesion as melanocytic (compared to nonmelanocytic lesions such as seborrheic keratosis), as melanocytic patterns such as reticular and globular pattern are immediately visible on dermoscopic examination. Numerous criteria have been proposed to identify features more specific for melanoma diagnosis. Some features that are highly sensitive but that lack specificity include atypical network and multicomponent dermoscopic pattern, as these features can also be seen in dysplastic nevi.[66,67] Some of the best validated dermoscopic features that have higher specificity for melanoma diagnosis include blue-white veil, shiny white structures, pseudopods, peppering/granularity, and irregular globules.[66,67]

Taking periodic photographs of nevi (often in combination with dermoscopic images) can help in tracking changes over time. One disadvantage of monitoring versus biopsy is that some patients are lost to follow-up; scheduling a shorter follow-up appointment (ie, 3 months) increases patient compliance.[68,69] Total body photography entails high-resolution imaging of the entire body surface as a reference for future examination. This technique is particularly useful for individuals with a large number of nevi, enabling precise monitoring for any changes. There is evidence that total body photography facilitates the detection of melanoma in high-risk individuals.[70] Dermoscopic imaging is often combined with photography; it has been shown that whole body dermoscopy has higher sensitivity for melanoma detection as compared to dermoscopy of selected/suspicious lesions.[71] Advances in technology have led to the development of digital mole mapping, which utilizes computer algorithms to map an individual's body moles, allowing for efficient tracking of changes in nevi over time. New technologies in this field include automated systems using artificial intelligence (AI) to analyze and flag atypical and/or changing nevi. Some exciting studies have demonstrated that neural networks can classify images of lesions on par with expert clinical dermatologists.[72] Overall, while there is strong evidence that these advanced approaches may increase sensitivity of diagnosing early melanoma, it has not been demonstrated that they are superior to conventional screening measures in improving patient outcomes.[73,74]

Clinical Monitoring and Management of Dysplastic Nevi

Up to 8% of patients exhibit clinically atypical nevi (the terms "atypical nevi" and "dysplastic nevi" are often used interchangeably).[75] These lesions have features that violate the ABCDE rules and often have size greater than 6 mm, slightly asymmetrical features, and can have abnormalities in dermoscopic pattern. On histopathological examination, these lesions often, but not always, exhibit signs of histologic dysplasia, which includes architectural disorder and cytologic atypia.[76] These lesions represent clinical challenges for several reasons.

First, historically clinically atypical nevi have been (to some extent) erroneously implicated as precancerous lesions. Two articles published in 1978 recognized that members of some melanoma prone families were prone to development of larger moles with atypical shapes and colors (atypical-mole melanoma syndrome or B-K mole syndrome).[77,78] Soon after, it was recognized that similar clinically atypical moles occur in sporadic fashion, and the term "dysplastic nevus syndrome" was utilized to describe patients with 2 or more histologically dysplastic nevi; it was noted that these patients were at an increased risk for melanoma and concern was raised that dysplastic nevi had an increased risk for transformation to melanoma.[79]

Over time, it has been appreciated that clinically atypical moles are quite common (up to 8% prevalence) and that these are associated with a spectrum of histopathologic features. Histopathologically, these lesions are often classified as mildly, moderately, or severely dysplastic. Mild and moderately atypical nevi been shown to have low yield for re-excision,[80] and the standard of care is shifting to excision only of lesions that exhibit evidence of severe cytologic atypia. There is variability of care for margins of excision (narrow excision vs 5 mm margin) even for severely dysplastic lesions.[81] Importantly, it has been demonstrated that diagnostic concordance among dermatopathologists is variable, and this may be a factor in driving variability of clinical care.[13] Similarly, one study showed that 88% of biopsies obtained from clinically benign nevi showed at least 1 histologic feature of dysplasia.[82] Overall, there is strong evidence that mildly or moderately dysplastic are not melanoma precursors and do not require re-excision when the diagnosis is certain (not a partial biopsy), while severely dysplastic nevi should be completely excised due to the overlap in histopathologic features with melanoma.

SUMMARY

Acquired melanocytic nevi, while considered benign lesions, harbor the seeds of potential malignancy and transform to melanoma at low frequency. The presence of oncogenic mutations in genes like BRAF and NRAS paralleled in both nevi and melanomas underlies the transformation of nevus to melanoma. However, the rarity of this transformation highlights the complexity and multifactorial nature of melanoma development. In clinical practice, surveillance of nevi by clinical examination, particularly of nevi with atypical features, remains a cornerstone in melanoma prevention. Emerging technologies in digital mole mapping and AI hold promise in enhancing the accuracy and efficiency of nevi surveillance. However, the traditional methods of clinical and self-examinations, photographic documentation, and dermoscopy remain standard of care, future studies will demonstrate the impact of new approaches on patient outcomes. Looking ahead, future research may allow the identification, both at the molecular level and clinical level, of nevi that might be at highest risk of transformation. Ultimately, these strategies will allow for effective prevention, early detection, and treatment of melanoma.

FUNDING

D.E. Fisher reports grants from the NIH (R01AR072304 , R01AR043369 , and P01CA163222); the Department of Defense (DoD W81XWH2220052 and DoD W81XWH2110981); and the Dr Miriam and Sheldon G. Adelson Medical Research

Foundation; and a financial interest in Soltego, a company developing salt-inducible kinase inhibitors for topical skin-darkening treatments that might be used for a broad set of human applications. D.E. Fisher also serves as a consultant for Coherent Medicines, Pierre Fabre, Tasca, Torqur, and Biocoz Inc. The interests of D.E. Fisher were reviewed and are managed by Massachusetts General Hospital and Partners Health-Care in accordance with their conflict-of-interest policies. D.E. Fisher gratefully acknowledges the Lancer Family for support of the Lancer Professorship at Harvard Medical School.

REFERENCES

1. Zalaudek I, Schmid K, Marghoob AA, et al. Frequency of dermoscopic nevus subtypes by age and body site: a cross-sectional study. Arch Dermatol 2011; 147:663–70.
2. Gallagher RP, Rivers JK, Yang CP, et al. Melanocytic nevus density in Asian, Indo-Pakistani, and white children: the Vancouver Mole Study. J Am Acad Dermatol 1991;25:507–12.
3. MacLennan R, Kelly JW, Rivers JK, et al. The Eastern Australian Childhood Nevus Study: site differences in density and size of melanocytic nevi in relation to latitude and phenotype. J Am Acad Dermatol 2003;48:367–75.
4. Wachsmuth RC, Gaut RM, Barrett JH, et al. Heritability and gene-environment interactions for melanocytic nevus density examined in a U.K. adolescent twin study. J Invest Dermatol 2001;117:348–52.
5. Bevona C, Goggins W, Quinn T, et al. Cutaneous melanomas associated with nevi. Arch Dermatol 2003;139:1620–4 [discussion 1624].
6. Pellacani G, Scope A, Ferrari B, et al. New insights into nevogenesis: in vivo characterization and follow-up of melanocytic nevi by reflectance confocal microscopy. J Am Acad Dermatol 2009;61:1001–13.
7. Reiter O, Kurtansky NR, Musthaq ST, et al. The long-term evolution of melanocytic nevi among high-risk adults. J Eur Acad Dermatol Venereol 2022;36:2379–87.
8. Paul E, Cochran AJ, Wen DR. Immunohistochemical demonstration of S-100 protein and melanoma-associated antigens in melanocytic nevi. J Cutan Pathol 1988;15:161–5.
9. Prieto VG, Shea CR. Immunohistochemistry of melanocytic proliferations. Arch Pathol Lab Med 2011;135:853–9.
10. Kiuru M, Tartar DM, Qi L, et al. Improving classification of melanocytic nevi: Association of BRAF V600E expression with distinct histomorphologic features. J Am Acad Dermatol 2018;79:221–9.
11. Kim CC, Berry EG, Marchetti MA, et al. Risk of Subsequent Cutaneous Melanoma in Moderately Dysplastic Nevi Excisionally Biopsied but With Positive Histologic Margins. JAMA Dermatol 2018;154:1401–8.
12. Bauer J, Garbe C. Acquired melanocytic nevi as risk factor for melanoma development. A comprehensive review of epidemiological data. Pigment Cell Res 2003;16:297–306.
13. Aydin Ulgen O, Yildiz P, Acar HC, et al. Analysis of interobserver reproducibility in grading dysplastic nevi: Results of the application of the 2018 World Health Organization grading criteria. J Cutan Pathol 2022;49:343–9.
14. Laughery MF, Brown AJ, Bohm KA, et al. Atypical UV photoproducts induce noncanonical mutation classes associated with driver mutations in melanoma. Cell Rep 2020;33. 108401.

15. Ruiz-Vega R, Chen CF, Razzak E, et al. Dynamics of nevus development implicate cell cooperation in the growth arrest of transformed melanocytes. Elife 2020;9.

16. Bennett DC. Review: Are moles senescent? Pigment Cell Melanoma Res 2024. https://doi.org/10.1111/pcmr.13163.

17. Dessinioti C, Geller AC, Stergiopoulou A, et al. A multicentre study of naevus-associated melanoma vs. de novo melanoma, tumour thickness and body site differences. Br J Dermatol 2021;185:101–9.

18. Patton EE, Widlund HR, Kutok JL, et al. BRAF mutations are sufficient to promote nevi formation and cooperate with p53 in the genesis of melanoma. Curr Biol 2005;15:249–54.

19. Tschandl P, Berghoff AS, Preusser M, et al. NRAS and BRAF mutations in melanoma-associated nevi and uninvolved nevi. PLoS One 2013;8:e69639.

20. Stark MS, Denisova E, Kays TA, et al. Mutation signatures in melanocytic nevi reveal characteristics of defective DNA Repair. J Invest Dermatol 2020;140:2093–2096 e2092.

21. Stark MS, Tan JM, Tom L, et al. Whole-exome sequencing of acquired nevi identifies mechanisms for development and maintenance of benign neoplasms. J Invest Dermatol 2018;138:1636–44.

22. Colebatch AJ, Ferguson P, Newell F, et al. Molecular genomic profiling of melanocytic nevi. J Invest Dermatol 2019;139:1762–8.

23. Tang J, Fewings E, Chang D, et al. The genomic landscapes of individual melanocytes from human skin. Nature 2020;586:600–5.

24. Sigg C, Pelloni F. Frequency of acquired melanonevocytic nevi and their relationship to skin complexion in 939 schoolchildren. Dermatologica 1989;179:123–8.

25. Synnerstad I, Nilsson L, Fredrikson M, et al. Frequency and distribution pattern of melanocytic naevi in Swedish 8-9-year-old children. Acta Derm Venereol 2004;84:271–6.

26. Harrison SL, Buettner PG, Nowak MJ. Sun-protective clothing worn regularly during early childhood reduces the number of new melanocytic nevi: the north queensland sun-safe clothing cluster randomized controlled trial. Cancers 2023;15. https://doi.org/10.3390/cancers15061762.

27. Luther H, Altmeyer P, Garbe C, et al. Increase of melanocytic nevus counts in children during 5 years of follow-up and analysis of associated factors. Arch Dermatol 1996;132:1473–8.

28. Koseoglu G, Akay BN, Kucuksahin O, et al. Dermoscopic changes in melanocytic nevi in patients receiving immunosuppressive and biologic treatments: results of a prospective case-control study. J Am Acad Dermatol 2015;73:623–9.

29. Duvic M, Lowe L, Rapini RP, et al. Eruptive dysplastic nevi associated with human immunodeficiency virus infection. Arch Dermatol 1989;125:397–401.

30. Grob JJ, Gouvernet J, Aymar D, et al. Count of benign melanocytic nevi as a major indicator of risk for nonfamilial nodular and superficial spreading melanoma. Cancer 1990;66:387–95.

31. Haenssle HA, Mograby N, Ngassa A, et al. Association of Patient Risk Factors and Frequency of Nevus-Associated Cutaneous Melanomas. JAMA Dermatol 2016;152:291–8.

32. Pandeya N, Kvaskoff M, Olsen CM, et al. Factors Related to Nevus-Associated Cutaneous Melanoma: A Case-Case Study. J Invest Dermatol 2018;138:1816–24.

33. Taylor NJ, Mitra N, Goldstein AM, et al. Germline Variation at CDKN2A and Associations with Nevus Phenotypes among Members of Melanoma Families. J Invest Dermatol 2017;137:2606–12.

34. Soura E, Eliades PJ, Shannon K, et al. Hereditary melanoma: Update on syndromes and management: Genetics of familial atypical multiple mole melanoma syndrome. J Am Acad Dermatol 2016;74:395–407 [quiz 408-310].

35. Duffy DL, Zhu G, Li X, et al. Novel pleiotropic risk loci for melanoma and nevus density implicate multiple biological pathways. Nat Commun 2018;9:4774.

36. Whiteman DC, Parsons PG, Green AC. p53 expression and risk factors for cutaneous melanoma: A case-control study. Int J Cancer 1998;77:843–8.

37. Sheen YS, Liao YH, Lin MH, et al. Clinicopathological features and prognosis of patients with de novo versus nevus-associated melanoma in Taiwan. PLoS One 2017;12:e0177126.

38. Tas F, Erturk K. De Novo and Nevus-Associated Melanomas: Different Histopathologic Characteristics but Similar Survival Rates. Pathol Oncol Res 2020;26: 2483–7.

39. Curtin JA, Fridlyand J, Kageshita T, et al. Distinct sets of genetic alterations in melanoma. N Engl J Med 2005;353:2135–47.

40. Yeh I. Melanocytic naevi, melanocytomas and emerging concepts. Pathology 2023;55:178–86.

41. Kanada KN, Merin MR, Munden A, et al. A prospective study of cutaneous findings in newborns in the United States: correlation with race, ethnicity, and gestational status using updated classification and nomenclature. J Pediatr 2012;161:240–5.

42. Jahnke MN, O'Haver J, Gupta D, et al. Care of Congenital Melanocytic Nevi in Newborns and Infants: Review and Management Recommendations. Pediatrics 2021;148. https://doi.org/10.1542/peds.2021-051536.

43. Stinco G, Argenziano G, Favot F, et al. Absence of clinical and dermoscopic differences between congenital and noncongenital melanocytic naevi in a cohort of 2-year-old children. Br J Dermatol 2011;165:1303–7.

44. Krengel S, Scope A, Dusza SW, et al. New recommendations for the categorization of cutaneous features of congenital melanocytic nevi. J Am Acad Dermatol 2013;68:441–51.

45. Bauer J, Curtin JA, Pinkel D, et al. Congenital melanocytic nevi frequently harbor NRAS mutations but no BRAF mutations. J Invest Dermatol 2007;127:179–82.

46. Charbel C, Fontaine RH, Malouf GG, et al. NRAS mutation is the sole recurrent somatic mutation in large congenital melanocytic nevi. J Invest Dermatol 2014; 134:1067–74.

47. Choi YS, Erlich TH, von Franque M, et al. Topical therapy for regression and melanoma prevention of congenital giant nevi. Cell 2022;185:2071–2085 e2012.

48. Ferrara G, Argenziano G, Soyer HP, et al. The spectrum of Spitz nevi: a clinicopathologic study of 83 cases. Arch Dermatol 2005;141:1381–7.

49. Requena C, Requena L, Kutzner H, et al. E. Spitz nevus: a clinicopathological study of 349 cases. Am J Dermatopathol 2009;31:107–16.

50. van Dijk MC, Bernsen MR, Ruiter DJ. Analysis of mutations in B-RAF, N-RAS, and H-RAS genes in the differential diagnosis of Spitz nevus and spitzoid melanoma. Am J Surg Pathol 2005;29:1145–51.

51. Damsky WE, Bosenberg M. Melanocytic nevi and melanoma: unraveling a complex relationship. Oncogene 2017;36:5771–92.

52. Vredeveld LC, Possik PA, Smit MA, et al. Abrogation of BRAFV600E-induced senescence by PI3K pathway activation contributes to melanomagenesis. Genes Dev 2012;26:1055–69.

53. Michaloglou C, Vredeveld LCW, Soengas MS, et al. BRAFE600-associated senescence-like cell cycle arrest of human naevi. Nature 2005;436:720–4.

54. Shain AH, Yeh I, Kovalyshyn I, et al. The Genetic Evolution of Melanoma from Precursor Lesions. N Engl J Med 2015;373:1926–36.
55. Bastian BC. The molecular pathology of melanoma: an integrated taxonomy of melanocytic neoplasia. Annu Rev Pathol 2014;9:239–71.
56. Shain AH, Joseph NM, Yu R, et al. Genomic and Transcriptomic Analysis Reveals Incremental Disruption of Key Signaling Pathways during Melanoma Evolution. Cancer Cell 2018;34:45–55 e44.
57. Huang FW, Hodis E, Xu MJ, et al. Highly recurrent TERT promoter mutations in human melanoma. Science 2013;339:957–9.
58. Horn S, Figl A, Rachakonda PS, et al. TERT promoter mutations in familial and sporadic melanoma. Science 2013;339:959–61.
59. Rashid S, Klebanov N, Lin WM, et al. Unsupervised Phenotype-Based Clustering of Clinicopathologic Features in Cutaneous Melanoma. JID Innov 2021;1:100047.
60. Shitara D, Tell-Martí G, Badenas C, et al. Mutational status of naevus-associated melanomas. Br J Dermatol 2015;173:671–80.
61. Kaddu S, Smolle J, Zenahlik P, et al. Melanoma with benign melanocytic naevus components: reappraisal of clinicopathological features and prognosis. Melanoma Res 2002;12:271–8.
62. Weatherhead SC, Haniffa M, Lawrence CM. Melanomas arising from naevi and de novo melanomas–does origin matter? Br J Dermatol 2007;156:72–6.
63. Abbasi NR, Shaw HM, Rigel DS, et al. Early diagnosis of cutaneous melanoma: revisiting the ABCD criteria. JAMA 2004;292:2771–6.
64. Titus LJ, Clough-Gorr K, Mackenzie TA, et al. Recent skin self-examination and doctor visits in relation to melanoma risk and tumour depth. Br J Dermatol 2013;168:571–6.
65. Duarte AF, Sousa-Pinto B, Azevedo LF, et al. Clinical ABCDE rule for early melanoma detection. Eur J Dermatol 2021;31:771–8.
66. Liopyris K, Navarrete-Dechent C, Marchetti MA, et al. Expert Agreement on the Presence and Spatial Localization of Melanocytic Features in Dermoscopy. J Invest Dermatol 2024;144:531–539 e513.
67. Williams NM, Rojas KD, Reynolds JM, et al. Assessment of Diagnostic Accuracy of Dermoscopic Structures and Patterns Used in Melanoma Detection: A Systematic Review and Meta-analysis. JAMA Dermatol 2021;157:1078–88.
68. Madigan LM, Treyger G, Kohen LL. Compliance with serial dermoscopic monitoring: An academic perspective. J Am Acad Dermatol 2016;75:1171–5.
69. Argenziano G, Mordente I, Ferrara G, et al. Dermoscopic monitoring of melanocytic skin lesions: clinical outcome and patient compliance vary according to follow-up protocols. Br J Dermatol 2008;159:331–6.
70. Ji-Xu A, Dinnes J, Matin RN. Total body photography for the diagnosis of cutaneous melanoma in adults: a systematic review and meta-analysis. Br J Dermatol 2021;185:302–12.
71. Seidenari S, Longo C, Giusti F, et al. Clinical selection of melanocytic lesions for dermoscopy decreases the identification of suspicious lesions in comparison with dermoscopy without clinical preselection. Br J Dermatol 2006;154:873–9.
72. Esteva A, Kuprel B, Novoa RA, et al. Dermatologist-level classification of skin cancer with deep neural networks. Nature 2017;542:115–8.
73. Ferris LK. Early Detection of Melanoma: Rethinking the Outcomes That Matter. JAMA Dermatol 2021;157:511–3.
74. Koh U, Cust AE, Fernández-Peñas P, et al. ACEMID cohort study: protocol of a prospective cohort study using 3D total body photography for melanoma imaging and diagnosis. BMJ Open 2023;13:e072788.

75. Drozdowski R, Spaccarelli N, Peters MS, et al. Dysplastic nevus part I: Historical perspective, classification, and epidemiology. J Am Acad Dermatol 2023;88:1–10.
76. Annessi G, Cattaruzza MS, Abeni D, et al. Correlation between clinical atypia and histologic dysplasia in acquired melanocytic nevi. J Am Acad Dermatol 2001;45: 77–85.
77. Clark WH Jr, Reimer RR, Greene M, et al. Origin of familial malignant melanomas from heritable melanocytic lesions. 'The B-K mole syndrome'. Arch Dermatol 1978;114:732–8.
78. Lynch HT, Frichot BC 3rd, Lynch JF. Familial atypical multiple mole-melanoma syndrome. J Med Genet 1978;15:352–6.
79. Elder DE, Goldman LI, Goldman SC, et al. Dysplastic nevus syndrome: a phenotypic association of sporadic cutaneous melanoma. Cancer 1980;46:1787–94.
80. Strazzula L, Vedak P, Hoang MP, et al. The utility of re-excising mildly and moderately dysplastic nevi: a retrospective analysis. J Am Acad Dermatol 2014;71: 1071–6.
81. Wall N, De'Ambrosis B, Muir J. The management of dysplastic naevi: a survey of Australian dermatologists. Australas J Dermatol 2017;58:304–7.
82. Klein LJ, Barr RJ. Histologic atypia in clinically benign nevi. A prospective study. J Am Acad Dermatol 1990;22:275–82.

Advances in Adjuvant and Neoadjuvant Therapy for Melanoma

Kailan Sierra-Davidson, MD, DPhil, Genevieve M. Boland, MD, PhD*

KEYWORDS

- Melanoma • Adjuvant therapy • Neoadjuvant therapy
- Immune checkpoint blockade • BRAF/MEK inhibitors • Talimogene laherparepvec
- Tumor-infiltrating lymphocytes • Cancer vaccines

KEY POINTS

- Adjuvant therapy with immune checkpoint blockade or targeted therapy with BRAF/MEK inhibitors is now standard of care for resectable stage III and IV melanoma.
- Recent clinical trials have demonstrated reduced disease recurrence with adjuvant programmed death-1 (PD-1) inhibitors in high-risk stage II patients without evidence of nodal disease by sentinel lymph node biopsy.
- Neoadjuvant-adjuvant compared with adjuvant only PD-1 therapy was associated with improved recurrence-free survival in stage IIIB-IV patients in a large randomized clinical trial and is now a reasonable option in this population.
- Early promising clinical trials have evaluated the role of limiting axillary dissection and tailoring adjuvant treatments in clinically node-positive patients who have a complete pathologic response to neoadjuvant therapy.
- Intralesional therapy with oncolytic viruses, cancer vaccines, and tumor-infiltrating lymphocytes therapy are additional emerging strategies in adjuvant or neoadjuvant therapy.

INTRODUCTION

Despite significant advances in treatment over the last 10 years, invasive cutaneous melanoma remains the one of the most common cancers in the United States, accounting for approximately 7990 deaths in 2023.[1] Surgical resection with wide local excision remains the cornerstone for curative treatment in patients with local disease. However, additional therapies are necessary in selected patients to manage disease spread to regional lymph nodes and distant sites. The development of paradigm-changing treatment with immune checkpoint blockade (ICB) and targeted therapies with BRAF/MEK inhibitors (BRAF/MEKi) led to improved survival in the metastatic

Department of Surgery, Massachusetts General Hospital, Boston, MA, USA
* Corresponding author. 55 Fruit Street, Yawkey 7B, Boston, MA 02114.
E-mail address: gmboland@mgh.harvard.edu

Hematol Oncol Clin N Am 38 (2024) 953–971
https://doi.org/10.1016/j.hoc.2024.05.007
0889-8588/24/© 2024 Elsevier Inc. All rights reserved.
hemonc.theclinics.com

setting.[2–6] These therapies have been evaluated in adjuvant therapy for patients with nodal disease with remarkable success.[7–9] Adjuvant ICB or targeted therapy with BRAF/MEKi in selected patients is a viable option for locally advanced melanoma.[10]

These trials have also led to renewed interest in neoadjuvant therapy for advanced resectable melanoma. There are several advantages for neoadjuvant therapy in the setting of melanoma.[11–13] Historically, neoadjuvant therapy was used for downstaging, which may lead to improved surgical resectability with greater likelihood of R0 resection and decreased morbidity. Additionally, pathologic responses to neoadjuvant therapy may be used to tailor adjuvant treatments by serving as a surrogate marker for relapse-free survival (RFS) or overall survival (OS). Interestingly, for neoadjuvant immunotherapy, exposure to therapy in the neoadjuvant setting with primary tumor intact may result in a more robust or broad tumor-specific immune responses compared with the adjuvant setting, which is an emerging benefit seen in the setting of neoadjuvant therapy that is distinct from other tumor-specific therapies. Theoretic concerns with neoadjuvant therapy include disease progression during therapy, treatment-related toxicities that may delay surgery and development of early resistance to treatment. Nonetheless, neoadjuvant therapy has a well-established role in multiple cancer phenotypes including breast,[14] rectal,[15] and esophageal cancers.[16] This is now a promising field of active investigation in the setting of advanced melanoma.

The aim of this article is to highlight important advances in adjuvant and neoadjuvant therapy for cutaneous melanoma, focusing on key clinical trials over the last 5 years (**Table 1**). The authors specifically discuss scientific developments in ICB therapies, targeted molecular therapies with BRAF/MEKi, oncolytic viruses, adoptive cellular therapy with tumor-infiltrating lymphocytes (TIL), and cancer vaccines. While this article is not exhaustive, the authors hope to provide a broad and useful overview for the practicing surgical oncologist.

IMMUNE CHECKPOINT BLOCKADE
Adjuvant Programmed Death-1 Therapy

Since the original work which demonstrated that blockade of cytotoxic T-lymphocyte-associated protein (CTLA-4) can lead to tumor regression in mice,[17] the treatment landscape for melanoma has changed dramatically. Ipilimumab, a monoclonal antibody against CTLA-4, improved survival for patients with metastatic melanoma and was approved in 2011.[2,3] The programmed death-1 (PD-1/programmed death ligand-1 [PD-L1]) pathway was identified as an additional checkpoint on the development of antitumor responses. Monoclonal antibodies against PD-1 including pembrolizumab and nivolumab improved survival in patients with metastatic disease compared with ipilimumab or chemotherapy with fewer toxicities.[4] Overall, this work in metastatic melanoma sparked clinical studies assessing the role of these therapies in the adjuvant setting.

Two pivotal randomized trials demonstrated that patients with resected stage III or IV disease benefited from adjuvant therapy with a PD-1–blocking antibody (nivolumab or pembrolizumab).[7,8] CheckMate 238 showed that adjuvant nivolumab versus ipilimumab in patients with resectable stage III or IV melanoma had significantly longer RFS at 12 month follow-up (70.5% vs 60.8%; HR 0.65, 97.56% CI 0.51–0.83). Furthermore, there were significantly fewer patients that discontinued therapy because of adverse events with adjuvant nivolumab versus ipilimumab (9.7% and 42.6%).[7] This pattern of improved efficacy over standard of care with tolerable safety profile with PD-1 inhibitors was also demonstrated in KEYNOTE-054.[8] In patients with resected stage III melanoma, pembrolizumab led to an improved RFS at 12 months (75.4%

Table 1
Summary of recent key trials in adjuvant and neoadjuvant therapy for melanoma

Therapy Modality	Trial Name	Phase	Melanoma Stage	Groups (n)	Primary Outcome (Results)	Notable Secondary Outcomes (Results)	Citation
Immune Checkpoint Blockade (Adjuvant)	Checkmate 238 (NCT02388906)	III	Resectable III and IV[a]	Adjuvant nivolumab (n = 453) vs adjuvant ipilimumab (n = 453)	RFS at 12 mo: 70.5% (95% CI 66.1–74.5) vs 60.8% (95% CI 56.0–65.2); HR 0.65, 97.56% CI 0.51–0.83, P<.001	Grade 3 or 4 adverse events: 14.4% vs 45.9%	Weber et al,[7] 2017
	Keynote 054 (NCT02362594)	III	Resectable III and IV[a]	Adjuvant pembrolizumab (n = 514) vs placebo (n = 505)	RFS at 12 mo: 75.4% (95% CI 71.3–78.9) vs 61.0% (95% CI 56.5–65.1); HR 0.57, 98.4% CI 0.43–0.74; P<.001. RFS at 12 mo in subgroup of patients with PD-L1 positive tumors: 77.1% (95% CI 72.7–80.9) vs 62.6% (95% CI 57.7–67.0); HR 0.54, 95% CI, 0.42–0.69, P<.001	Grade 3–5 adverse events: 14.7% vs 3.4%. One treatment-related death occurred with pembrolizumab.	Eggermont et al,[8] 2018
	Keynote 716 (NCT03553836)	III	IIB and IIC	Adjuvant pembrolizumab (n = 487) vs placebo (n = 489)	RFS First interim analysis (median follow-up 14 mo): 89% vs 83% (HR 0.65 [95% CI 0.46–0.92]) Second interim analysis (median follow-up 20 mo): 85% vs 76% (HR 0.61 [95% CI 0.45–0.82]) Luke et al., Lancet 2022	DMFS Third interim analysis: (median follow-up 27 mo): median DMFS not reached; HR 0.64, 95% CI 0.47–0.88, P = .0029. Grade 3 or 4 adverse events: 10% vs 2% Long et al., Lancet Oncology 2022	Luke et al,[25] 2022; Long et al,[68] 2022

(continued on next page)

Table 1
(continued)

Therapy Modality	Trial Name	Phase	Melanoma Stage	Groups (n)	Primary Outcome (Results)	Notable Secondary Outcomes (Results)	Citation
	CheckMate 76K (NCT04099251)	III	IIB and IIC	Adjuvant nivolumab (n = 524) vs placebo (n = 264)	RFS at 12 mo: 89.0% vs 79.4%; HR 0.42, 95% CI 0.30–0.59; P<.0001	DMFS: HR 0.47; 95% CI 0.30–0.72). Grade 3 or 4 adverse events: in 10.3% vs 2.3%. One treatment-related death occurred with nivolumab.	Kirkwood et al,[27] 2023

Therapy Modality	Trial Name	Phase	Melanoma Stage	Groups (n)	Primary Outcome (Results)	Notable Secondary Outcome (Results)	Citation
Immune Checkpoint Blockade (Neoadjuvant)	NCT02519322	II	Resectable IIIB-IV	Combined neoadjuvant ipilimumab/ nivolumab plus adjuvant nivolumab (n = 11) vs neoadjuvant-adjuvant nivolumab (n = 12)	pCR: 45% vs 25%	ORR: 73% vs 25% Grade 3 or 4 adverse events: 73% vs 8%	Amaria et al,[28] 2018
	OpACIN (NCT02437279)	II	Resectable IIIB/C	Neoadjuvant-adjuvant ipilimumab/ nivolumab (n = 10) vs adjuvant ipilimumab/ nivolumab (n = 10)	Grade 3 or 4 adverse events: 90% in both arms Immune-activating capacity: neoadjuvant-adjuvant therapy expanded more tumor-resident clones compared to adjuvant therapy alone using tetramer staining	MPR in neoadjuvant arm: 7/9 Only 1/10 patients in neoadjuvant arm received all four courses	Blank et al,[29] 2018

	Phase	Resectable	Neoadjuvant			
PRADO (NCT02977052)	II	Resectable IIIB and IIIC	Neoadjuvant ipilimumab/ nivolumab (n = 99), then evaluated ILN In patients with MPR (<10% viable tumor), CLND + adjuvant therapy omitted (n = 60) In patients with pPR (>10 to ≤50% viable tumor), CLND only (n = 11) In patients with pNR (>50% viable tumor), CLND + adjuvant systemic therapy ± synchronous radiotherapy (n = 19)	Confirmation of pPR (ILN at week 6): 72% Grade 3 or 4 adverse events during neoadjuvant phase: 22% patients.	24-mo RFS: In patients with MPR 93% In patients with pPR 64% In patients with pNR 71%	Reijers et al,[43] 2022
SWOG 1801	III	Resectable III and IV	Neoadjuvant-adjuvant pembrolizumab (3 doses neoadjuvant- 15 doses adjuvant) vs adjuvant only (18 doses)	RFS at 2 y: 72% (95% CI 64–80) vs 49% (95% CI 41–59)	Grade 3 or 4 adverse events: 12% vs 14%	Patel et al,[32] 2023
NCT02519322	Ib	Resectable III and IV	Nivolumab and relatlimab: 2 neoadjuvant doses, surgery, 10 adjuvant doses (n = 30, single arm)	pCR rate: 57%	pRR: 70% Among patients with any pathologic response: 1 y RFS 100%, 2-y RFS 92% No grade 3 or 4 adverse events	Amaria et al,[38] 2022.

(continued on next page)

Table 1
(continued)

Therapy Modality	Trial Name	Phase	Melanoma Stage	Groups (n)	Primary Outcome (Results)	Notable Secondary Outcome (Results)	Citation
BRAFi/MEKi	COMBI-AD (5-y analysis)	III	Resectable III (with BRAF V600 mutation)	Adjuvant dabrafenib/ trametinib (n = 438) vs placebo (n = 432)	RFS at 5 y: 52% (95% CI 48–58) vs 36% (95% CI 32–41); HR 0.51, 95% CI 0.42–0.61	5-y DMFS: 65% (95% CI 61–71) vs 54% (95% CI 49–60); HR 0.55, 95% CI 0.44–0.70	Dummer et al,[50] 2020
	NCT02231775	II	Resectable III (with BRAF V600 mutation)	Neoadjuvant-adjuvant dabrafenib/ trametinib (n = 14) vs upfront surgery and consideration of adjuvant therapy (n = 7)	Trial terminated early after 25% accrual Median follow-up (18 mo): 10/14 vs 0/7 were alive without disease progression RFS at 12 mo: 19.7 mo [95% CI 16.2-not estimable] vs 2.9 mo [95% CI 1.7-not estimable]; HR 0·016, 95% CI 0·00,012–0·14, P<0·0001)	Grade 3 or 4 adverse events: 2/14 patients	Amaria et al,[67] 2018
	NeoCombi	II	Resectable III (with BRAF V600 mutation)	Neoadjuvant-adjuvant dabrafenib/ trametinib therapy (n = 35, single arm)	pRR at 12 wk: 100%; pCR at 12 wk: 49% (95% CI 31–66) Radiographic response according to RECIST at 12 wk: 30/35 (86%); complete response 16/35 (46%, 95% CI 29–63); partial response 14/35 (40%, 24–58); 5/35 stable disease (14%, 95% CI 5–30). No patient progressed.	Grade 3 or 4 adverse events: 29%	Long et al,[68] 2019; Menzies et al,[70] 2022

	Trial	Phase	Stage	Treatment	Outcome	Outcome	Reference
Oncolytic Viruses (TVEC)	Masterkey 265/ KEYNOTE-034	III	Unresectable IIIB-IVM1c	T-VEC-pembrolizumab (n = 346) vs placebo-pembrolizumab (n = 346)	PFS at 2 y: HR 0.86, 95% CI 0.71–1.04, P=.13 OS at 2 y: HR 0.96, 95% CI 0.76–1.22, P=.74	ORR: 48.6 (95% CI 43.3–53.8) vs 41.3% (95% CI 36.1–45.5)	Chesney et al,[82] JCO 2023
	NCT02211131	II	Resectable IIIB-IVM1a	Neoadjuvant T-VEC + surgery (n = 76) vs upfront surgery (n = 74)	RFS at 2 y: 29.5% vs 16.5% (HR 0.75, 80% CI 0.58–0.96)	OS at 2 y: 88.9% vs 77.4% (HR = 0.49, 80% CI 0.30–0.79).	Dummer et al,[83] 2021
TIL	NCT02278887	III	Unresectable IIIC-IV	TIL therapy (n = 84) vs ipilimumab (n = 84)	PFS (median follow-up 33 mo): 7.2 mo (95% CI 4.2–13.1) vs 3.1 mo (95% CI 3.0–4.3); HR 0.50, 95% CI 0.35–0.72, P<.001	OS (median follow-up 33 mo): 25.8 mo (95% CI 18.2-not reached) vs 18.9 mo (95% CI 13.8–32.6)	Rohaan et al,[91] 2022
Cancer Vaccines	KEYNOTE-942 (NCT03897881)	II	Resectable IIIB-IV	mRNA-4157/V940 in combination with pembrolizumab (n = 107) vs pembrolizumab alone (n = 50)	RFS at 12 mo: 78.6% vs 62.2%, HR 0.56; 95% CI: (0.309, 1.017	DMFS at 12 mo: HR 0.347; 95% CI: (0.145, 0.828)	AACR, Unpublished; Moderna release, 2023

Abbreviations: CI, confidence interval; HR, hazard ratio; MPR, major pathologic response; ORR, objective response rate; OS, overall survival; pCR, complete pathologic response; pPR, pathologic partial response; pRR, pathologic response rate; RECIST, response evaluation criteria in solid tumors; RFS, Relapse-free survival; Progression-free survival.
[a] Trials with inclusion criteria based on AJCC 7th edition.

vs 61.0%, HR 0.57, 98.4% CI 0.43–0.74). There was a similar rate of grade 3 or higher adverse events as previously seen with PD-1 inhibitors.[7] Interestingly, sub-group analysis demonstrated similar RFS in patients with PD-L1 positive versus negative tumors.[8] While multiple trials have investigated the combination PD-1 inhibitors with CTLA-4 for resected stage III/IV disease,[18–20] the rate of grade 3 or higher adverse events with combination therapy has been exceedingly high (71% in one study),[19] and thus, this combination is not routinely used in the adjuvant setting for cutaneous melanoma.

Long-term follow-up combined with correlative studies arising from these studies has enabled more detailed analysis of potential clinical biomarkers. Four- and 5-year follow-up data of CheckMate-238 demonstrated sustained RFS and distant metastasis-free survival (DMFS) with nivolumab compared with ipilimumab with no notable difference in overall survival.[21,22] Generally, RFS was sustained across subgroup analysis, including tumor PD-L1 expression and BRAF mutation status, and the American Joint Committee on cancer (AJCC) 8th edition staging. Interestingly, high tumor mutational burden (TMB), higher levels of a tumor interferon-gamma (IFNγ)-associated gene signature and lower levels of serum C-reactive peptide were associated with favorable RFS but with limited predicted clinical utility in this cohort.[22] Five-year analysis of KEYNOTE-054 also showed a long-term sustained benefit in RFS and DMFS compared with placebo.[23] This is particularly interesting as approximately 70% of patients in the placebo arm received pembrolizumab at the time of locoregional recurrence, supporting the early use of adjuvant ICB in disease progression. While data regarding clinically useful biomarkers are lacking in this cohort, the occurrence of immune-related adverse events were associated with RFS,[24] in line with previous associations between potential shared mechanisms of autoimmunity and antitumor responses.

More recent studies have investigated the use of adjuvant PD-1 therapy in the setting of high-risk stage II disease.[25–27] Patients with stage IIB or IIC disease (≥T3b, N0) have historically had a greater risk of disease recurrence compared with those with stage IIIA (N1a) disease based on the AJCC 8th edition, despite the absence of regional lymph node involvement based on sentinel lymph node biopsy. Yet, these patients were excluded from earlier trials.[7,8] Landmark trial KEYNOTE-716 demonstrated that adjuvant pembrolizumab significantly reduced the risk of recurrence over placebo by 46% at 27 months in patients with resected stage IIB or C (HR 0.64, 95% CI 0.50–0.84).[25,26] Of note, distant metastasis were more common in these patients than local, regional, or locoregional disease as the first recurrence in the placebo group (16% vs 11%), supporting the argument for early systemic therapy in this high-risk population.[26] CheckMate 76K demonstrated similar findings with adjuvant nivolumab in stage IIB and C disease. At median follow-up of 15 months, adjuvant nivolumab reduced the risk of disease recurrence or death by 58% at over placebo (HR 0.42, 95% CI 0.30–0.59).[27] Adjuvant pembrolizumab or nivolumab is now a National Comprehensive Cancer Network (NCCN) category I recommendation for patients with stage IIB or C disease,[10] though its impact on OS remains to be seen.

Neoadjuvant Programmed Death-1 Therapy

Improved recurrence-free survival with adjuvant PD-1 therapy in advanced resectable melanoma has encouraged multiple clinical trials evaluating neoadjuvant ICB.[28–32] There are several advantages to neoadjuvant therapy as discussed earlier. A key hypothesis unique for immunotherapy in the neoadjuvant setting is that neoadjuvant ICB boosts the antitumor adaptive immune response and reduces the burden of mircometastases compared with adjuvant therapy. The mechanism of action of

PD-1 inhibitors relies on pre-existing tumor-specific T cells,[33,34] and the surgical resection of tumor and tumor-infiltrating lymphocytes may blunt the generation of these responses. This is supported by preclinical work that demonstrated increased number of circulating tumor-specific CD8$^+$ T cells with neoadjuvant compared with adjuvant therapy.[35]

Several phase I or II clinical trials have demonstrated improved antitumor T cell responses with neoadjuvant PD-1 therapy, though with variable safety profiles. In a small Phase II trial, combination neoadjuvant nivolumab and ipilimumab was associated with higher overall response rates (ORR) and pathologic complete responses (pCRs) but with significant toxicities compared with neoadjuvant nivolumab alone (ORR 73% vs 25%, grade 3 adverse events 73% vs 8%).[28] Biomarker analysis revealed higher numbers of tumor-infiltrating CD8 T cells in responders in both groups. The OpACIN trial evaluated neoadjuvant versus adjuvant combination ICB and re-demonstrated high toxicities.[29] Neoadjuvant therapy expanded more T cells compared with adjuvant therapy,[29] and high TMB and IFN-γ score were associated with RFS at 2 years.[36,37] An extension of this trial (OpACIN-neo) aimed to identify a tolerable neoadjuvant nivolumab or ipilimumab dosing schedule that lead to a pathologic response in a high proportion of patients.[30] Yet remarkably in other studies, a single dose of pembrolizumab induced a complete or major pathologic response in approximatelt 30% patients with stage III or IV melanoma.[31] As anticipated, the presence of tumor-infiltrating CD8$^+$ T cells was associated with RFS. Pre-treatment transcriptional analysis of the tumor demonstrated increased expression in genes associated with T cell activation, adaptive immune response, and T cell migration in patients with improved RFS,[31] supporting potential selection of patients who might best benefit from neoadjuvant.

SWOG 1801 was the first randomized trial that evaluated neoadjuvant or adjuvant versus adjuvant-only pembrolizumab in advanced resectable melanoma.[32] The experimental schema was very simple, changing only the timing of 3 doses of adjuvant therapy to be administered in the neoadjuvant setting versus standard-of-care adjuvant pembrolizumab. A total of 313 patients with resectable stage IIIB to IVC disease underwent randomized to either 3 doses of neoadjuvant pembrolizumab, surgery, and 15 doses of adjuvant pembrolizumab (neoadjuvant–adjuvant group) or to surgery followed by 18 doses of adjuvant pembrolizumab (adjuvant-only group). At 2 years, RFS was significantly lower in the neoadjuvant-adjuvant versus adjuvant-only group 72% (95% CI 64%–80%) versus 49% (95% CI 41%–59%). Given tolerable safety profile and substantial improvement in DFS, neoadjuvant pembrolizumab is now a reasonable treatment option in this population. This study was the first to address the impact of the timing of therapy compared with the adjuvant setting, and solidified the superiority of neoadjuvant immunotherapy over adjuvant resulting in a dramatic change in clinical practice.

Overall, the case for neoadjuvant ICB in high-risk node-positive disease is building.[11–13] However, there are several outstanding questions. First, there is no consensus regarding the optimal agents and duration of neoadjuvant therapy. SWOG 1801 had an acceptable safety profile with single-agent pembrolizumab, but it is unclear if different agents, doses or timing could improve pCR rates. Indeed, emerging checkpoint inhibitors against the lymphocyte-activation gene 3 have shown great promise.[38,39] Second, the impact on OS remains unclear. Long-term analysis should inform this, though early data are encouraging.[40] Third, the role of neoadjuvant therapy in patient with thick melanomas (>T3b) but no clinically positive nodes are unknown. Finally, ongoing work is investigating de-escalation of surgery or adjuvant therapy based on pathologic response. Early work demonstrated the feasibility of magnetic seed localization to assess the response to neoadjuvant therapy in a single pathologic index lymph node (ILN) in order to potentially spare patients with pCR from a complete lymph node dissection (CLND).[41,42] In the PRADO extension cohort of the OpACIN-neo trial, patients with stage IIIB-D disease who received neoadjuvant ipilimumab or nivolumab underwent magnetic seed localization of the ILN.[43] If there was evidence of a major pathologic response (MPR; pCR; or <10% viable tumor), CLND and adjuvant therapy were omitted. At 2 years, RFS and DMFS was 93% and 98%, respectively, in patients with MPR, suggesting that there is a population of patients who may benefit from de-escalation of therapy. However, patients who had a partial response in this trial did not receive adjuvant therapy, suggesting that the authors must be cautious in interpreting these outcomes. While cross-trial analysis suggests that de-escalation of care may not affect RFS or DFMS,[44] randomized clinical trials will be necessary to test response-directed personalized treatment following neoadjuvant therapy.

BRAF/MEK INHIBITORS

Pathogenic *BRAF* mutations are found in approximately 60% of melanomas and are associated with constitutive activation of the MAP kinase signal-transduction pathway.[45] Identification of *BRAF* V600 E and V600 K as the most frequent variants lead to the development of small molecule-targeted therapies.[46] Promising survival data in the setting of unresectable metastatic melanoma with BRAF inhibitors[5,6] along with further understanding of resistance mechanisms[47–49] encouraged clinical trials in the adjuvant setting. The COMBI-AD trial randomized patients with resected stage III melanoma with *BRAF* V600 E/K mutations to 12 months of adjuvant therapy with dabrafenib plus trametinib (BRAF/MEKi) or placebo.[9] Recently published long-term analysis showed sustained RFS in the treatment arm at 5 years (52% vs 36%; HR 0.51, 95% CI 0.42–0.61).[50] Given the overall reasonable safety profile, adjuvant dabrafenib plus trametinib is now a reasonable option for patients advanced resectable *BRAF*-mutated melanoma.

It is unclear whether patients with *BRAF* V600 mutations would benefit from adjuvant targeted therapy or ICB as first-line treatment. There are no randomized clinical trials comparing the 2 options in advanced resectable melanoma. Retrospective analysis of patients with *BRAF*-mutant melanoma suggests that adjuvant targeted therapy was associated with improved RFS with comparable OS compared with PD-1 therapy at 3 years.[51] In the metastatic setting, nivolumab or ipilimumab appears to have improved 2-year OS compared with dabrafenib or trametinib in patients with *BRAF* V600-mutant melanoma in a randomized prospective trial.[52] This is line with general observations that targeted therapy leads to higher ORR, while ICB leads to more durable responses. However, it is unclear how to extrapolate these findings to neoadjuvant or adjuvant clinical-decision making. Thus far, there are no clinically useful tumors or patient characteristics to help further define which patients with BRAF-mutated melanoma would benefit the most from targeted therapy. Biomarker analysis of COMBI-AD suggests that patients with low TMB may derive greater benefit from targeted therapy compared with placebo,[53] in contrast to historically poor responses to ICB in this group, albeit in the setting of metastatic melanoma.[54–56] At this time, the choice of adjuvant therapy is largely driven by the different toxicity profiles of both therapies.[57] While side effects from dabrafenib or trametinib can mitigated by dose-interruption,[58] ICB can induce long-term immune-related adverse events even years off therapy.[59,60] Of note, combined "triple" therapy with ICB (against either PD-1 or PD-L1), BRAF/MEKi in the metastatic setting has been associated with mixed improvements in progression-free survival (PFS), substantial toxicity, and no clear durable survival benefit.[61–66] Ultimately, the choice of adjuvant BRAF/MEKi or ICB in

BRAF-mutated melanoma remains an individual patient-physician choice, in the absence of randomized clinical data.

Two key small trials have looked at neoadjuvant targeted therapy. Amaria *and colleagues* randomized patients to neoadjuvant plus adjuvant dabrafenib or trametinib or upfront surgery and consideration for adjuvant therapy. The trial was stopped early given impressive results: 10/14 versus 0/7 patients were alive without disease progression at 18 months.[67] The NeoCombi trial was a single-arm trial that evaluated neoadjuvant plus adjuvant dabrafenib or trametinib. Short-term results were promising with pCR in 17/35 patients.[68] This is in line with the REDUCTOR trial, which enrolled patients with previously deemed unresectable melanoma and showed that 17/21 patients were able to proceed with R0 resection following treatment with BRAF/MEKi.[69] While long-term analysis of the NeoCombi trial shows high risk of recurrence with 5-year RFS of 40%,[70] neoadjuvant BRAF/MEK inhibition remains a promising strategy.

ONCOLYTIC VIRUSES

Oncolytic viruses are a newer and understudied class of immunotherapy that utilizes genetically modified viruses to treat cancer.[71] Talimogene laherparepvec (T-VEC) is a modified herpes simplex virus type 1 expressing granulocyte-macrophage colony-stimulating factor (GM-CSF).[72] It is currently the only oncolytic virus to be approved for the treatment of melanoma in the United States. Intralesional T-VEC therapy aims to promote preferential viral replication in tumor cells via deletion of the *ICP34.5* gene, which leads to cell lysis, release of tumor-derived antigens, and subsequent activation of tumor-specific $CD8^+$ T cells.[73–75] Additional genetic modifications with the deletion of *ICP47* and insertion of the gene encoding GM-CSF lead to preferential loading of tumor antigen on major histocompatibility complex class I molecules and dendritic cell recruitment, respectively.[75,76] Food and Drug Administration (FDA) approval in 2015 was based on findings from the OPTIM trial, which demonstrated improved durable response rates (ORR > 6 months) in patients with unresectable melanoma patients who received intralesional T-VEC (16.3%) compared with GM-CSF (2.1%).[77] Durable responses have been seen even 5 years following therapy with 17% in the T-VEC arm achieving CR.[78]

Randomized clinical trials combined with real-world experience have helped us refine the clinical indications for T-VEC and how oncolytic immunotherapy therapy could be incorporated into the treatment of resectable disease.[79–83] Recent work has evaluated T-VEC with concurrent ICB. The rationale is to combine the enhanced intratumoral infiltration of adaptive immune cells induced by T-VEC with blockade of immune inhibitor checkpoint receptors.[84] The Masterkey 265/KEYNOTE-034 was a Phase III clinical trial that evaluated pembrolizumab with and without T-VEC in patients with unresectable Stage IIIB-IVM1c melanoma.[82] T-VEC-pembrolizumab did not significantly improve progression free survival (PFS) (HR 0.86; 95% CI 0.71–1.04) or OS (HR 0.96; 95% CI 0.76–1.22) compared with pembrolizumab alone. Notably, 41% patients in this trial had M1c disease and the trial group had overall more advanced than the original OPTIM study, which excluded patients with extensive visceral disease,[77] possibly highlighting its application to upfront therapy, specific patient populations (such as those with in-transit disease), or borderline resectable disease.

Neoadjuvant T-VEC is a promising strategy. The goal is to both induce a local response to improve resectability, as well as a durable systemic immune response in the setting of an existing tumor.[85] In recent important trial, Dummer *and colleagues* randomized patients with resectable IIIB-IVM1a disease to neoadjuvant T-VEC followed by surgery versus upfront surgery. The neoadjuvant T-VEC arm had improved PFS (29.5%

vs 16.5%, HR 0.75, 80% CI 0.58–0.96) and OS (88.9% vs 77.4%, HR 0.49, 80% CI 0.30–0.79) at 2 years, overall leading to a 25% reduction in disease recurrence.[83] Interestingly, significant differences in PFS, OS, and DMFS persisted at 5 years, suggestive of a durable systemic response induced by local intralesional therapy.[86] Pathology analysis revealed 17.1% pCR in the neoadjuvant T-VEC arm and increased CD8+ T cell infiltration in good responders.[83] Of note, adjuvant therapy was investigator-driven in both arms, and as such it is difficult to determine the optimal combination of this therapy with standard-of-care treatments. Future trials evaluating neoadjuvant T-VEC and ICB, as well as neoadjuvant T-VEC in high-risk stage II disease should shed light on how oncolytic viruses can fit in the large arsenal of available therapies.[87]

TUMOR-INFILTRATING LYMPHOCYTE THERAPY

Rosenberg and colleagues first demonstrated the clinical activity of adoptive cellular therapy with TIL in the 1980s.[88] This process involves tumor resection, *in vitro* expansion of TIL with interleukin-2, followed by intravenous administration in the setting of lymphodepleting chemotherapy.[89] Subsequent work demonstrated durable responses in up to 30% of patients with metastatic melanoma,[90] though this was before widespread use of ICB therapy. Recent work has highlighted the importance of TIL therapy in the current landscape of systemic treatments. A large multicenter phase III clinical compared TIL therapy versus ipilimumab in patients with unresectable metastatic melanoma, of which the vast majority (89%) had failed PD-1 therapy. PFS was significantly improve in the TIL arm (7.2 vs 3.1 months, HR 0.50, 95% CI 0.35–0.72) with a complete response in 20% patients.[91] Widespread availability of TIL therapy, now with the expected FDA approval of Lifileucel (Iovance Biotherapeutics),[92] will enable further understanding of the antitumor T cell response and how this therapy could be used in the adjuvant setting for patients who may not benefit from ICB or BRAF/MEKi. Furthermore, TIL therapy may provide durable benefits to patients with mucosal melanoma, a group that historically has not responded well to ICB.[93]

CANCER VACCINES

Cancer vaccines are another form of personalized immunotherapy that has made significant progress in the last 5 years.[94] The goal of therapeutic cancer vaccines is to induce a robust antitumor immune response in patients with established disease by targeting neoantigens that are either shared (common across tumor type) or private (predicted for each individual patient). As in conventional vaccines against pathogens, cancer vaccines can include various components of the antigen (deoxyribonuclease [DNA], ribonucleic acid [RNA], protein, and whole cells), as well as different adjuvants (Toll-like receptors agonist, and water-in-oil emulsions) to boost an adaptive immune response.

Early work with personalized cancer vaccines has demonstrated that this is safe strategy that can generate *de novo* neoantigen-specific CD8+ T cells with promising clinical efficacy.[95–98] A recent Phase II trial, KEYNOTE-942, evaluated the role of mRNA-4157 (also known as V940) in combination with pembrolizumab in the adjuvant setting.[99] This novel personalized cancer vaccine is made up of a synthetic mRNA molecule encoding up to 34 patient-specific neoantigens based on whole-genome sequencing of matched tumor- and normal-cell DNA, followed by computational prediction of human leukocyte antigens-binding peptides.[95] KEYNOTE-942 evaluated adjuvant pembrolizumab with and without mRNA-4157 following surgical resection in patients with stage IIIB-IV disease. In a small cohort, combination therapy with mRNA-4157 and pembrolizumab reduced the risk of recurrence or death by 44% compared with pembrolizumab alone

(RFS 78.6% vs 62.2%, HR 0.56, 95% CI 0.31–1.02).[99] Interestingly, this combination therapy had similar efficacy in patients with low TMB, a group that historically has not responded well to ICB alone.[54–56] Based on these results and a tolerable safety profile, mRNA-4157 combined with pembrolizumab received breakthrough designation from the FDA in February 2023, and a multicenter, randomized Phase III trial is currently underway (V940–001; NCT05933577).[100] Ongoing progress with other vaccines in the metastatic setting such as BNT111 (Melanoma FixVac)[98,101] demonstrates that therapeutic cancer vaccines may become an emerging option in the treatment of melanoma.

CONCLUSIONS/FUTURE DIRECTIONS

Over the last decade, the arsenal of adjuvant therapy options for melanoma has exploded. Cancer immunotherapy has provided new ways to augment pre-existing tumor-specific T cells and generate *de novo* responses. Advances in high-throughput whole genome sequencing made targeted therapy with BRAF/MEKi into a treatment reality. Furthermore, the clinical indications for these tools have expanded with early success in the neoadjuvant setting and for patients with high-risk stage II disease. As large clinical trials continue to assess different treatment modalities, systematic tumor banking and multi-omics biomarker analysis will be important in elucidating mechanisms of response and treatment resistance. This will ultimately be critical in helping clinicians determine the optimal therapy for melanoma patients in a rapidly changing treatment landscape.

CLINICS CARE POINTS

- Adjuvant pembrolizumab or nivolumab in stage IIIB-IV melanoma patients is associated with sustained recurrence-free survival and DMFS compared with placebo.
- Adjuvant pembrolizumab or nivolumab is also now an NCCN category I recommendation for patients with stage IIB or C disease, though its long-term impact remains to be seen.
- Neoadjuvant-adjuvant pembrolizumab should be considered in patients with stage IIIB-IV disease given improved recurrence free survival at 2 years.
- Targeted therapy with BRAF/MEKi is associated with improved recurrence free and overall survival in the adjuvant setting in patients with BRAF V600 E/K mutations.
- It is unclear whether patients with BRAF V600 mutations would benefit from adjuvant targeted therapy or ICB as first-line treatment, as there are no randomized clinicals comparing the 2 options, and thus the choice remains a personalized decision.
- Neoadjuvant T-VEC is a promising strategy to both induce a local and durable systemic immune response in the setting of an existing tumor and has shown early success in small clinical trials.

FUNDING

G.M.B. acknowledges research support from the Adelson Medical Research Foundation (AMRF), the Patricia K. Donahoe Award from the Huiying Foundation, and the Emma and Bill Roberts MGH Scholar Award.

DISCLOSURE

G.M. Boland has sponsored research agreements through her institution with: Olink Proteomics, Teiko Bio, InterVenn Biosciences, Palleon Pharmaceuticals. She served on advisory boards for: Iovance, Merck, Nektar Therapeutics, Novartis, and Ankyra Therapeutics. She consults for: Merck, InterVenn Biosciences, Iovance, and Ankyra Therapeutics. She holds equity in Ankyra Therapeutics.

REFERENCES

1. Melanoma Cancer Statistics. Surveillance, epidemiology, and end results (SEER) research program. National Cancer Institute; 2023. Available at: https://seer.cancer.gov/statfacts/html/melan.html.
2. Hodi FS, O'Day SJ, McDermott DF, et al. Improved survival with ipilimumab in patients with metastatic melanoma. N Engl J Med 2010;363:711–23.
3. Robert C, Thomas L, Bondarenko I, et al. Ipilimumab plus dacarbazine for previously untreated metastatic melanoma. N Engl J Med 2011;364:2517–26.
4. Robert C, Schachter J, Long GV, et al. Pembrolizumab versus ipilimumab in advanced melanoma. N Engl J Med 2015;372:2521–32.
5. Chapman PB, Hauschild A, Robert C, et al. Improved survival with vemurafenib in melanoma with BRAF V600E mutation. N Engl J Med 2011;364:2507–16.
6. Hauschild A, Grob JJ, Demidov LV, et al. Dabrafenib in BRAF-mutated metastatic melanoma: a multicentre, open-label, phase 3 randomised controlled trial. Lancet 2012;380:358–65.
7. Weber J, Mandala M, Del Vecchio M, et al. Adjuvant nivolumab versus ipilimumab in resected stage III or IV melanoma. N Engl J Med 2017;377:1824–35.
8. Eggermont AMM, Blank CU, Mandala M, et al. Adjuvant pembrolizumab versus placebo in resected stage III melanoma. N Engl J Med 2018;378:1789–801.
9. Long GV, Hauschild A, Santinami M, et al. Adjuvant dabrafenib plus trametinib in stage III BRAF-mutated melanoma. N Engl J Med 2017;377:1813–23.
10. National Cancer Comprehensive Network. Melanoma: cCutaneous (Version 3.2023).
11. Witt RG, Erstad DJ, Wargo JA. Neoadjuvant therapy for melanoma: rationale for neoadjuvant therapy and pivotal clinical trials. Ther. Adv. Med. Oncol 2022;14.
12. Garbe C, Dummer R, Amaral T, et al. Neoadjuvant immunotherapy for melanoma is now ready for clinical practice. Nat Med 2023;29:1310–2.
13. Hieken TJ, Kreidieh F, Aedo-Lopez V, et al. Neoadjuvant immunotherapy in melanoma: the paradigm shift. Am Soc Clin Oncol Educ Book 2023;e390614.
14. Fisher B, Brown A, Mamounas E, et al. Effect of preoperative chemotherapy on local-regional disease in women with operable breast cancer: findings from National Surgical Adjuvant Breast and Bowel Project B-18. J Clin Oncol 1997;15:2483–93.
15. Conroy T, Bosset JF, Etienne PL, et al. Neoadjuvant chemotherapy with FOLFIRINOX and preoperative chemoradiotherapy for patients with locally advanced rectal cancer (UNICANCER-PRODIGE 23): a multicentre, randomised, open-label, phase 3 trial. Lancet Oncol 2021;22:702–15.
16. van Hagen P, Hulshof MCCM, van Lanschot JJB, et al. Preoperative Chemoradiotherapy for esophageal or junctional cancer. N Engl J Med 2012;366:2074–84.
17. Leach DR, Krummel MF, Allison JP. Enhancement of antitumor immunity by CTLA-4 blockade. Science 1996;271:1734–6.
18. Livingstone E, Zimmer L, Hassel JC, et al. Adjuvant nivolumab plus ipilimumab or nivolumab alone versus placebo in patients with resected stage IV melanoma with no evidence of disease (IMMUNED): final results of a randomised, double-blind, phase 2 trial. Lancet 2022;400:1117–29.

19. Zimmer L, Livingstone E, Hassel JC, et al. Adjuvant nivolumab plus ipilimumab or nivolumab monotherapy versus placebo in patients with resected stage IV melanoma with no evidence of disease (IMMUNED): a randomised, double-blind, placebo-controlled, phase 2 trial. Lancet 2020;395:1558–68.

20. Weber JS, Schadendorf D, Del Vecchio M, et al. Adjuvant Therapy of Nivolumab Combined With Ipilimumab Versus Nivolumab Alone in Patients With Resected Stage IIIB-D or Stage IV Melanoma (CheckMate 915). J Clin Oncol 2023;41:517–27.

21. Ascierto PA, Del Vecchio M, Mandalá M, et al. Adjuvant nivolumab versus ipilimumab in resected stage IIIB–C and stage IV melanoma (CheckMate 238): 4-year results from a multicentre, double-blind, randomised, controlled, phase 3 trial. Lancet Oncol 2020;21:1465–77.

22. Larkin J, Del Vecchio M, Mandalá M, et al. Adjuvant nivolumab versus ipilimumab in resected stage III/IV Melanoma: 5-year efficacy and biomarker results from checkmate 238. Clin Cancer Res 2023;29:3352–61.

23. Eggermont Alexander MM, Kicinski M, Blank CU, et al. Five-year analysis of adjuvant pembrolizumab or placebo in stage III melanoma. NEJM Evidence 2022;1. EVIDoa2200214.

24. Eggermont AMM, Kicinski M, Blank CU, et al. Association between immune-related adverse events and recurrence-free survival among patients with stage III melanoma randomized to receive pembrolizumab or placebo: a secondary analysis of a randomized clinical trial. JAMA Oncol 2020;6:519–27.

25. Luke JJ, Rutkowski P, Queirolo P, et al. Pembrolizumab versus placebo as adjuvant therapy in completely resected stage IIB or IIC melanoma (KEYNOTE-716): a randomised, double-blind, phase 3 trial. Lancet 2022;399:1718–29.

26. Long GV, Luke JJ, Khattak MA, et al. Pembrolizumab versus placebo as adjuvant therapy in resected stage IIB or IIC melanoma (KEYNOTE-716): distant metastasis-free survival results of a multicentre, double-blind, randomised, phase 3 trial. Lancet Oncol 2022;23:1378–88.

27. Kirkwood JM, Del Vecchio M, Weber J, et al. Adjuvant nivolumab in resected stage IIB/C melanoma: primary results from the randomized, phase 3 Check-Mate 76K trial. Nat Med 2023;29:2835–43.

28. Amaria RN, Reddy SM, Tawbi HA, et al. Neoadjuvant immune checkpoint blockade in high-risk resectable melanoma. Nat Med 2018;24:1649–54.

29. Blank CU, Rozeman EA, Fanchi LF, et al. Neoadjuvant versus adjuvant ipilimumab plus nivolumab in macroscopic stage III melanoma. Nat Med 2018;24:1655–61.

30. Rozeman EA, Menzies AM, van Akkooi ACJ, et al. Identification of the optimal combination dosing schedule of neoadjuvant ipilimumab plus nivolumab in macroscopic stage III melanoma (OpACIN-neo): a multicentre, phase 2, randomised, controlled trial. Lancet Oncol 2019;20:948–60.

31. Huang AC, Orlowski RJ, Xu X, et al. A single dose of neoadjuvant PD-1 blockade predicts clinical outcomes in resectable melanoma. Nat Med 2019;25:454–61.

32. Patel SP, Othus M, Chen Y, et al. Neoadjuvant–adjuvant or adjuvant-only pembrolizumab in advanced melanoma. N Engl J Med 2023;388:813–23.

33. Tumeh PC, Harview CL, Yearley JH, et al. PD-1 blockade induces responses by inhibiting adaptive immune resistance. Nature 2014;515:568–71.

34. Herbst RS, Soria JC, Kowanetz M, et al. Predictive correlates of response to the anti-PD-L1 antibody MPDL3280A in cancer patients. Nature 2014;515:563–7.

35. Liu J, Blake SJ, Yong MCR, et al. Improved efficacy of neoadjuvant compared to adjuvant immunotherapy to eradicate metastatic disease. Cancer Discov 2016; 6:1382–99.

36. Rozeman EA, Hoefsmit EP, Reijers ILM, et al. Survival and biomarker analyses from the OpACIN-neo and OpACIN neoadjuvant immunotherapy trials in stage III melanoma. Nat Med 2021;27:256–63.

37. Reijers ILM, Rao D, Versluis JM, et al. IFN-γ signature enables selection of neoadjuvant treatment in patients with stage III melanoma. J Exp Med 2023;220.

38. Amaria RN, Postow M, Burton EM, et al. Neoadjuvant relatlimab and nivolumab in resectable melanoma. Nature 2022;611:155–60.

39. Tawbi HA, Schadendorf D, Lipson EJ, et al. Relatlimab and nivolumab versus nivolumab in untreated advanced melanoma. N Engl J Med 2022;386:24–34.

40. Sharon CE, Tortorello GN, Ma KL, et al. Long-term outcomes to neoadjuvant pembrolizumab based on pathological response for patients with resectable stage III/IV cutaneous melanoma. Ann Oncol 2023;34:806–12.

41. Schermers B, Franke V, Rozeman EA, et al. Surgical removal of the index node marked using magnetic seed localization to assess response to neoadjuvant immunotherapy in patients with stage III melanoma. Br J Surg 2019;106:519–22.

42. Reijers ILM, Rawson RV, Colebatch AJ, et al. Representativeness of the index lymph node for total nodal basin in pathologic response assessment after neoadjuvant checkpoint inhibitor therapy in patients with stage III melanoma. JAMA Surg 2022;157:335–42.

43. Reijers ILM, Menzies AM, van Akkooi ACJ, et al. Personalized response-directed surgery and adjuvant therapy after neoadjuvant ipilimumab and nivolumab in high-risk stage III melanoma: the PRADO trial. Nat Med 2022;28:1178–88.

44. Reijers ILM, Menzies AM, Versluis JM, et al. The impact of response-directed surgery and adjuvant therapy on long-term survival after neoadjuvant ipilimumab plus nivolumab in stage III melanoma: Three-year data of PRADO and OpACIN-neo. J Clin Orthod 2023;41:101.

45. Davies H, Bignell GR, Cox C, et al. Mutations of the BRAF gene in human cancer. Nature 2002;417:949–54.

46. Cancer Genome Atlas Network. Genomic classification of cutaneous melanoma. Cell 2015;161:1681–96.

47. Robert C, Grob JJ, Stroyakovskiy D, et al. Five-year outcomes with dabrafenib plus trametinib in metastatic melanoma. N Engl J Med 2019;381:626–36.

48. Long GV, Stroyakovskiy D, Gogas H, et al. Combined BRAF and MEK inhibition versus BRAF inhibition alone in melanoma. N Engl J Med 2014;371:1877–88.

49. Flaherty KT, Infante JR, Daud A, et al. Combined BRAF and MEK inhibition in melanoma with BRAF V600 mutations. N Engl J Med 2012;367:1694–703.

50. Dummer R, Hauschild A, Santinami M, et al. Five-year analysis of adjuvant dabrafenib plus trametinib in stage III melanoma. N Engl J Med 2020;383:1139–48.

51. Bai X, Shaheen A, Grieco C, et al. Dabrafenib plus trametinib versus anti-PD-1 monotherapy as adjuvant therapy in BRAF V600-mutant stage III melanoma after definitive surgery: a multicenter, retrospective cohort study. eClinicalMedicine 2023;65.

52. Atkins MB, Lee SJ, Chmielowski B, et al. Combination dabrafenib and trametinib versus combination nivolumab and ipilimumab for patients with advanced BRAF-mutant melanoma: The DREAMseq trial-ECOG-ACRIN EA6134. J Clin Oncol 2023;41:186–97.

53. Dummer R, Brase JC, Garrett J, et al. Adjuvant dabrafenib plus trametinib versus placebo in patients with resected, BRAFV600-mutant, stage III

melanoma (COMBI-AD): exploratory biomarker analyses from a randomised, phase 3 trial. Lancet Oncol 2020;21:358–72.

54. Hugo W, Zaretsky JM, Sun L, et al. Genomic and transcriptomic features of response to anti-PD-1 therapy in metastatic melanoma. Cell 2016;165:35–44.

55. Van Allen EM, Miao D, Schilling B, et al. Genomic correlates of response to CTLA-4 blockade in metastatic melanoma. Science 2015;350:207–11.

56. Goodman AM, Kato S, Bazhenova L, et al. Tumor mutational burden as an independent predictor of response to immunotherapy in diverse cancers. Mol Cancer Therapeut 2017;16:2598–608.

57. Mooradian MJ, Sullivan RJ. The case for adjuvant BRAF-targeted therapy versus adjuvant anti-PD-1 therapy for patients with resected, high-risk melanoma. Cancer 2023;129:2117–21.

58. Schadendorf D, Robert C, Dummer R, et al. Pyrexia in patients treated with dabrafenib plus trametinib across clinical trials in BRAF-mutant cancers. Eur J Cancer 2021;153:234–41.

59. Patrinely JR, Johnson R, Lawless AR, et al. Chronic immune-related adverse events following adjuvant anti-PD-1 therapy for high-risk resected melanoma. JAMA Oncol 2021;7:744–8.

60. Wang DY, Salem JE, Cohen JV, et al. Fatal toxic effects associated with immune checkpoint inhibitors: a systematic review and meta-analysis. JAMA Oncol 2018;4:1721–8.

61. Callahan MK, Chapman PB. PD-1 or PD-L1 blockade adds little to combination of BRAF and MEK inhibition in the treatment of BRAF V600–mutated melanoma. J Clin Orthod 2022;40:1393–5.

62. Sullivan RJ, Hamid O, Gonzalez R, et al. Atezolizumab plus cobimetinib and vemurafenib in BRAF-mutated melanoma patients. Nat Med 2019;25:929–35.

63. Ribas A, Lawrence D, Atkinson V, et al. Combined BRAF and MEK inhibition with PD-1 blockade immunotherapy in BRAF-mutant melanoma. Nat Med 2019;25: 936–40.

64. Ascierto PA, Ferrucci PF, Fisher R, et al. Dabrafenib, trametinib and pembrolizumab or placebo in BRAF-mutant melanoma. Nat Med 2019;25:941–6.

65. Gutzmer R, Stroyakovskiy D, Gogas H, et al. Atezolizumab, vemurafenib, and cobimetinib as first-line treatment for unresectable advanced BRAFV600 mutation-positive melanoma (IMspire150): primary analysis of the randomised, double-blind, placebo-controlled, phase 3 trial. Lancet 2020;395:1835–44.

66. Ascierto PA, Stroyakovskiy D, Gogas H, et al. Overall survival with first-line atezolizumab in combination with vemurafenib and cobimetinib in BRAFV600 mutation-positive advanced melanoma (IMspire150): second interim analysis of a multicentre, randomised, phase 3 study. Lancet Oncol 2023;24:33–44.

67. Amaria RN, Prieto PA, Tetzlaff MT, et al. Neoadjuvant plus adjuvant dabrafenib and trametinib versus standard of care in patients with high-risk, surgically resectable melanoma: a single-centre, open-label, randomised, phase 2 trial. Lancet Oncol 2018;19:181–93.

68. Long GV, Saw RPM, Lo S, et al. Neoadjuvant dabrafenib combined with trametinib for resectable, stage IIIB-C, BRAFV600 mutation-positive melanoma (NeoCombi): a single-arm, open-label, single-centre, phase 2 trial. Lancet Oncol 2019;20:961–71.

69. Blankenstein SA, Rohaan MW, Klop WMC, et al. Neoadjuvant cytoreductive treatment with BRAF/MEK inhibition of prior unresectable regionally advanced melanoma to allow complete surgical resection, REDUCTOR: A Prospective, Single-arm, Open-label Phase II Trial. Ann Surg 2021;274:383–9.

70. Menzies AM, Saw RP, Lo SN, et al. Neoadjuvant dabrafenib and trametinib (D+T) for stage III melanoma: Long-term results from the NeoCombi trial. J Clin Orthod 2022;40:9580.

71. Shalhout SZ, Miller DM, Emerick KS, et al. Therapy with oncolytic viruses: progress and challenges. Nat Rev Clin Oncol 2023;20:160–77.

72. Ferrucci PF, Pala L, Conforti F, et al. Talimogene laherparepvec (T-VEC): an intralesional cancer immunotherapy for advanced melanoma. Cancers 2021;13.

73. Kaufman HL, Shalhout SZ, Iodice G. Talimogene Laherparepvec: Moving From First-In-Class to Best-In-Class. Front Mol Biosci 2022;9:834841.

74. Liu BL, Robinson M, Han ZQ, et al. ICP34.5 deleted herpes simplex virus with enhanced oncolytic, immune stimulating, and anti-tumour properties. Gene Ther 2003;10:292–303.

75. Kohlhapp FJ, Kaufman HL. Molecular pathways: mechanism of action for talimogene laherparepvec, a new oncolytic virus immunotherapy. Clin Cancer Res 2016;22:1048–54.

76. Bowne WB, Wolchok JD, Hawkins WG, et al. Injection of DNA encoding granulocyte-macrophage colony-stimulating factor recruits dendritic cells for immune adjuvant effects. Cytokines Cell Mol Ther 1999;5:217–25.

77. Andtbacka RHI, Kaufman HL, Collichio F, et al. Talimogene laherparepvec improves durable response rate in patients with advanced melanoma. J Clin Oncol 2015;33:2780–8.

78. Andtbacka RHI, Collichio F, Harrington KJ, et al. Final analyses of OPTiM: a randomized phase III trial of talimogene laherparepvec versus granulocyte-macrophage colony-stimulating factor in unresectable stage III-IV melanoma. J Immunother Cancer 2019;7:145.

79. Perez MC, Miura JT, Naqvi SMH, et al. Talimogene laherparepvec (TVEC) for the treatment of advanced melanoma: a single-institution experience. Ann Surg Oncol 2018;25:3960–5.

80. van Akkooi ACJ, Haferkamp S, Papa S, et al. A retrospective chart review study of real-world use of talimogene laherparepvec in unresectable stage IIIB-IVM1a melanoma in four european countries. Adv Ther 2021;38:1245–62.

81. Louie RJ, Perez MC, Jajja MR, et al. Real-world outcomes of talimogene laherparepvec therapy: a multi-institutional experience. J Am Coll Surg 2019;228:644–9.

82. Chesney JA, Ribas A, Long GV, et al. Randomized, double-blind, placebo-controlled, global phase iii trial of talimogene laherparepvec combined with pembrolizumab for advanced melanoma. J Clin Oncol 2023;41:528–40.

83. Dummer R, Gyorki DE, Hyngstrom J, et al. Neoadjuvant talimogene laherparepvec plus surgery versus surgery alone for resectable stage IIIB-IVM1a melanoma: a randomized, open-label, phase 2 trial. Nat Med 2021;27:1789–96.

84. Ribas A, Dummer R, Puzanov I, et al. Oncolytic Virotherapy Promotes Intratumoral T Cell Infiltration and Improves Anti-PD-1 Immunotherapy. Cell 2017;170:1109–19.e10.

85. Kaufman HL, Kim DW, DeRaffele G, et al. Local and distant immunity induced by intralesional vaccination with an oncolytic herpes virus encoding GM-CSF in patients with stage IIIc and IV melanoma. Ann Surg Oncol 2010;17:718–30.

86. Dummer R, Gyorki DE, Hyngstrom JR, et al. Final 5-year follow-up results evaluating neoadjuvant talimogene laherparepvec plus surgery in advanced melanoma: a randomized clinical trial. JAMA Oncol 2023;9:1457–9.

87. Rohaan MW, Stahlie EHA, Franke V, et al. Neoadjuvant nivolumab + T-VEC combination therapy for resectable early stage or metastatic (IIIB-IVM1a) melanoma

with injectable disease: study protocol of the NIVEC trial. BMC Cancer 2022; 22:851.

88. Rosenberg SA, Packard BS, Aebersold PM, et al. Use of Tumor-Infiltrating Lymphocytes and Interleukin-2 in the Immunotherapy of Patients with Metastatic Melanoma. N Engl J Med 1988;319:1676–80.
89. Yang JC, Rosenberg SA. Adoptive T-cell therapy for cancer. Adv Immunol 2016; 130:279–94.
90. Goff SL, Dudley ME, Citrin DE, et al. Randomized, prospective evaluation comparing intensity of lymphodepletion before adoptive transfer of tumor-infiltrating lymphocytes for patients with metastatic melanoma. J Clin Oncol 2016;34:2389–97.
91. Rohaan MW, Borch TH, van den Berg JH, et al. Tumor-infiltrating lymphocyte therapy or ipilimumab in advanced melanoma. N Engl J Med 2022;387:2113–25.
92. Tumour-infiltrating lymphocyte cancer therapy nears FDA finish line. Available at: https://www.nature.com/articles/d41573-023-00206-6.
93. Chesney J, Lewis KD, Kluger H, et al. Efficacy and safety of lifileucel, a one-time autologous tumor-infiltrating lymphocyte (TIL) cell therapy, in patients with advanced melanoma after progression on immune checkpoint inhibitors and targeted therapies: pooled analysis of consecutive cohorts of the C-144-01 study. J Immunother Cancer 2022;10.
94. Lin MJ, Svensson-Arvelund J, Lubitz GS, et al. Cancer vaccines: the next immunotherapy frontier. Nature Cancer 2022;3:911–26.
95. Ott PA, Hu Z, Keskin DB, et al. An immunogenic personal neoantigen vaccine for patients with melanoma. Nature 2017;547:217–21.
96. Sahin U, Derhovanessian E, Miller M, et al. Personalized RNA mutanome vaccines mobilize poly-specific therapeutic immunity against cancer. Nature 2017;547:222–6.
97. Ott PA, Hu-Lieskovan S, Chmielowski B, et al. A Phase Ib trial of personalized neoantigen therapy plus anti-PD-1 in patients with advanced melanoma, non-small cell lung cancer, or bladder cancer. Cell 2020;183:347–62.e24.
98. Sahin U, Oehm P, Derhovanessian E, et al. An RNA vaccine drives immunity in checkpoint-inhibitor-treated melanoma. Nature 2020;585:107–12.
99. Moderna and Merck Announce mRNA-4157/V940, an Investigational Personalized mRNA Cancer Vaccine, in Combination with KEYTRUDA® (Pembrolizumab), Met Primary Efficacy Endpoint in Phase 2b KEYNOTE-942 Trial. https://www.merck.com/news/moderna-and-merck-announce-mrna-4157-v940-an-investigational-personalized-mrna-cancer-vaccine-in-combination-with-keytruda-pembrolizumab-met-primary-efficacy-endpoint-in-phase-2b-keynote-94/.
100. Personalized anti-cancer vaccine combining mRNA and immunotherapy tested in melanoma trial. Available at: https://www.nature.com/articles/d41591-023-00072-0.
101. Lorentzen CL, Haanen JB, Met Ö, et al. Clinical advances and ongoing trials of mRNA vaccines for cancer treatment. Lancet Oncol 2022;23:e450–8.

Targeted Therapy Innovations for Melanoma

Dahiana Amarillo, MD[a], Keith T. Flaherty, MD[b,*],
Ryan J. Sullivan, MD[c]

KEYWORDS

- Melanoma • Genetics • Oncogenes • Immune checkpoint inhibitors • Resistance

KEY POINTS

- Recent whole-genome analyses have provided deeper insight into the genetic heterogeneity of melanoma, revealing mutations in pathways such as mitogen-activated protein kinase (MAPK), phosphoinositide-3-kinase (PI3K), and cyclin D-cyclin-dependent kinase 4/6 (CDK4/6) that offer new therapeutic targets.
- Innovations in targeting NRAS-mutant melanoma, which lacks direct inhibitors, include using MAPK kinase (MEK) inhibitors and strategies targeting downstream effectors such as extracellular signal-regulated protein kinase. Moreover, identifying new targets, such as the SHP2 phosphatase, CDK4/6, and components of the PI3K pathway, has broadened the therapeutic horizon. CDK4/6 and MEK inhibitors have shown promise in preclinical studies and early phase clinical trials.
- Agents targeting the immune-suppressive microenvironment, such as LAG-3 or PD-1/PD-L1 inhibitors, have been proposed to synergize with targeted therapies, potentially reversing resistance and improving patient outcomes.
- Importantly, novel biomarker-driven clinical trials aim to personalize therapy and improve the selection of patients likely to benefit from specific treatment combinations.

INTRODUCTION

Melanoma is a tumor originating from melanocytes, cells responsible for producing the pigment melanin which leads to skin, hair, and eye coloration. While predominantly located in the skin, melanocytes exist in other body parts, including the eyes, gastrointestinal system, leptomeninges, and mucous membranes (genital region, sinonasal passages, and mouth).[1] Incidence rates of melanoma are increasing, especially in Western countries, and in 2023, over 97,000 new cases of cutaneous melanomas in

[a] Oncóloga Médica, Departamento Básico de Medicina, Universidad de la República, Montevideo, Uruguay; [b] Mass General Cancer Center, Massachusetts General Hospital, Harvard Medical School, Boston, MA, USA; [c] Mass General Cancer Center, Harvard Medical School, 55 Fruit Street, Boston, MA 02114, USA
* Corresponding author.
E-mail address: kflaherty@mgh.harvard.edu

Hematol Oncol Clin N Am 38 (2024) 973–995
https://doi.org/10.1016/j.hoc.2024.05.006
0889-8588/24/© 2024 Elsevier Inc. All rights reserved.

the United States were expected.[2] While a significant portion of cutaneous melanomas results from ultraviolet radiation (UVR) exposure, the less common acral cutaneous subtype, as well as mucosal and uveal melanoma is not associated with UVR exposure.[3] Among Caucasian populations, non-acral cutaneous melanoma is the most common, accounting for over 90% of cases, while mucosal and uveal melanomas represent only 1% to 5% of diagnoses. On the other hand, in non-Caucasian populations, the acral type of melanoma is most prevalent.[4]

Melanoma is diverse in its driving and common contributing genetic alterations and underlying activated pathways. Additionally, different subtypes of melanomas, such as non-acral cutaneous, acral, uveal, and mucosal arise from different anatomic sites and typically have different driving genetic alterations.[5] The most commonly altered oncogenic pathways in melanoma are the mitogen-activated protein kinase (MAPK) and the phosphoinositide-3-kinase (PI3K) pathways, while alterations in genetic regulators of the telomerase (telomerase reverse transcriptase [TERT]), and cell cycle and survival, including p53, CDKN2A, CCND1, and cyclin D-cyclin-dependent kinase 4 (CDK4), are also common. The MAPK pathway, which plays a pivotal role in melanoma development, is activated in most melanomas. Specifically, NRAS or BRAF mutations trigger this activation, with NRAS mutations found in approximately 15% to 20% of skin melanomas and BRAF mutations in around 40% to 50%. These genetic alterations are present in invasive and metastatic melanoma stages, as well as in benign melanocytic nevi.[6] Other mutations result in the loss of phosphatase and tensin homolog (PTEN), a key regulator of the PI3K pathway, which often co-occur with BRAF-V600E mutations. However, both BRAFV600 and/or PTEN mutations rarely coincide with NRAS mutations, as typically they are mutually exclusive events. Additionally, mutations in the receptor tyrosine kinase (RTK) c-KIT are frequently observed in mucosal and acral melanomas, with a prevalence of around 20%.[7]

The clinical relevance of these genetic alterations is clear in the BRAFV600-mutant population, since there are Food and Drug Administration (FDA) approved MAPK pathway inhibitors including combinations of BRAF and MEK inhibitors, which lead to responses in most patients with metastatic melanoma and improve relapse-free survival (RFS) in patients with resected stage III melanoma when given as adjuvant therapy. General MAPK inhibition in NRAS-mutant populations as well as in uveal melanoma patients has led to less profound clinical benefit, as has the use of cKIT (tyrosine-protein kinase KIT, CD117) inhibitors in c-KIT-mutant melanoma. Finally, in the limited number of patients with neurotrophic tyrosine receptor kinase (NTRK) mutations in melanoma may also benefit from FDA-approved NTRK inhibitors.

This review provides an overview of melanoma gene alteration, explicitly focusing on the melanoma pathways that can be effectively targeted. Additionally, it highlights the emerging combination therapies that show the most potential for achieving successful outcomes in harder to treat populations.

MITOGEN-ACTIVATED PROTEIN KINASE PATHWAY

The mitogen-activated protein kinase pathway (MAPK) signaling pathway plays a critical role in the development of various types of cancer, especially non-small cell lung cancer (NSCLC), colorectal cancer (CRC), thyroid cancer, and melanoma. This pathway is activated when growth factors attach to specific cell surface receptors, known as RTKs. RTKs that associate with RAS and other entities within the RAS superfamily encompass a broad and varied spectrum (eg, cKIT epidermal growth factor receptor [EGFR], platelet-derived growth factor receptor [PDGFR], vascular endothelial growth factor receptors [VEGFRs], and fibroblast growth factor receptor).[8] RAS proteins, classified as small GTPases, are inherent within cellular structures, transitioning between an active guanosine triphosphate (GTP)-bound configuration and its passive guanosine diphosphate (GDP)-bound counterpart. Activating RTK signaling promotes a transition to the activated RAS configuration. This transitory phase is mediated by guanine nucleotide exchange factors such as SOS1, SOS2, and RASGRF10, supplemented by adaptor molecules such as GRB2. The reversion to the inactive RAS configuration is facilitated by the enzymatic action of GTPase-activating proteins. RAS GTPases regulate various cellular functions in their operative state, encompassing cell proliferation, viability, differentiation, apoptosis, and cellular interaction dynamics.[8–10]

MAPK and PI3K cascades are central to the downstream effects governed by RAS.[8] In physiologically normal melanocytes, a pronounced affinity between NRAS and its effector molecule, BRAF, steers the signaling predominantly through BRAF activation instead of alternative RAF isoforms such as CRAF.[7] The activation of RAF instigates a signaling cascade culminating in the phosphorylation of MAPK kinase (MEK) which phosphorylates and activated the extracellular signal-regulated protein kinase (ERK) 1/2, a kinase responsible for regulating many substrates. One of the functions of ERK is to augment cell proliferation via the stabilization of FOS, thereby fostering the genesis of AP-1 complexes.[11] The transcriptional prowess of AP-1 enhances D-type cyclin expression, streamlining the transition of the cell cycle from the G1 to the S phase. The resultant complex of CDK4 instigates hyperphosphorylation, subsequently inactivating the retinoblastoma protein and liberating E2F-mediated transcription. This cascade results in upregulating E-type cyclins (comprising cyclin E1 and E2), which synergistically operate with CDKs (CDK1, 2, 3).[8–10,12]

Concurrently, RAS activation is also integral to the PI3K pathway, a crucial component for cell cycle progression and metabolic synchronization during the cell's S phase. Its major regulator PTEN acts in opposition to PI3K. Subsequently, the signal is transmitted to AKT3 (RAC-gamma serine/threonine-protein kinase) and culminates in activating the mitochondrial antiapoptotic protein, BCL2, and the cellular growth regulator, mammalian target of rapamycin (mTOR). Notably, the suppression of PI3K signaling is associated with an extended S phase.[13,14]

Melanoma and Mitogen-activated Protein Kinase Pathway Mutation

In melanoma, mutations in RAS are detected in approximately 15% to 30%, the great majority are NRAS mutations, although a minority of these are KRAS mutations. These are present in approximately 30% of cutaneous melanoma, less than 20% in mucosal and acral melanomas, and essentially nonexistent in uveal melanoma.[5] The predominant NRAS mutations in melanoma hinder the enzyme's capacity to convert GTP to GDP. Consequently, the mutated NRAS remains primarily in its GTP-bound state. These cause constitutive activation of the MAPK and PI3K pathways.[9]

The most common alteration in the MAPK pathway in melanoma arises in the BRAF oncogene, encoding the BRAF protein. Such mutations are observed in approximately 50% of all melanomas.[15] They are more prevalent in cutaneous melanoma (almost 45%), less so in acral and mucosal melanoma (<20% and 10% respectability), and like NRAS, essentially nonexistent in uveal melanoma.[16,17] These mutations result in constitutive BRAF activation independent of RTK binding, leading to perpetual activation of MEK and ERK, thereby promoting uncontrolled cell proliferation.[11,18] The predominant mutation is the BRAFV600E, a valine to glutamic acid single-nucleotide substitution, which is present in around 90% of BRAF-mutated melanomas. The BRAF V600K mutation, where lysine replaces valine, is the next most frequent, accounting for an additional 5% to 6% of BRAF-mutated melanoma. Other rarer mutations include BRAF V600D and BRAF V600R. Intriguingly, around 80% of melanocytic nevi have BRAF mutations, indicating its potential early role in tumor development. Nonetheless, only a fraction of these nevi eventually evolve into melanoma.[11,19] BRAF non-V600 mutations are less frequent, and their prognostic and predictive role is, to date, still challenging to elucidate. The so-called class II BRAF mutations, including L597, K601, and G469 mutations, are associated with an increased kinase catalytic activity through constitutive dimerization of RAF, as opposed to the monomeric signaling that occurs with BRAFV600, or class 1 BRAF mutations. While these class 2 mutations do not confer the same sensitivity to BRAF inhibitors as class 1 mutations, they activate downstream target proteins and have reported sensitivity to MEK inhibitors. [20]

The PI3K pathway is mutated in 30% to 60% of melanomas, mainly due to the loss of the tumor suppressor protein PTEN (10%–7% in cutaneous and acral melanoma), which is often accompanied by BRAF mutations.[5,21] In addition, 40% to 60% of melanomas have activated or amplified the serine/threonine protein kinase AKT3. The signaling pathway of this pathway can be described as RTK-RAS-PI3K-(PTEN)-AKT3, leading to the activation of the mitochondrial antiapoptotic protein BCL2 and the cellular growth regulator, mTOR.[21] Additionally, these alterations may serve as a potential mechanism of resistance to BRAFV600 inhibition.[22,23]

Mutations in the TERT promoter are commonly observed in melanoma. These mutations predominantly occur in mutated subtypes such as BRAF, NRAS, and NF1. This suggests a potential association between MAPK pathway activation and TERT expression. Activation of the MAPK pathway facilitates the phosphorylation and subsequent activation of the ETS1 transcription factor via ERK, given that the mutated TERT promoter possesses ETS-binding domains.[24]

OTHER GENETIC ALTERATIONS
KIT

c-KIT, also known as CD117, it is a transmembrane RTK. Its ligands include the cellular receptor for stem cell factor, also named c-kit ligand, mast cell growth factor, and steel factor.[25] Mutations in the KIT gene are found in approximately 3% of all melanomas. When categorized by subtype, these mutations are present in 10% to 20% of acral melanomas and 20% to 40% of mucosal melanomas and occur with low frequency in melanomas that develop on chronically sun-damaged skin. However, KIT mutations typically are not observed in cutaneous melanomas arising in skin without chronic sun damage.[5,26]

Neurotrophic Tyrosine Receptor Kinase Fusions

Fusions involving the NTRK are recognized as crucial drivers of oncogenesis. These fusion events, although rare, have been observed in cases of melanoma. Three distinct NTRK genes, each situated on a separate chromosome, are responsible for encoding the respective tropomyosin receptor kinases (TRKs): TRKA, TRKB, and TRKC. The encoding of these proteins is facilitated by the corresponding NTRK1, 2, and 3 genes. The engagement of a specific neurotrophin with the extracellular domain triggers downstream pathways, notably phospholipase C-γ, MAPK, and PI3K. TRKA, B, and C play a pivotal role in the maturation of the central and peripheral nervous systems and significantly influence cellular viability regulation.[27] TRK fusion proteins form from merging an NTRK gene with a distinct gene during DNA repair via a nonhomologous end connection. Such a fusion perpetuates a consistently activated TRK, leading to an unchecked synthesis of TRK fusion proteins, which promotes enhanced proliferation and migration capabilities in melanoma cells, resulting in unrestrained cellular growth.[28] The prevalence of NTRK fusions is less than 1% in both cutaneous and mucosal melanoma. However, acral melanoma exhibits a higher frequency of NTRK fusions, with a rate of 2.5%. It is observed that these fusion proteins and prevalent oncogenic drivers such as BRAF, NRAS, HRAS, GNAQ, and GNA11 are mutually exclusive.[29]

GNAQ and GNA11

G-protein-coupled receptors (GPCRs) are a diverse group of transmembrane receptors that play a vital role in transmitting signals. They have various functions, including sensory perception, neurologic and endocrine signaling, and organ development. Because of their importance in maintaining homeostasis, any changes, or alterations in GPCR activity can lead to cancer development.[30] Mutations in GPCRs have been found in approximately 20% of human cancers. Certain tumors have mutations that increase the activity of G-alpha (Gα) subunits, stimulating downstream signals that promote cell growth.[31] Gα proteins have 2 domains: a RAS-like GTPase domain and an α-helical bundle relevant to their function. Mutations in critical residues within these switch regions are responsible for much of the aberrant signaling. Within this general structure, there are at least 17 distinct types of Gα proteins that are classified into 4 mammalian families: Gαs, Gαi/o, Gαq/11, and Gα11/12. These families are grouped based on the degree of shared amino acid sequence homology and have distinct tissue distribution and signaling roles. For example, GNAQ and GNA11, the genes that encode Gαq and Gα11, are 90% homologous at the amino acid level. The highest prevalence of GNAQ mutations is found in uveal melanomas (33%), blue nevi (32%), and cutaneous melanomas (1.4%). GNA11 mutations are found in 39% of uveal melanomas, 3% to 5% of blue nevi, and 1.3% of cutaneous melanomas.[32]

TARGET THERAPIES IN MELANOMA
BRAF–MEK Inhibitors in Cutaneous Melanoma

Advances in the understanding of the MAPK pathway and the mutations that activate it led to the recognition of the potential for therapeutic targeting in cancer. In melanoma, this has resulted in the formulation of highly specific BRAF and MEK inhibitors. The initial development of BRAF-specific inhibitors selectively targeted the mutated BRAF kinase, through favored inhibition of monomeric signally, and subsequent attenuation of signal propagation through the MAPK pathway. The approved use of these inhibitors as single-agent therapy is limited to cutaneous melanoma. In 2011, vemurafenib was the first BRAF inhibitor approved based on data from the BRIM-3 trial.[33] This study included 675 patients with advanced or nonresectable BRAF V600-mutant melanoma who had not been previously treated. The overall response rate (ORR) was 48% with vemurafenib, compared to 5% with dacarbazine. The median overall survival (OS) was 13.6 months for those randomized to vemurafenib versus 9.7 months for those in the dacarbazine group. Further analysis showed that vemurafenib OS rates at 3 and 4 years were 21% and 17%, respectively. It is worth noting that 84 out of the 338 patients on dacarbazine were switched to vemurafenib during the study.[34] Analogous efficacy outcomes have been observed with other approved BRAF inhibitors, dabrafenib[35] and encorafenib.[36]

Although BRAF inhibitors can lead to significant tumor regression in patients with advanced melanoma, treatment resistance often develops within 5 to 7 months.[34–36] Combining a MEK inhibitor (trametinib, cobimetinib, binimetinib), a downstream component of the MAPK pathway, with BRAF inhibition, delays the onset of this resistance. Clinical trials have shown that combination therapy with dabrafenib/trametinib, vemurafenib/

cobimetinib, or encorafenib/binimetinib leads to better ORR, progression-free survival (PFS), and OS as compared to using single-agent treatment with BRAF or MEK inhibitors.[36–40] Therefore, the current standard of care recommends using combination-targeted therapy for eligible patients whose tumors harbor a mutation in BRAF. To date, there has not been any direct comparison among these combination regimens, and thus, treatment choices are typically based on toxicity predictions, treatment availability, and individual preferences.

In the COMBI-d study,[37,38] 423 untreated patients with unresectable stage IIIC or metastatic (advanced) melanoma harboring a mutation in BRAFV600E/K were randomized to receive combination dabrafenib plus trametinib versus dabrafenib alone. The results of this trial have been updated multiple times with mature follow-ups since the original report in 2014, maintaining the benefits of combination therapy. The reported ORR is 68% for the combination versus 55% for monotherapy. Median PFS was 11.0 months for the combination and 8.8 months for monotherapy. In another phase 3 trial called COMBI-v, dabrafenib and trametinib were compared with vemurafenib alone, and similar efficacy results were seen. Given the constrained duration of progression typically seen with targeted treatments, a pooled analysis from both COMBI-d and COMBI-v trials revealed that the median PFS and OS were 11.1 and 25.9 months, respectively. Several factors contributed to improved prognosis, including age, gender, BRAF status, normal lactate dehydrogenase (LDH) levels, and fewer metastatic sites.[41]

The coBRIM phase 3 trial juxtaposed a combined regimen of vemurafenib and cobimetinib against vemurafenib with a placebo.[39] According to the latest follow-up, the combination targeted therapy resulted in a PFS of 12.3 months and a median OS of 22.3 months. The OS rate after 2 years was 48.3%. Patients with normal baseline LDH levels had a longer median PFS. The OS benefits were predicted by their baseline LDH levels and the longest diameters of target lesions.[40]

Finally, the COLUMBUS trial, an open-label phase 3 study, compared the combination targeted therapy using BRAF inhibitor, encorafenib, and MEK inhibitor, binimetinib, with BRAF inhibitors alone. Encorafenib showcases a distinctive pharmacokinetic profile, marked by a dissociation half-life surpassing 30 hours, which markedly exceeds either dabrafenib or vemurafenib, facilitating sustained target modulation. The combined approach exhibited a median OS of 33.6 months, in contrast to vemurafenib, 16.9 months. The combination treatment also demonstrated superior PFS results, with a median value of 14.9 against 7.3 months. A confirmed ORR was discerned in 64% of individuals subjected to the combination protocol.[36]

The combination of anti-BRAF and anti-MEK also has been evaluated as adjuvant therapy in patients with resected stage III melanoma. The COMBI-AD study was a double-blind, placebo-controlled, phase 3 trial that assessed the RFS through the combination of dabrafenib and trametinib versus placebo, administered over 12 months, for patients with resected stage III cutaneous melanoma, as classified by the American Joint Committee on Cancer (7th edition) and manifesting BRAF V600E/K mutations [42] For inclusion, stage IIIA patients were mandated to present with lymph node metastases exceeding 1 mm. Of the 870 randomized participants, a substantial majority (81%) were categorized under stage IIIB or IIIC. At 5 years, the percentage of patients alive without relapse was 52% with dabrafenib plus trametinib and 36% with placebo. The percentage of patients alive without distant metastasis was 65% with dabrafenib plus trametinib and 54% with placebo. During the preliminary assessment of the initial interim analysis of OS, the 3 year OS projection was 83% for the combination regimen and 77% for the placebo. Still, this variance did not meet the stipulated conservative interim threshold for statistical significance.

In subsequent evaluations, the event count necessary for the ensuing preordained OS interim analysis was yet to be achieved.[43]

BRAF–MEK inhibitors with immunotherapy

Immune checkpoint inhibitors (ICIs), such as ipilimumab (anti-CTLA-4 antibody), nivolumab, and pembrolizumab (anti-PD-1 antibodies), are the new standard of care in metastatic melanoma. Nivolumab and ipilimumab showed in clinical trials an OS rate of 5 years superior to 50%.[44] A combination of nivolumab with a LAG-3 inhibitor relatlimab recently become a new combination strategy.[45] These combinations are effective regardless of BRAF mutational status.

Previous studies have reported that BRAF mutations can lead to immune evasion. Targeted BRAF and MEK inhibitors have shown potential in promoting antigen processing and presentation, T cell priming and infiltration, and immune microenvironment regulation.[46] Therefore, combining targeted therapy with immunotherapy, and more specifically ICI, is a promising strategy to maximize therapeutic benefits while minimizing toxicity. Despite ongoing explorations, there is currently no evidence to support OS benefits in clinical trials.

In the IMspire150 phase III trial, a randomized, placebo-controlled study, 514 patients with advanced BRAF V600-mutant melanoma without prior treatment were randomized to receive vemurafenib and cobimetinib with either atezolizumab or placebo. The median PFS was 15 months in the triplet arm compared to 11 months in the placebo group. The initial reports did not validate the statistical significance of these findings through an independent review.[47] The OS displayed statistically comparable outcomes between both groups (eg, differences were not statistically significant), with median OS values of 39 months for the combination treatment and 26 months for the targeted therapy alone.[48] The 2 year OS rates were 62% for the combined approach and 53% for the targeted therapy. The ORR was 67% for the combination therapy and 65% for targeted therapy.

A second randomized phase III trial, COMBI-i, evaluated the efficacy of combining the PD-1 inhibitor spartalizumab with dabrafenib and trametinib. This study involved 532 patients diagnosed with advanced, unresectable BRAF V600-mutant melanoma. It revealed that adding spartalizumab to the targeted treatment improved PFS (16 compared to 12 months), but this difference did not meet the prespecified level of statistical significance. The ORR was recorded at 69% for the triplet therapy and 64% for BRAF/MEK inhibitor doublet. Moreover, while the median duration of response was not reached for the combination group, it was 21 months for the targeted therapy group. Importantly, incorporating spartalizumab increased grade ≥3 toxicities (55% vs 33%).

Sequencing of BRAF–MEK inhibitors and immunotherapy

Trials about the efficacy of immunotherapy as an initial treatment show durable responses, substantiate long-term OS benefits, and are associated with extended treatment-free survival intervals for patients.[44,45,49] Targeted therapy can quickly offer an initial treatment response but often with a limited duration. Further, there is retrospective evidence that immunotherapy tends to be less effective when given after targeted therapy.[50] However, until recent data became available, there remained an unanswered question about whether frontline BRAF-targeted therapy or ICI was more effective.

A recently reported randomized phase III trial has provided the first data about the optimal sequencing of ICI and BRAF-targeted therapy. The DREAMseq (ECOG-ACRIN EA6134) was an open-label phase III trial that randomized 265 patients, all treatment-naive and with advanced BRAFV600-mutant melanoma, to receive either immunotherapy—comprising an initial regimen of nivolumab plus ipilimumab, succeeded by maintenance nivolumab—or BRAF-targeted therapy with dabrafenib plus trametinib. By treatment design, at disease progression, patients were offered to receive the alternative regimen. The strategy of initiating treatment with immunotherapy followed by targeted therapy was superior, evidenced by improved 2 year OS rate, the primary endpoint of the trial, of 72% for patients randomized immunotherapy versus 52% for those randomized to BRAF-targeted therapy. Further, the sequence also tended to augment PFS with a median of 11.8 versus 8.5 months, a 2 year PFS of 42 versus 19%, and an extended median duration of response (not reached, as opposed to 13 months). Among initial immunotherapy responders, 88% retained remission status at a median follow-up of 28 months versus 48% of patients with a response to BRAF-targeted therapy. The ORR was lower for patients who received immunotherapy following targeted therapy (30%) than those who received initial immunotherapy (46%). In contrast, ORR was similar for targeted therapy whether given as initial therapy (43%) or following disease progression on immunotherapy (48%)[51]

Thus, the implication of these data is that the frontline standard of care therapy for patients with advanced, BRAFV600 melanoma should be combination immunotherapy. That said, a subset of patients with clinically aggressive disease had improved outcomes with frontline BRAF-targeted therapy in the DREAMseq study, and thus, this remains an option for this patient population as well as those patients in whom combined ICI is contraindicated.

Resistance to BRAF–MEK Inhibitors

Many patients who show either partial or complete response to immunotherapy can survive long term. However, this is not typically the case with patients who start with targeted therapies. To improve outcomes in patients with BRAF mutations, it is essential to investigate the resistance mechanisms to current therapies and explore molecular pathways currently being studied in preclinical and clinical trials.

Multiple mechanisms have been identified to resist BRAF–MEK inhibitors, including genetics and epigenetic abnormalities, including alterations in tumor microenvironment.

Reactivation of the mitogen-activated protein kinase pathway

It has been shown that the MAPK pathway reactivates in many BRAF-mutant melanomas resistant to BRAF and MEK inhibitors. BRAF amplification and activating mutations in NRAS and MEK2 are the most observed acquired mutations that lead to this resistance. These mutations are frequently seen in preclinical and clinical scenarios.[52,53] Constitutive activation of mutated RAS increased BRAF dimerization and subsequent reactivation of MAPK (including dimerization of BRAF and CRAF).[54]

BRAF alterations have been described, too, including overexpression of mutated BRAF gene or splicing alterations that favor dimerization.[55] The activation of ARAF and CRAF also can lead to resistance to BRAF inhibitors because all RAF isoforms have the same capability of regulating the stability of RAF and forming a complex to target BRAF degradation.[56] Additionally, hyperactivation of RTKs promotes resistance by activating parallel pathways or directly activating RAS, involving receptors such as PDGFRb, EGFR, KIT, and IGF-1R.[57] Further, it has been described that BRAF inhibition triggers a resetting event in the ERK1/2 pathway and reduces SPRY2, DUSP, and SPRY expression, resulting in RAS reactivation. Thus, BRAF inhibition leads to downstream ERK activity, partially restoring RAS activity and inducing the formation of BRAF dimers by RAS which then reactivate ERK. Similar to upstream

RAS-activating mutations, NF1 loss can result in unopposed RAS activation.[54] As described earlier, mutations in MEK1/MEK2 activate downstream of BRAF inhibition and reactivate ERK, leading to resistance.[58] Finally, activation of an alternative MAPK, COT, can also reactivate MEK downstream of BRAF inhibition and reactivate downstream ERK expression.[59]

Other mechanisms

Continuous targeted inhibition may lead to abnormal activation of downstream pathways via bypass tracks. The PI3K/AKT/mTOR pathway interacts with MAPK pathways at multiple points. Adaptive PI3K/AKT activity can occur when ERK signaling is blocked, leading to permanent PI3K/AKT signaling. Overexpression of PDGFRβ, IGFR1, and EGFR also can reactivate this pathway leading to BRAFi resistance. Mutations in the PI3K/AKT genes induce AKT phosphorylation, increasing antiapoptotic signaling and expression of crucial proliferation genes independent of BRAF. These changes enable melanoma cells to proliferate independently of BRAF and are involved in adaptive resistance to BRAFi.[60]

The Hippo pathway is essential for the growth and spread of cancer stem cells. YAP and TAZ proteins regulate this pathway. When melanoma cells are resistant to BRAFi, YAP and TAZ increase, promoting cell cycle expression. Lowering YAP or TAZ levels can decrease melanoma cell viability. The activation of the YAP/TAZ pathway leads to BRAFi resistance, linked with continuous ERK1/2 activity.[61]

JNK/c-Jun pathway regulates cell proliferation, metabolism, and death. JNKs increase the transcription of cyclin D1, promoting the G1-S cell cycle transition in melanoma. Upregulation of p-c-Jun leads to vemurafenib resistance. Combining vemurafenib with JNK inhibitors such as JNK-IN-8 preclinically results in synergistic cell killing.[54]

Aberrant WNT pathways, activated by WNT5A, are identified in melanoma. Increased WNT5A levels are seen in BRAFi-resistant cells and its loss reduces cell viability. WNT5A signaling promotes melanoma cell resistance to BRAFi via RYK and FZD7 receptors and PI3K/AKT activation.[62]

Epigenetic alterations are changes that can modify gene transcription without altering the DNA sequence. Several epigenetic mechanisms such as DNA methylation, noncoding RNAs, histone modifications, and histone-modifying enzymes play a vital role in BRAFi resistance.[63] DNA methylation can lead to genomic instability and transcriptional repression. Transcriptomic analysis revealed that drug resistance is related to transcriptomic and methylomic alterations. Differences in mRNA expression in genes connected with differential methylation at CpG clusters and short CG-rich DNA sequences that remain unmethylated suggest a connection between drug resistance and epigenetic regulation of DNA methylation. Mutations in DNMTs such as DNMT3B have a role in tumor progression, and low global DNA methylation levels appeared in drug-tolerant melanoma cells following targeted treatment.[64]

Histone-modifying enzymes and post-translational modifications can promote either transcriptional activation or repression of targeted genes by remodeling their chromatin structures.[64] The expression of histone demethylases such as KDM6A and KDM6B is elevated in melanoma with a drug-tolerant state, which is accompanied by increased levels of H3K9me3 and lower levels of H3K4me3 and H3K27me3, indicating selected gene silencing and epigenetic activation. Histone methyltransferases, SETDB1 and SETDB2, are also upregulated after treatment with BRAFi and MEKi, and their knockdown restored drug sensitivity. Additionally, the histone deacetylase SIRT6 was downregulated in BRAFi-resistant melanoma cells, leading to upregulation of the IGF-1R and subsequent AKT pathway activation.[65]

KIT ALTERATION

KIT mutations are the driving oncogene in melanomas in a subset of patients, most prominent in those with melanoma arising from mucosal regions, acral skin, and skin with sun damage.[26] After discovering KIT mutations in melanoma, multiple studies have been initiated to identify patients who would benefit most from KIT inhibition. Imatinib emerged as the inaugural targeted therapy for KIT-mutated melanoma, given its successful application in other malignancies possessing KIT mutations. Although initial case reports showcased the clinical potency of KIT inhibitors, such as imatinib and dasatinib, early investigations involving imatinib did not yield substantial efficacy. This may be due to the lack of selection for specific molecular subtypes of melanoma that is more likely to have the relevant target.[66]

A clinical study was conducted on 25 patients with c-KIT mutations and/or amplification, which resulted in an ORR of 16%. The PFS was 12 weeks, with the median OS of 46.3 weeks. Remarkably, the 4 patients with durable responses retained disease control for a year.[67] A phase 2 imatinib trial was conducted in China, assessing 43 patients. They recorded an ORR of 23.3%, with a median PFS of 3.5 months. The comprehensive 1 year OS rate was 51%, with the disease control rate at 53.5%. Though dose escalation was allowed for patients who exhibited progression, it showed limited success.[68] Other phase II trial shows similar results. A systematic review included 19 single-arm studies with an overall sample size of 601 patients. The studies investigated imatinib ($n = 8$), nilotinib ($n = 7$), dasatinib ($n = 3$), and sunitinib ($n = 1$). The pooled ORR for all inhibitors was 15%. Subgroup analysis revealed the highest ORR (20%) for nilotinib. The ORR for mucosal melanoma was 14% and 22% for acral lentiginous melanoma. Cumulatively, these studies hint at the potential of achieving durable responses in a subset of patients with KIT-mutant melanoma via imatinib treatment. However, nearly all patients inevitably develop resistance to therapy and have disease progression. The underlying reasons for this disparate response between KIT-mutant melanoma and GIST, which commonly has KIT mutations, remain elusive even when harboring identical mutations. This discrepancy suggests the presence of alternative pathways in treatment resistance that warrants further investigation. High-quality trials are urgently needed to investigate putative combinations of these specific targeted therapies, including combinations with immunotherapy.[66]

NRAS MUTATION

MEK suppression has been considered for treating NRAS-mutant melanoma due to challenges in directly targeting NRAS and understanding RAS activation's downstream effects. Binimetinib, a MEK 1/2 inhibitor, yielded a relatively modest 20% response rate, exclusively partial responses, in NRAS-mutant melanoma.[9] The NEMO trial was a phase 3 clinical trial of 402 with NRAS-mutant stage IIIC or IV melanoma, including previously untreated patients and those exhibiting progression post-immunotherapy patients. Patients were randomized in a 2:1 ratio to receive either an oral dose of binimetinib 45 mg twice daily or dacarbazine. The ORR for binimetinib was 15%. The median PFS was 2.8 months for binimetinib, in contrast to 1.5 months for dacarbazine. However, the median OS was comparable across both treatment modalities.[69]

Considering these outcomes, binimetinib might offer a therapeutic alternative for some patients with NRAS-mutant melanoma who experience disease progression following primary immunotherapy, especially when other actionable mutations are absent or specific clinical trials are inaccessible.

TARGETED THERAPY INNOVATIONS FOR MELANOMA
Atypical BRAF Mutation

Melanomas with atypical BRAF mutations have diverse genetic alterations and are divided into 2 categories: BRAF V600 and non-V600 mutants. Rare BRAF V600 mutations include V600R/D/M/L, which are kinase-activating monomers typically found in older male patients with a history of chronic sun damage. Non-V600 mutants can be categorized as class II (L597P/Q/R/S, K601E, G469R/S/A) or III (G596R, D594Y/N/G/E, D287Y) depending on the formation of dimers to activate RAF kinases or heterodimers that impair kinase activity entirely, resulting in paradoxic activation of ERK signaling, respectively. Typically, class II and III tumors exhibit a more aggressive clinical course and are associated with a poorer prognosis.[70]

While BRAF/MEK inhibitor combination therapy is well established in patients with BRAFV600 E/K mutations, the clinical data for the approximately 5% of melanomas with non-V600 BRAF mutations mainly consists of case reports due to their rarity and genetic heterogeneity. Based on preclinical evidence indicating a reduction in phospho-ERK signaling after MEK inhibition, a phase I trial was conducted, which resulted in a partial radiographic response. The treatment was given to a patient with a BRAF mutation and lasted for 24 weeks using a MEK inhibitor (TAK 773).[20] Patients with atypical BRAF mutations or fusions treated with trametinib achieved an ORR of 33% (3 of 9 patients), with the best treatment response (87% reduction, PFS 19.2 months) occurring in a patient who harbored a class III non-V600 (BRAF T470R). During the phase I trial, 41 patients were evaluated for response. Of these patients, 2 (5%) with cutaneous melanoma showed partial responses, one of whom had BRAF L597R-mutant melanoma. The maximum tolerated dose of TAK-733 was generally well tolerated with a manageable toxicity profile. The pharmacodynamic effect of sustained inhibition of ERK phosphorylation was as expected. However, the antitumor activity was limited, and further investigation is not currently planned.[71] A more extensive retrospective cohort study assessed the clinical responses of patients with atypical BRAF mutations treated with a BRAF inhibitor, an MEK inhibitor, or a combination of BRAF and MEK inhibitors. Of the 103 patients, 58 (56%) had tumors with a rare V600 mutation, 38 (37%) had a non-V600 mutation, and 7 had both V600E and a rare BRAF mutation. Ninety-six patients in the study received BRAF inhibitor, MEK inhibitor, or combination treatment. The response rate depended on the BRAF genotype, with the best treatment response seen in non-V600/KE/K BRAF-mutated melanomas when given BRAF plus MEK inhibitors (ORR 56%, median PFS 8.0 months). Patients with non-V600 mutations achieved an ORR of 28% (5 of 18) when treated with BRAF and MEK inhibitors.[72]

BRAF kinase fusions, which typically function such as class 2 BRAF mutations (eg, activation of ERK), have been targeted using MEK inhibitors. These fusions are commonly found in younger patients and tumors with spitzoid histopathologic features.[73] In vitro data from 6 melanoma cell lines with representative fusion kinases demonstrated different responses to RAF/MEK inhibition based on the specific features of translocation. Translocations that yield a higher expression level are associated with more resistance. A combination of a third-generation (αC-IN/DFG-OUT) RAF and MEK inhibitors demonstrated preclinical therapeutic efficacy in the most resistant cell lines, both in vitro and in vivo.[74] A 2015 case series (with 2 patients) reported clinical activity of the MEK inhibitor trametinib in pretreated patients with BRAF fusion-positive metastatic melanoma. Both patients reported symptomatic improvement, and one patient demonstrated a 90% reduction in extracranial disease burden.[75] A patient with advanced melanoma and SKAP2-BRAF fusion had a partial response to MEK inhibitor monotherapy after failing immunotherapy and dacarbazine. However, the response was not durable, and the disease progressed.[76]

In an international, retrospective study, there was no antitumoral activity in patients harboring non-V600 mutations with BRAF inhibitors, whereas MEK inhibition with or without BRAF inhibitors demonstrated clinical activity with an ORR of 28% to 40%, suggesting that MEK inhibition may be the primary therapeutic agent.[77] In contrast, patients with atypical (non-E/K) V600 mutations demonstrated promising responses to BRAF inhibitor monotherapy or combined BRAF and MEK inhibitors in select phase II studies.[72]

Collectively, the findings suggest that there may be a potential use of BRAF and MEK inhibitors for patients who have an activating non-V600 mutation and who are either unsuitable or have failed immunotherapy. However, further research is required to better identify which patients with non-V600-mutated melanoma would benefit from MEK inhibitors with or without BRAF inhibition.

Next-Generation RAF Inhibitors

Next-generation RAF inhibitors are being developed as an alternative approach to prevent or overcome resistance and the paradoxic activation of BRAF-specific inhibitors. This approach may be especially useful in patients with BRAF-WT and NRAS mutations, as well as in patients with acquired resistance to BRAFV600E mutations. Although all RAF inhibitors are ATP-competitive kinase inhibitors, they differ in the conformation of the αC-helix and DFG motif they form. BRAF-selective inhibitors, such as dabrafenib and vemurafenib, bind in the DFG-in/αC-helix-out conformation, while "pan-RAF" inhibitors bind in a DFG-out conformation.[78] This achieves inhibition of BRAF and CRAF without paradoxic activation, through dimer inhibition (and thus these inhibitors will be denoted dBRAF dimer RAF inhibitors hereafter), thereby inhibiting the activity of both BRAFV600-mutant and NRAS-mutant disease in preclinical models. Further preclinical studies undertaken with LY3009120, a dRAF inhibitor, demonstrated inhibition of all 3 RAF isoforms with similar affinity for inhibition of RAF dimers.[79] In vivo studies using colorectal, lung, and melanoma (NRASQ61K SKMel-30) models showed dose-dependent tumor growth inhibition across KRAS- and NRAS-mutated tumors.[80]

Several phase I trials with different dRAF inhibitors have shown only modest to no activity despite strong preclinical evidence of their efficacy against melanoma.

To establish the maximum tolerated dose and antitumoral efficacy of pan-RAF inhibition as monotherapy, a first-in-human phase I multicenter trial of RAF265 (NCT00304525) was conducted. The trial found that tolerable doses of pan-RAF inhibitors resulted in an antitumor response of 12.1%, regardless of BRAF mutation status. A higher proportion of patients (20.7%) demonstrated a metabolic response and changes in angiogenesis modulators.[81] Lifirafenib (BGB-283), a dRAF and EGFR kinase inhibitor, was assessed in a phase I trial that included patients with various advanced solid tumors. Antitumoral activity was observed among patients with melanoma with BRAF mutations, with 8 of 53 (15.1%) achieving PR and 27 of 53 patients with stable disease.[82] In another study, LY3009120 was investigated in a phase I dose–escalation/confirmation study (NCT02014116) in patients with metastatic melanoma, CRC, and NSCLC. The patients were divided into 3 study cohorts, 2 included patients with melanoma (advanced melanoma with BRAFV600 mutations that had relapsed after treatment with BRAF, MEK, or BRAF/MEK combination therapy or advanced melanoma harboring an NRASQ61X mutation). Although adequate plasma concentrations associated with tumor regression in preclinical models were achieved, no partial or complete responders were seen in any group. Only 8 patients in the trial had stable disease, with 5 of the 8 in the non-melanoma cohort.[83]

There have been studies of combination therapy approaches with these dRAF inhibitors to overcome acquired resistance to MAPK inhibition in BRAF and NRAS-mutant melanoma. Preclinical data support the use of dRAF and MEK inhibitors in several models of MAPK inhibition resistance in NRAS-mutant, BRAFV6000E-mutant, and NF1-mutant cell lines. This approach has been shown to overcome resistance in vivo with dRAF/MEK inhibitors, partly due to CD8 + TIL-mediated tumor regression with concomitant expansion of central memory T cells and regression of T-reg compartments.[84] The addition of PD-L1 inhibition has extended the duration of the response. Moreover, pan-RAF inhibitor therapy has sensitized KRAS-, NRAS-, or BRAF-mutated tumors to CDK4/6 inhibitors both in vitro and in vivo.[85] Several early-stage trials are underway to investigate different pan-RAF inhibitors in combination with other agents. Two early phase studies are exploring the combination of a pan-RAF inhibitor with a MEK inhibitor.

During the 2023 AACR Annual Meeting, it was reported that a promising dRAF inhibitor, BGB-3245, showed early positive results for patients with advanced or refractory solid tumors that contain MAPK pathway mutations. These findings were documented in a phase 1a/1b trial (NCT04249843).[86] Patients must meet specific criteria having a confirmed advanced or metastatic solid tumor harboring a BRAF or KRAS mutation. At the time of the presentation, 42 patients had enrolled in the study, and 9 patients were still undergoing treatment. The confirmed ORR was 18%, while stable disease was observed in 61% of these patients. The most common treatment emergent adverse events were consistent with inhibitors of the MAP kinase pathway and included rash, fever, thrombocytopenia, and ALT elevation. Antitumor activity was observed across various disease types, mutations, and dose levels. Additionally, this agent is now being evaluated in combination with the MEK inhibitor mirdametinib (identified by PD-0325901) for patients with advanced solid tumors (NCT05580770).

Data with the combination of lifirafenib and mirdametinib (PD-0325901) (NCT03905148) were also presented in AACR 2023 and showed antitumor activity in patients with RAS and RAF mutations across several solid tumor types.[87] Tovorafenib is another dRAF inhibitor evaluated as a single agent and combined with the MEK inhibitor pimasertib. In the phase I trial, 68 patients were evaluated, and 10 (15%) of them showed positive responses to the treatment.[88] The largest study of dRAF inhibitor combination is a phase II, open-label study (NCT04417621) in patients with either BRAFV600 melanoma previously treated with BRAF-targeted therapy or NRAS-mutant melanoma who were randomized to receive the dRAF inhibitor naporafenib with either LTT462 (an oral ERK1/2 inhibitor), trametinib, or ribociclib. At ESMO 2022, preliminary data were presented. Grade 3/4 TRAEs occurred in 46% of patients; rash (7%) was most common. The best overall response was seen in patients receiving LXH254 + LTT462 (29 patients).[88] A phase 1b trial (NCT04835805) is underway to determine the effectiveness of combining belvarafenib and cobimetinib with or without nivolumab in patients with NRAS-mutated melanoma. However, the challenge with these and similar combinations has been a high rate of cutaneous toxicity, likely related to multilevel inhibition of MAPK in the skin, which may limit the use of these combinations.

Targeting NRAS

Despite being prevalent and important in melanoma, direct targeting of RAS has been historically difficult due to a lack of a readily targetable pocket. The high affinity of RAS for GTP and high intracellular concentrations of GTP limited the creation of GTP-competitive drugs. Stopping cell modifications after creating proteins using farnesyltransferase inhibitors has ineffective.[89] In laboratory experiments, RAS-targeting siRNA has been found to make melanoma cells more sensitive to BRAF inhibitors, but it has not been very successful in real-life applications. Recently, a new drug called sotorasib, which inhibits KRASG12C, was approved for treating NSCLC.[90] However, finding a good inhibitor for NRAS-mutant melanoma is still a challenge because there are many downstream effectors with varying levels of activation once the pathway is activated.[89]

Owing to the technical difficulties of targeting RAS, researchers have started focusing on targeting other downstream RAS pathways. MEK inhibitors have been used in RAS-mutated cancer with some success.[91,92] As described earlier, the NEMO study showed that MEK inhibition was associated with a statistically significant but not clinically significant improvement of PFS compared to patients treated with dacarbazine. However, other MEK and ERK inhibitors have been studied in this treatment population. Tunlametinib (also known as HL-085) is a novel, potent, selective, oral MEK1/2 inhibitor that exhibited higher inhibitory activity against MEK1/2 than selumetinib and binimetinib, both in vitro and in vivo.[91] In patients with NRAS-mutant melanoma, tunlametinib showed a favorable PK profile, acceptable tolerability, and encouraging antitumor activity at the recommended phase II dose level in a phase I study.[92] In the large phase II trial which enrolled 100 patients, tunlametinib (NCT05217303) was associated with a confirmed ORR of 34.7% and a median PFS of 4.2 months, and a 1 year survival rate was 57.2%.[93] Similarly, another first-in-human study evaluated FCN-159, a potent oral MEK1/2 inhibitor shown to be 10 times more selective than trametinib, which demonstrated improved tolerability when compared to historical rates of adverse events of binimetinib and pimasertib and had promising antitumoral activity. The objective response and clinical benefit rates were 19.0% (4 partial responses) and 52.4%, respectively. The median duration of response and PFS was 4.8 months (2.8 not reached) and 3.8 months (1.8–5.6), respectively.[94]

ERK Inhibition

Various examples of ERK inhibitors are currently undergoing clinical trials in multiple tumor types. Ulixertinib (BVD-523) demonstrated robust antitumor activity in the preclinical models of the BRAF-mutated tumor. A phase I dose-escalation and expansion study included 135 patients with advanced solid tumors. Among patients with melanoma who had previously been treated with and progressed on BRAF and/or MEK inhibitors, 3 of 19 patients (15%) achieved a PR (including a durable response in one patient that remained on study for over 38 months), 6 patients had stable disease, and 10 patients had progressive disease. Objective responses were also observed among patients with atypical BRAF non-V600E mutations.[95] Cutaneous toxicity was frequently observed in patients receiving ERK inhibitors, with incidences reported as high as 79% and 76% of patients treated with ulixertinib. The most reported dermatologic adverse events included acneiform and maculopapular rashes.[96] Interestingly, ERK inhibition with ulixertinib (BVD-523) did not demonstrate any clinical activity in patients with metastatic uveal melanoma (NCT03417739).[97]

It has been observed that resistance to ERK inhibition occurs in cell lines that have BRAF/RAS mutations. This resistance is caused by acquired mutations that inhibit binding to ERK and ERK2 amplification. One important mutation was identified in the DFG motif, which is highly conserved. It is worth noting that even though these mutated cells become resistant to ERK inhibition, they remain sensitive to MEK inhibition. Therefore, a combination therapy of ERK/MEK could be an effective treatment option. To test this hypothesis, MK-8353, a selective ERK1/2 inhibitor that had limited evidence for drug efficacy as a single agent, is currently being investigated in combination with selumetinib (MEK1/2 inhibitor) in 30 patients (NCT03745989) had acceptable safety and tolerability, and no responses were observed.[98]

CDK4/6 + MEK Inhibition

Fifty percent of melanomas with NRAS mutations exhibit genetic abnormalities in genes related to cell cycle, providing justification for the combination of MEK inhibitors with CDK4/6 inhibitors.[24,99] A preclinical study using NRAS-mutant human melanoma cell lines demonstrated that synergistic effects on apoptosis and cell cycle arrest led to corresponding tumor regression. Patients who had a co-mutation in the D-cyclin-CDK4/6-INK4a-Rb pathway exhibited improved outcomes with an ORR of 32.5% compared to 10% in patients who did not have such alterations, suggesting a synergistic antitumoral effect of the combined MEK and CKD4/6 inhibition in this genetically defined population. Recently, a phase II trial evaluating the efficacy of pan-RAF inhibitor naporafenib combined with ribociclib in patients with unresectable or metastatic NRAS-mutated melanoma (NCT04417621) showed in ESMO 2022.[88] Abemaciclib, a selective CDK4/6 inhibitor, was evaluated in patients with brain metastasis of melanoma and lung cancer and showed limited activity.[100]

Heat Shock Protein 90

Heat shock protein 90 (HSP90) chaperone complex has been suggested to be essential in coordinating cancer-specific proteome and alternated signaling pathways. HSP90 is a family of 5 members, including HSP90α and HSP90β (both of which are cytoplasmic), GRP94 (a glucose-regulated protein 94 located in the ER), TRAP1 (a tumor necrosis factor receptor-associated protein-1 located in the mitochondria), and isoform HSP90N. HSP90 forms an HSP90 chaperone machine with other co-chaperones, which is responsible for protein folding and maturation, intracellular disposition, and proteolytic turnover of several crucial regulators for cellular metabolic functions, including cell proliferation, differentiation, and survival.[101]

Several proteins that can cause and drive cancer, such as RTKs (EGFR, HER2, and VEGFR), signal transduction proteins (BRAF and AKT), transcription factors (HIF1α and p53), cell cycle regulatory proteins (CDK4 and cyclin D), antiapoptotic proteins (BCL2 and surviving), and telomerase (hTERT) are reliant on the HSP90 complex.[102]

Ganetespib is a second-generation HSP90 inhibitor that has been shown to be more effective than single-agent vemurafenib in melanoma cell lines driven by mutant BRAFV600. Several clinical trials exploring the effects of combining BRAF and/or MEK inhibitors to increase efficacy and overcome acquired resistance have been run. XL-888 is an orally available inhibitor of HSP90, displaying selective inhibition of HSP90α and HSP90β. A clinical trial tested a combination therapy of vemurafenib and XL888 on 25 patients with advanced melanoma. The therapy was found to be as effective as BRAF and MEK inhibitors. The dose-escalation design identified the maximum tolerated dose of XL888 as 60 mg, with 3 DLTs observed in 12 patients. Seventy-six percent of the patients had objective responses, and the treatment was associated with an increase in immune cells and a decrease in melanoma cell population.[103] A subsequent phase II clinical trial evaluated the effectiveness of XL888 when taken orally along with vemurafenib and cobimetinib in individuals with BRAF-mutated melanoma. The trial's primary objective is to assess the combination safety and tolerability. Nineteen patients (76%) showed positive responses to treatment, while the median PFS was 7.6 months, and the 5 year PFS rate was 20%. The median OS was 41.7 months, with a 5 year OS rate of 37%. However, vemurafenib and cobimetinib in combination with an unspecified drug caused significant toxicity and required frequent dose reductions. This might have contributed to the relatively low PFS, despite the high response rate of tumors.[103]

Targeting Autophagy

Autophagy is a process in which organelles and proteins are enclosed in autophagic vesicles and degraded in the lysosome. The lysosomal degradation of autophagic material helps recycle nutrients, further fueling cancer cell growth. Autophagy is a crucial adaptive resistance mechanism for cancers with BRAFV600 mutations treated with BRAF and/or BRAF and MEK inhibitors.[104]

A multicenter clinical trial was conducted to evaluate the effectiveness of hydroxychloroquine in combination with dabrafenib and trametinib in patients with advanced BRAFV600-mutant melanoma who had previously not received BRAF-targeted therapy. In the 34 evaluable patients, the 1 year PFS rate was found to be 48.2%, the median PFS was 11.2 months, and the ORR was 85%. The complete response rate was 41%, and the median OS was 26.5 months. A randomized trial of this triplet compared to BRAF/MEK inhibitor combination was closed due to poor accrual.

BCL-2 Family Inhibitors

Navitoclax is a BH3-mimetic that inhibits the antiapoptotic BCL-2 family members BCL-2, BCL-w, and BCL-xL that has been evaluated in combination with dabrafenib and trametinib. After determining the safety and preliminary efficacy in patients with advanced BRAFV600-mutant solid tumors, a randomized phase II clinical trial was launched (NCT01989585).[105] Patients with BRAF-mutated advanced melanoma who were previously untreated with BRAF-targeted therapy were randomized to either the triplet of dabrafenib, trametinib, and navitoclax or dabrafenib and trametinib. The ORR was very high for each arm, 84% for triplet and 80% for doublet. With a median follow-up of 25.9 months, there was a trend for improved OS with the triplet (median 36 vs 25 months, $P = .07$).

While it remains to be determined whether any of these approaches, HSP90 inhibition, autophagy inhibition, or apoptosis targeting will be further developed, these 3 approaches provide a proof of principle that targeting other cellular processes in combination with BRAF and MEK inhibition is feasible and associated with benefit. It is anticipated that further studies of these and other combinations will be launched in the future and build upon the preliminary success of these efforts.

SUMMARY

The role of targeted therapy in melanoma has changed radically since the initial development of vemurafenib for BRAF-mutant melanoma 15 years ago. In particular, there is a deeper understanding of the targets (eg, BRAFV600E/K, BRAFV600 non-R/K, class 2 and 3 BRAF mutations, BRAF fusions, NRAS, NF1 loss, KIT, and NTRK) and the development of next-generation agents to inhibit these targets. While the next standard-of-care targeted therapy regimen is uncertain, the gains that have been made over the past decade are substantial and ongoing progress is expected.

REFERENCES

1. Shain AH, Bastian BC. From melanocytes to melanomas. Nature Rev Cancer 2016;16(6):345–58.
2. Siegel RL, Miller KD, Wagle NS, et al. Cancer statistics, 2023. CA Cancer J Clin 2023;73(1):17–48.

3. Pehamberger H, Okamoto I, Rauscher S, et al. Human determinants and the role of melanocortin-1 receptor variants in melanoma risk independent of UV radiation exposure. JAMA Dermatol 2016;152(7):776.

4. Arnold M, Singh D, Laversanne M, et al. Global burden of cutaneous melanoma in 2020 and projections to 2040. JAMA Dermatol 2022;158(5):495. Available at: https://jamanetwork.com/journals/jamadermatology/fullarticle/2790344.

5. Newell F, Johansson PA, Wilmott JS, et al. Comparative genomics provides etiologic and biological insight into melanoma subtypes. Cancer Discov 2022; 12(12):2856–79.

6. Sullivan RJ, Flaherty K. MAP kinase signaling and inhibition in melanoma. Oncogene 2013;32(19):2373–9. Available at: https://www.nature.com/articles/onc2012345.

7. Fecher LA, Amaravadi RK, Flaherty KT. The MAPK pathway in melanoma. Curr Opin Oncol 2008;20(2):183–9. Available at: https://journals.lww.com/00001622-200803000-00007.

8. Simanshu DK, Nissley DV, McCormick F. RAS Proteins and Their Regulators in Human Disease. Cell 2017;170(1):17. Available at:http://pmc/articles/PMC5555610/.

9. Randic T., Kozar I., Margue C., et al., NRAS mutant melanoma: towards better therapies. Vol. 99, Cancer Treatment Reviews, 2021, W.B. Saunders Ltd. Available at: https://www.cancertreatmentreviews.com/article/S0305-7372(21)00086-4/fulltext. Accessed June 30, 2024.

10. Song Y., Bi Z., Liu Y., et al., Targeting RAS–RAF–MEK–ERK signaling pathway in human cancer: current status in clinical trials. Vol. 10, Genes and Diseases, 2023, KeAi Communications Co, 76–88. Available at: https://www.sciencedirect.com/science/article/pii/S2352304222001404?via%3Dihub. Accessed June 30, 2024.

11. Ottaviano M, Giunta EF, Tortora M, et al. BRAF Gene and Melanoma: Back to the Future. Int J Mol Sci 2021;22(7):22. Available at:http://pmc/articles/PMC8037827/.

12. Patton EE, Mueller KL, Adams DJ, et al. Melanoma models for the next generation of therapies. Cancer Cell 2021;39(5):610. Available at:http://pmc/articles/PMC8378471/.

13. Vanhaesebroeck B, Guillermet-Guibert J, Graupera M, et al. The emerging mechanisms of isoform-specific PI3K signalling. Nat Rev Mol Cell Biol 2010; 11(5):329–41.

14. Papa A, Pandolfi PP. The PTEN–PI3K Axis in Cancer. Biomolecules 2019;9(4). Available at:http://pmc/articles/PMC6523724/.

15. Rahhali N, Chalem Y, Arkoub H, et al. Epidemiology of BRAFV600-mutated metastatic melanoma in Europe: A systematic review. Value Health 2017;20(9):A413. Available at: http://ovidsp.ovid.com/ovidweb.cgi?T=JS&CSC=Y&NEWS=N&PAGE=fulltext&D=emexb&AN=619025997%0Ahttp://sfx.nottingham.ac.uk:80/sfx_local?genre=article&atitle=Epidemiology+of+BRAFV600-mutated+metastatic+melanoma+in+Europe%3A+A+systematic+review&title=Value+in+He.

16. Lim SY, Shklovskaya E, Lee JH, et al. The molecular and functional landscape of resistance to immune checkpoint blockade in melanoma. Nat Commun 2023;14(1).

17. Hayward NK, Wilmott JS, Waddell N, et al. Whole-genome landscapes of major melanoma subtypes. Nature 2017;545(7653):175–80.

18. Sullivan RJ, Flaherty KT. BRAF in Melanoma: Pathogenesis, Diagnosis, Inhibition, and Resistance. J Skin Cancer 2011;2011:1–8.

19. Sullivan RJ, Flaherty KT. Resistance to BRAF-targeted therapy in melanoma. Eur J Cancer 2013;49(6):1297–304. Available at: https://linkinghub.elsevier.com/retrieve/pii/S095980491200915X.

20. Dahlman KB, Xia J, Hutchinson K, et al. BRAFL597 mutations in melanoma are associated with sensitivity to MEK inhibitors. Cancer Discov 2012;2(9):791–7.

21. Sun J, Carr MJ, Khushalani NI. Principles of Targeted Therapy for Melanoma. Surg Clin 2020;100:175–88. W.B. Saunders.

22. Shi H, Hugo W, Kong X, et al. Acquired resistance and clonal evolution in melanoma during BRAF inhibitor therapy. Cancer Discov 2014;4(1):80–93.

23. Van Allen EM, Wagle N, Sucker A, et al. The genetic landscape of clinical resistance to RAF inhibition in metastatic melanoma. Cancer Discov 2013;4(1):94–109. Available at: https://www.ncbi.nlm.nih.gov/pmc/articles/pmid/24265153/?tool=EBI.

24. Akbani R, Akdemir KC, Aksoy BA, et al. Genomic classification of cutaneous melanoma. Cell 2015;161(7):1681–96. Available at: http://www.cell.com/article/S0092867415006340/fulltext.

25. Radu A, Bejenaru C, Țolea I, et al. Immunohistochemical study of CD117 in various cutaneous melanocytic lesions. Exp Ther Med 2021;21(1). Available at:.

26. Pham DM, Guhan S, Tsao H. KIT and melanoma: biological insights and clinical implications. Yonsei Med J 2020;61(7):562–71. Available at: https://pubmed.ncbi.nlm.nih.gov/32608199/.

27. Kheder ES, Hong DS. Emerging targeted therapy for tumors with NTRK fusion proteins. Clin Cancer Res 2018;24(23):5807–14.

28. Forschner A, Forchhammer S, Bonzheim I. NTKR gene fusions in melanoma: detection, prevalence and potential therapeutic implications. JDDG J der Deutschen Dermatol Gesellschaft 2020;18(12):1387–92.

29. Forschner A, Forchhammer S, Bonzheim I. NTRK gene fusions in melanoma: detection, prevalence and potential therapeutic implications. Journal der Deutschen Dermatologischen Gesellschaft 2020;18(12):1387–92. Available at: https://onlinelibrary.wiley.com/doi/10.1111/ddg.14160.

30. O'Hayre M, Vázquez-Prado J, Kufareva I, et al. The emerging mutational landscape of G proteins and G-protein-coupled receptors in cancer. Nat Rev Cancer 2013;13(6):412–24. Available at: https://www.nature.com/articles/nrc3521.

31. Larribère L, Utikal J. Update on GNA Alterations in Cancer: Implications for Uveal Melanoma Treatment. Cancers (Basel) 2020;12(6):1524. Available at: https://www.mdpi.com/2072-6694/12/6/1524.

32. Shoushtari AN, Carvajal RD. GNAQ and GNA11 mutations in uveal melanoma. Melanoma Res 2014;24(6):525–34. Available at: https://journals.lww.com/00008390-201412000-00001.

33. Chapman PB, Hauschild A, Robert C, et al. Improved Survival with Vemurafenib in Melanoma with BRAF V600E Mutation. N Engl J Med 2011;364(26):2507–16. Available at: https://www.nejm.org/doi/full/10.1056/nejmoa1103782.

34. Chapman PB, Robert C, Larkin J, et al. Vemurafenib in patients with BRAFV600 mutation-positive metastatic melanoma: Final overall survival results of the randomized BRIM-3 study. Ann Oncol 2017;28(10):2581–7.

35. Hauschild A, Grob JJ, Demidov LV, et al. Dabrafenib in BRAF-mutated metastatic melanoma: A multicentre, open-label, phase 3 randomised controlled trial. Lancet 2012;380(9839):358–65.

36. Dummer R, Ascierto PA, Gogas HJ, et al. Overall survival in patients with BRAF-mutant melanoma receiving encorafenib plus binimetinib versus vemurafenib or

encorafenib (COLUMBUS): a multicentre, open-label, randomised, phase 3 trial. Lancet Oncol 2018;19(5):1315–27.

37. Long GV, Flaherty KT, Stroyakovskiy D, et al. Dabrafenib plus trametinib versus dabrafenib monotherapy in patients with metastatic BRAF V600E/K-mutant melanoma: long-term survival and safety analysis of a phase 3 study. Ann Oncol 2017;28(7):1631–9.

38. Long GV, Weber JS, Infante JR, et al. Overall survival and durable responses in patients with BRAF V600-mutant metastatic melanoma receiving dabrafenib combined with trametinib. J Clin Oncol 2016;34(8):871–8.

39. Garbe C, Sovak MA, Ribas A, et al. Combined vemurafenib and cobimetinib in BRAF -mutated melanoma. N Engl J Med 2014;371(20):1867–76.

40. Ascierto PA, McArthur GA, Dréno B, et al. Cobimetinib combined with vemurafenib in advanced BRAFV600-mutant melanoma (coBRIM): updated efficacy results from a randomised, double-blind, phase 3 trial. Lancet Oncol 2016;17(9): 1248–60.

41. Robert C, Grob JJ, Stroyakovskiy D, et al. Five-Year Outcomes with Dabrafenib plus Trametinib in Metastatic Melanoma. N Engl J Med 2019;381(7):626–36. Available at: https://www.nejm.org/doi/full/10.1056/NEJMoa1904059.

42. Dummer R, Hauschild A, Santinami M, et al. Five-year analysis of adjuvant dabrafenib plus trametinib in stage iii melanoma. N Engl J Med 2020;383(12): 1139–48.

43. Long GV, Hauschild A, Santinami M, et al. Adjuvant dabrafenib plus trametinib in stage III BRAF -mutated melanoma. N Engl J Med 2017;377(19):1813–23. Available at: https://www.nejm.org/doi/full/10.1056/NEJMoa1708539.

44. Wolchok JD, Chiarion-Sileni V, Gonzalez R, et al. Overall survival with combined nivolumab and ipilimumab in advanced melanoma. N Engl J Med 2017;377(14): 1345–56.

45. Tawbi HA, Schadendorf D, Lipson EJ, et al. Relatlimab and nivolumab versus nivolumab in untreated advanced melanoma. N Eng J Med 2022;386(1): 24–34. Available at: https://www.nejm.org/doi/full/10.1056/nejmoa2109970.

46. Rager T, Eckburg A, Patel M, et al. Treatment of metastatic melanoma with a combination of immunotherapies and molecularly targeted therapies. Cancers (Basel) 2022;14(15). Available at:http://pmc/articles/PMC9367420/.

47. Gutzmer R, Stroyakovskiy D, Gogas H, et al. Atezolizumab, vemurafenib, and cobimetinib as first-line treatment for unresectable advanced BRAFV600 mutation-positive melanoma (IMspire150): primary analysis of the randomised, double-blind, placebo-controlled, phase 3 trial. Lancet 2020;395(10240): 1835–44.

48. Ascierto PA, Stroyakovskiy D, Gogas H, et al. Overall survival with first-line atezolizumab in combination with vemurafenib and cobimetinib in BRAFV600 mutation-positive advanced melanoma (IMspire150): second interim analysis of a multicentre, randomised, phase 3 study. Lancet Oncol 2023;24(1):33–44. Available at: https://pubmed.ncbi.nlm.nih.gov/36460017/.

49. Schachter J, Ribas A, Long GV, et al. Pembrolizumab versus ipilimumab for advanced melanoma: final overall survival results of a multicentre, randomised, open-label phase 3 study (KEYNOTE-006). Lancet 2017;390(10105):1853–62.

50. Borcoman E, Nandikolla A, Long G, et al. Patterns of response and progression to immunotherapy. American Society of Clinical Oncology Educational Book; 2018. p. 169–78. Available at: https://ascopubs.org/doi/10.1200/EDBK_200643.

51. Atkins MB, Lee SJ, Chmielowski B, et al. Combination Dabrafenib and Trametinib Versus Combination Nivolumab and Ipilimumab for Patients With Advanced

BRAF-Mutant Melanoma: The DREAMseq Trial ECOG-ACRIN EA6134. J Clin Oncol 2023;41(2):186–97. Available at: https://ascopubs.org/doi/10.1200/JCO.22.01763.

52. Moriceau G, Hugo W, Hong A, et al. Tunable-Combinatorial Mechanisms of Acquired Resistance Limit the Efficacy of BRAF/MEK Cotargeting but Result in Melanoma Drug Addiction. Cancer Cell 2015;27(2):240–56. Available at: http://www.cell.com/article/S1535610814004693/fulltext.

53. Long GV, Fung C, Menzies AM, et al. Increased MAPK reactivation in early resistance to dabrafenib/trametinib combination therapy of BRAF-mutant metastatic melanoma. Nat Commun 2014;5:1–9. Available at: https://www.nature.com/articles/ncomms6694.

54. Bartnik E, Fiedorowicz M, Czarnecka AM. Mechanisms of melanoma resistance to treatment with BRAF and MEK inhibitors. Nowotwory Journal of Oncology 2019;69(3–4):133–41. Available at: https://journals.viamedica.pl/nowotwory_journal_of_oncology/article/view/NJO.2019.0025.

55. Johnson DB, Menzies AM, Zimmer L, et al. Acquired BRAF inhibitor resistance: a multicenter meta-analysis of the spectrum and frequencies, clinical behavior, and phenotypic associations of resistance mechanisms. Eur J Cancer 2015;51(18):2792. Available at:http://pmc/articles/PMC4666799/.

56. Saei A, Palafox M, Benoukraf T, et al. Loss of USP28-mediated BRAF degradation drives resistance to RAF cancer therapies. J Exp Med 2018;215(7):1913–28. Available at: https://pubmed.ncbi.nlm.nih.gov/29880484/.

57. Leung GP, Feng T, Sigoillot FD, et al. Hyperactivation of MAPK Signaling Is Deleterious to RAS/RAF-mutant Melanoma. Mol Cancer Res 2019;17(1):199–211.

58. Wu PK, Park JI. MEK1/2 inhibitors: molecular activity and resistance mechanisms. Semin Oncol 2015;42(6):849–62.

59. Sharma V, Young L, Cavadas M, et al. Registered Report: COT drives resistance to RAF inhibition through MAP kinase pathway reactivation. Elife [Internet] 2016;5(MARCH2016). Available at:http://pmc/articles/PMC4811761/.

60. Caporali S, Alvino E, Lacal PM, et al. Targeting the PI3K/AKT/mTOR pathway overcomes the stimulating effect of dabrafenib on the invasive behavior of melanoma cells with acquired resistance to the BRAF inhibitor. Int J Oncol 2016;49(3):1164–74. Available at: https://pubmed.ncbi.nlm.nih.gov/27572607/.

61. Kim MH, Kim J, Hong H, et al. Actin remodeling confers BRAF inhibitor resistance to melanoma cells through YAP/TAZ activation. EMBO J 2016;35(5):462–78. Available at: https://www.embopress.org/doi/10.15252/embj.201592081.

62. Anastas JN, Kulikauskas RM, Tamir T, et al. WNT5A enhances resistance of melanoma cells to targeted BRAF inhibitors. J Clin Invest 2014;124. Available at: http://www.jci.org.

63. Hugo W, Shi H, Sun L, et al. Non-genomic and Immune Evolution of Melanoma Acquiring MAPKi Resistance. Cell 2015;162(6):1271–85. Available at: http://www.cell.com/article/S0092867415010405/fulltext.

64. Emran A Al, Marzese DM, Menon DR, et al. Distinct histone modifications denote early stress-induced drug tolerance in cancer. Oncotarget 2017;9(9):8206–22. Available at: https://www.oncotarget.com/article/23654/text/.

65. Strub T, Ballotti R, Bertolotto C. The "ART" of Epigenetics in Melanoma: From histone "Alterations, to Resistance and Therapies.". Theranostics 2020;10(4):1777. Available at:http://pmc/articles/PMC6993228/.

66. Steeb T, Wessely A, Petzold A, et al. c-Kit inhibitors for unresectable or metastatic mucosal, acral or chronically sun-damaged melanoma: a systematic review and one-arm meta-analysis. Eur J Cancer 2021;157:348–57.

67. Carvajal RD. KIT as a Therapeutic Target in Metastatic Melanoma. JAMA 2011; 305(22):2327. Available at: http://jama.jamanetwork.com/article.aspx?doi=10. 1001/jama.2011.746.

68. Guo J, Si L, Kong Y, et al. Phase II, open-label, single-arm trial of imatinib mesylate in patients with metastatic melanoma harboring c-kit mutation or amplification. J Clin Oncol 2011;29(21):2904–9. Available at: https://ascopubs.org/doi/10. 1200/JCO.2010.33.9275.

69. Dummer R, Schadendorf D, Ascierto PA, et al. Binimetinib versus dacarbazine in patients with advanced NRAS-mutant melanoma (NEMO): a multicentre, open-label, randomised, phase 3 trial. Lancet Oncol 2017;18(4):435–45. Available at: http://www.thelancet.com/article/S1470204517301808/fulltext.

70. Dumaz N, Jouenne F, Delyon J, et al. Atypical BRAF and NRAS Mutations in Mucosal Melanoma. Cancers 2019;11:1133. Available at: https://www.mdpi. com/2072-6694/11/8/1133/htm.

71. Adjei AA, LoRusso P, Ribas A, et al. A phase I dose-escalation study of TAK-733, an investigational oral MEK inhibitor, in patients with advanced solid tumors. Invest New Drugs 2017;35(1):47. Available at:http://pmc/articles/PMC5306265/.

72. Nebhan CA, Johnson DB, Sullivan RJ, et al. Efficacy and safety of trametinib in non-V600 BRAF mutant melanoma: a phase II study. Oncologist 2021;26(9): 731e1498. Available at: https://pubmed.ncbi.nlm.nih.gov/33861486/.

73. Sun C, Wang L, Huang S, et al. Reversible and adaptive resistance to BRAF(V600E) inhibition in melanoma. Nature 2014;508(7494):118–22. Available at: https:// pubmed.ncbi.nlm.nih.gov/24670642/.

74. Botton T, Talevich E, Mishra VK, et al. Genetic Heterogeneity of BRAF Fusion Kinases in Melanoma Affects Drug Responses. Cell Rep 2019;29(3):573–88.e7. Available at: https://pubmed.ncbi.nlm.nih.gov/31618628/.

75. Menzies AM, Yeh I, Botton T, et al. Clinical activity of the MEK inhibitor trametinib in metastatic melanoma containing BRAF kinase fusion. Pigment Cell Melanoma Res 2015;28(5):607–10. Available at: https://pubmed.ncbi.nlm.nih.gov/26072686/.

76. Chew SM, Lucas M, Brady M, et al. SKAP2-BRAF fusion and response to an MEK inhibitor in a patient with metastatic melanoma resistant to immunotherapy. BMJ Case Rep 2021;14(6). Available at: https://pubmed.ncbi.nlm.nih.gov/34167970/.

77. Menzer C, Menzies AM, Carlino MS, et al. Targeted Therapy in Advanced Melanoma With Rare BRAF Mutations. J Clin Oncol 2019;37(33):3142–51. Available at: https://pubmed.ncbi.nlm.nih.gov/31580757/.

78. Liu L, Lee MR, Kim JL, et al. Purinylpyridinylamino-based DFG-in/αC-helix-out B-Raf inhibitors: Applying mutant versus wild-type B-Raf selectivity indices for compound profiling. Bioorg Med Chem 2016;24(10):2215–34.

79. Peng S Bin, Henry JR, Kaufman MD, et al. Inhibition of RAF Isoforms and Active Dimers by LY3009120 Leads to Anti-tumor Activities in RAS or BRAF Mutant Cancers. Cancer Cell 2015;28(3):384–98. Available at: https://pubmed.ncbi. nlm.nih.gov/26343583/.

80. Wood K, Nussbaum D, Martz C, et al. Mediator Kinase Inhibition Impedes Transcriptional Plasticity and Prevents Resistance to ERK/MAPK-Targeted Therapy in KRAS-Mutant Cancers. Res Sq [Internet] 2023. Available at: http://www. ncbi.nlm.nih.gov/pubmed/37961649.

81. Izar B, Sharfman W, Hodi FS, et al. A first-in-human phase I, multicenter, open-label, dose-escalation study of the oral RAF/VEGFR-2 inhibitor (RAF265) in locally advanced or metastatic melanoma independent from BRAF mutation status. Cancer Med [Internet] 2017;6(8):1904–14. Available at: https://pubmed. ncbi.nlm.nih.gov/28719152/.

82. Desai J, Gan H, Barrow C, et al. Phase I, Open-Label, Dose-Escalation/Dose-Expansion Study of Lifirafenib (BGB-283), an RAF Family Kinase Inhibitor, in Patients With Solid Tumors. J Clin Oncol [Internet] 2020;38(19):2140–50. Available at: https://pubmed.ncbi.nlm.nih.gov/32182156/.

83. Sullivan RJ, Hollebecque A, Flaherty KT, et al. A Phase I Study of LY3009120, a Pan-RAF Inhibitor, in Patients with Advanced or Metastatic Cancer. Mol Cancer Ther 2020;19(2):460–7. Available at: https://pubmed.ncbi.nlm.nih.gov/31645440/.

84. Hong A, Piva M, Liu S, et al. Durable suppression of acquired mek inhibitor resistance in cancer by sequestering mek from erk and promoting antitumor t-cell immunity. Cancer Discov 2021;11(3):714–35.

85. Chen SH, Gong X, Zhang Y, et al. RAF inhibitor LY3009120 sensitizes RAS or BRAF mutant cancer to CDK4/6 inhibition by abemaciclib via superior inhibition of phospho-RB and suppression of cyclin D1. Oncogene 2018;37(6):821–32. Available at: https://pubmed.ncbi.nlm.nih.gov/29059158/.

86. Schram AM, Subbiah V, Sullivan R, et al. A first-in-human, phase 1a/1b, open-label, dose-escalation and expansion study to investigate the safety, pharmacokinetics, and antitumor activity of the RAF dimer inhibitor BGB-3245 in patients with advanced or refractory tumors. AACR Annual Meeting 2023. April 14-19, 2023; Orlando, FL Abstract CT031.

87. Solomon B, Gao B, Subbiah V, et al. Abstract CT033: Safety, pharmacokinetics, and antitumor activity findings from a phase 1b, open-label, dose-escalation and expansion study investigating RAF dimer inhibitor lifirafenib in combination with MEK inhibitor mirdametinib in patients with advanced or refractory solid tumors. Cancer Res [Internet] 2023;83(8_Supplement):CT033.

88. Lebbe C, Long GV, Robert C, et al. Phase II study of multiple LXH254 drug combinations in patients (pts) with unresectable/metastatic, BRAF V600- or NRAS-mutant melanoma. Ann Oncol 2022;33(suppl_7):S808–69.

89. Al Mahi A, Ablain J. RAS pathway regulation in melanoma. Dis Model Mech 2022;15(2). Available at: https://pubmed.ncbi.nlm.nih.gov/35234863/.

90. Hong DS, Fakih MG, Strickler JH, et al. KRASG12C Inhibition with Sotorasib in Advanced Solid Tumors. N Engl J Med 2020;383(13):1207–17. Available at: https://pubmed.ncbi.nlm.nih.gov/32955176/.

91. Wang X, Luo Z, Chen J, et al. First-in-human phase I dose-escalation and dose-expansion trial of the selective MEK inhibitor HL-085 in patients with advanced melanoma harboring NRAS mutations. BMC Med 2023;21(1):1–12. Available at: https://bmcmedicine.biomedcentral.com/articles/10.1186/s12916-022-02669-7.

92. Shi YK, Zheng Y, Chen J, et al. Efficacy and safety of tunlametinib (HL-085) combined with vemurafenib in patients with advanced BRAF V600-mutated solid tumors: A multicenter, phase I study. Ann Oncol 2023;34:S790. Available at: http://www.annalsofoncology.org/article/S0923753423032489/fulltext.

93. Si L, Zou Z, Zhang W, et al. Efficacy and safety of tunlametinib in patients with advanced NRAS-mutant melanoma: A multicenter, open-label, single-arm, phase 2 study. 2023;41(16_suppl):9510–9510. Available at: https://ascopubs.org/doi/10.1200/JCO.2023.41.16_suppl.9510.

94. Mao L, Guo J, Zhu L, et al. A first-in-human, phase 1a dose-escalation study of the selective MEK1/2 inhibitor FCN-159 in patients with advanced NRAS-mutant melanoma. Eur J Cancer 2022;175:125–35. Available at: https://pubmed.ncbi.nlm.nih.gov/36113242/.

95. Sullivan RJ, Infante JR, Janku F, et al. First-in-Class ERK1/2 Inhibitor Ulixertinib (BVD-523) in Patients with MAPK Mutant Advanced Solid Tumors: Results of a

Phase I Dose-Escalation and Expansion Study. Cancer Discov 2018;8(2): 184–95. Available at: https://pubmed.ncbi.nlm.nih.gov/29247021/.

96. Wu J, Liu D, Offin M, et al. Characterization and management of ERK inhibitor associated dermatologic adverse events: analysis from a nonrandomized trial of ulixertinib for advanced cancers. Invest New Drugs 2021;39(3):785–95. Available at: https://link.springer.com/article/10.1007/s10637-020-01035-9.

97. Buchbinder EI, Cohen JV, Haq R, et al. A phase II study of ERK inhibition by ulixertinib (BVD-523) in metastatic uveal melanoma. Cancer Res Commun 2020; 38(15_suppl):10036. Available at: https://ascopubs.org/doi/10.1200/JCO.2020. 38.15_suppl.10036.

98. Stathis A, Tolcher AW, Wang JS, et al. Results of an open-label phase 1b study of the ERK inhibitor MK-8353 plus the MEK inhibitor selumetinib in patients with advanced or metastatic solid tumors. Invest New Drugs 2023;41(3):380–90. Available at: https://link.springer.com/article/10.1007/s10637-022-01326-3.

99. Posch C, Sanlorenzo M, Ma J, et al. MEK/CDK4,6 co-targeting is effective in a subset of NRAS, BRAF and "wild type" melanomas. Oncotarget 2018;9(79): 34990–5. Available at: https://pubmed.ncbi.nlm.nih.gov/30405888/.

100. Sahebjam S, Le Rhun E, Queirolo P, et al. A phase II study of abemaciclib in patients (pts) with brain metastases (BM) secondary to non-small cell lung cancer (NSCLC) or melanoma (MEL). Ann Oncol 2019;30:v117. Available at: http:// www.annalsofoncology.org/article/S0923753419585532/fulltext.

101. Mayer MP. Hsp70 chaperone dynamics and molecular mechanism. Trends Biochem Sci 2013;38(10):507–14. Available at: http://www.cell.com/article/S0968 000413001321/fulltext.

102. Trepel J, Mollapour M, Giaccone G, et al. Targeting the dynamic HSP90 complex in cancer. Nat Rev Cancer 2010;10:537–49. Available at: https://www. nature.com/articles/nrc2887.

103. Eroglu Z., Chen Y.A., Smalley I., et al., Combined BRAF, MEK, and heat-shock protein 90 (HSP90) inhibition in advanced BRAF V600-mutant melanoma, *Cancer*, 2023, Available at: https://acsjournals.onlinelibrary.wiley.com/doi/10.1002/ cncr.35029. Accessed June 30, 2024.

104. Thorburn A, Morgan MJ. Targeting autophagy in BRAF-mutant tumors. Cancer Discov 2015;5(4):353–4.

105. Eroglu Z, Mehnert JM, Giobbie-Hurder A, et al. Randomized phase II trial of dabrafenib and trametinib with or without navitoclax in patients (pts) with BRAF-mutant (MT) metastatic melanoma (MM) (CTEP P9466). J Clin Oncol 2023;41(16_suppl): 9511.

Progress in Immune Checkpoint Inhibitor for Melanoma Therapy

Celine Boutros, MD[a], Hugo Herrscher, MD[b],
Caroline Robert, MD, PhD[a,c,d],*

KEYWORDS

- Melanoma • Neoadjuvant • Adjuvant • Metastatic • Therapy • Immunotherapy
- RNA vaccine

KEY POINTS

- Ipilimumab combined with nivolumab has emerged as the most effective treatment in the metastatic setting to date, including brain metastasis.
- A highly innovative strategy combining a tumor-specific RNA vaccine with pembrolizumab has recently shown promising results in macroscopic stage III resected patients versus pembrolizumab alone.
- After the success of immune checkpoint inhibitors in both the adjuvant and metastatic settings, a neoadjuvant approach has emerged in patients with macroscopic stage III melanoma.
- Patients with a high lactase dehydrogenase level and/or symptomatic brain metastases remain a high medical need.

INTRODUCTION

Melanoma, comprising only 1% of skin cancers, is responsible for over 70% of skin cancer-related deaths. Two main strategies have profoundly modified metastatic melanoma prognosis: targeted anti-BRAF-based therapy for BRAF V600 E/K-mutant melanoma accounting for about 50% of patients and immune checkpoint inhibitors (ICI; **Fig. 1**) This review will focus on the latter strategy, but sequencing and combining immunotherapy with targeted agents will also be mentioned. It is indeed largely thanks to the use of immunotherapy that melanoma has transitioned from being a disease

[a] Department of Medicine, Gustave Roussy Cancer Campus, 114 Rue Edouard Vaillant, 94805 Villejuif, France; [b] Oncology Unit, Clinique Sainte-Anne, Groupe Hospitalier Saint Vincent, rue Philippe Thys, 67000 Strasbourg, France; [c] Faculty of Medicine, University Paris-Saclay, 63 Rue Gabriel Péri, 94270 Kremlin-Bicêtre, France; [d] INSERM Unit U981, 114 Rue Edouard Vaillant, 94805 Villejuif, France
* Corresponding author.
E-mail address: Caroline.robert@gustaveroussy.fr

Hematol Oncol Clin N Am 38 (2024) 997–1010
https://doi.org/10.1016/j.hoc.2024.05.016
0889-8588/24/© 2024 Elsevier Inc. All rights reserved, including those for text and data mining, AI training, and similar technologies.

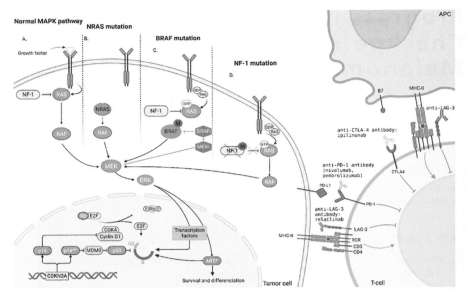

Fig. 1. Mechanism of action of targeted therapies and immunotherapy in melanoma. (Created with BioRender.com.).

almost always deadly to a potentially curable one with a 5 fold increase in the median overall survival (OS) for this patient population over the past 12 years.

A DECADE OF SUCCESS FOR DRUGS DEVELOPMENT IN METASTATIC MELANOMA

Cytotoxic T-lymphocyte-associated antigen 4 (CTLA-4) was the first immune check-point receptor to be targeted with the development of melanoma (**Table 1**).

Ipilimumab, a fully humanized monoclonal antibody, was approved by the Food and Drug Administration (FDA) for the treatment of metastatic melanoma in March 2011 and by the European Medicines Agency (EMEA) in July 2011.

In a first-line treatment study, ipilimumab in combination with the cytotoxic chemotherapy dacarbazine was found to lower the risk of death by 28% compared to dacarbazine alone. While the objective response rate of ipilimumab is modest, ranging between 10% and 15%, ipilimumab was able to provide long-lasting responses in some patients. This marked the first time in the history of metastatic melanoma that a significant improvement in OS was observed.[1]

Shortly after the introduction of ipilimumab, attention turned toward targeting the PD-1 molecule, leading to the development of 2 antibodies: nivolumab and pembrolizumab.[2] Both therapies demonstrated historic results in their phase I development stages, with an unusually large number of patients enrolled, a rare occurrence for early-stage trials. Notably, pembrolizumab was able to obtain accelerated market authorization based on the remarkable results of its phase I trial.[2]

Indeed, these 2 drugs were able to achieve objective responses in approximately 30% to 40% of patients, with even complete responses (CR) in 15% to 20% of them. One remarkable finding was the prolonged duration of response which persisted even after treatment was discontinued in some cases.

Following the positive results from early trials, several phase III studies were conducted. In one study, nivolumab was compared to dacarbazine chemotherapy, while

Table 1
Main outcomes of major immunotherapy-based clinical trials in patients with melanoma

Study Type	N	Treatment	Median OS (mo)	Median PFS (mo)	Median Follow-Up (mo)	CR (%)	PR (%)	SD (%)	PD (%)
KEYNOTE-006[51]	556	Pembrolizumab	32.7	9.4	85.3	17	34	33	16
CheckMate-067[5]	314	Ipilimumab + nivolumab	72.1	11.5	57.5	21	116	38	74
	316	Nivolumab	36.9	6.9	36	18	85	30	121
	315	Ipilimumab	19.9	2.9	18.6	5	44	68	159
CheckMate-204[18]	101	Ipilimumab + nivolumab (asymptomatic MBM)	36-mo OS: 71.9%	36-mo PFS: 54.1%	34.3	17	35	4	26
	18	Ipilimumab + nivolumab (symptomatic MBM)	36-mo OS: 36.6%	36-mo PFS: 25.9%	7.5	1	3	0	10
C-144-01[53]	156	Lifileucel	13.9	4.1	27.6	5	26	46	18
RELATIVITY-047[7]	355	Relatlimab + nivolumab	NR	10.1	13.2	-	-	-	-

in another study, pembrolizumab was compared to ipilimumab, which had become the new standard.[3,4] In both trials, the anti-PD1 antibodies demonstrated greater efficacy and a very favorable benefit-to-risk ratio, with serious side effects present in only approximately 15% of patients.[3,4]

The combined blockade of CTLA-4 and PD-1 with ipilimumab and nivolumab has emerged as the most effective treatment in the metastatic setting to date, with 49% of patients alive after 6.5 years and a median OS of 72.1 months.[5] However, this combination comes with significant toxicity, with 60% of treated patients experiencing severe adverse events (AEs), including rare but potentially fatal side effects such as myocarditis and encephalitis.[2]

ANTI-LYMPHOCYTE ACTIVATION GENE-3: A THIRD IMMUNE CHECKPOINT INHIBITOR

Another co-inhibitor of lymphocytes is the lymphocyte activation gene 3 (LAG-3), which can induce T-cell exhaustion and decrease T-cell activation.[6] The anti-LAG-3 monoclonal antibody relatlimab has been evaluated in combination with nivolumab in a phase II/III randomized controlled trial (RCT) for patients with metastatic melanoma, and has been found to have a hazard ratio (HR) of 0.75 for progression-free survival (PFS) compared to nivolumab alone, with an ORR of 43.1%. The combination is associated with a tolerable toxicity profile, with only 18% of patients experiencing grade 3 or more AEs, which is much lower than the rate associated with nivolumab and ipilimumab.[7,8] This combination has been approved by the FDA in March 2022.

COMBINATION OF IMMUNE CHECKPOINT INHIBITORS AND TARGETED THERAPY

Two large RCTs have investigated the combination of anti-PD1 or anti-PDL-1 with a BRAF inhibitor and a MEK inhibitor. The trials compared dabrafenib plus trametinib plus spartalizumab (an anti-PD1) or vemurafenib plus cobimetinib plus atezolizumab (an anti-PD-L1 that is not approved for melanoma) to the respective targeted therapies plus an ICI placebo. The trials showed very similar benefits in terms of PFS with HRs in favor of the triplet combination versus targeted therapies (0.78 and 0.8, respectively).[9,10] However, only the difference in the second trial reached statistical significance, leading to the approval of vemurafenib plus cobimetinib plus atezolizumab for treating patients with BRAF V600 mutant melanoma.[10] It would, however, have been critical to evaluate this triple combination against ICI single or combination immunotherapies, which currently represent the most effective approved therapies in metastatic melanoma.

CHOICE OF FIRST-LINE TREATMENT AND OPTIMAL SEQUENCES OF TREATMENTS IN ADVANCED MELANOMA

The choice of first-line treatment is based on multiple factors including BRAF status, metastasis location, symptoms, comorbidities, and in particular autoimmune diseases (**Fig. 2**).

Nivolumab plus relatlimab showed PFS benefits compared to nivolumab monotherapy.[7] Ipilimumab combined with nivolumab also tends to demonstrate superior efficacy versus nivolumab although the checkmate 067 was not powered to compare these 2 arms. Nivolumab plus relatlimab has a lower rate of irAEs (22% grade 3–4) than nivolumab plus ipilimumab (55% grade 3–4). However, nivolumab plus ipilimumab has shown substantial activity in patients with asymptomatic central nervous system (CNS) metastases, whereas CNS efficacy has not been formally evaluated for nivolumab plus relatlimab.[11] The HRs for PFS benefit of nivolumab plus ipilimumab and nivolumab plus relatlimab (0.89 and 0.82 respectively) versus nivolumab monotherapy are similar in patients with BRAF wild-type melanoma, but based on HR comparisons, nivolumab plus ipilimumab might have greater activity relative to nivolumab in patients with BRAF-mutant melanoma (HR, 0.59 vs 0.78). Neither combination regimen showed enhanced benefit over monotherapy in patients with tumors expressing PD-L1 greater than 1%.[12,13]

Based on these data, nivolumab plus ipilimumab may be considered as a first-line therapy in patients with CNS metastases and in asymptomatic BRAF-mutant

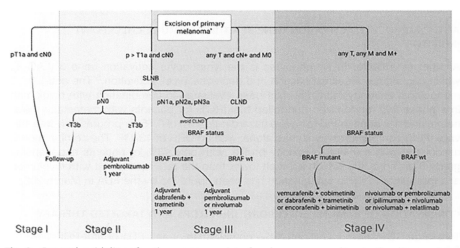

Fig. 2. General guidelines for the management of melanoma according to the disease staging. (Created with BioRender.com.).

melanoma, whereas nivolumab plus relatlimab could be considered in patients with BRAF wild-type melanoma lacking CNS metastases or those not felt to be able to tolerate nivolumab plus ipilimumab due to comorbidities.[13] Anti–PD-1 monotherapy may be considered in patients with low tumor burden, poor performance status, no CNS metastasis, or autoimmune disorders.

In patients with advanced BRAF V600 E/K-mutant melanoma, the question of which therapy, ICIs or targeted therapy, to start in priority was recently addressed by the DREAMSeq and SECOMBIT trials.[14,15] The DREAMSeq trial evaluated the optimal treatment sequencing for patients with BRAF V600 E/K-mutant melanoma, performance status (PS) of 1 to 2, no active CNS metastases, and no prior immunotherapy or history of autoimmune disease by comparing ipilimumab/nivolumab followed by dabrafenib/trametinib at progression against dabrafenib/trametinib followed by ipilimumab/nivolumab at progression.[14] Ipilimumab/nivolumab was associated with higher 2 year OS and durability of disease response versus the inverse sequence, confirming that ipilimumab/nivolumab should be considered the preferred first-line therapy for the majority of patients.[14] The SECOMBIT trial evaluated the combination of ipilimumab/nivolumab, encorafenib/binimetinib, or encorafenib/binimetinib for 8 weeks, followed by ipilimumab/nivolumab (sandwich regimen).[15] In patients with a high lactase dehydrogenase (LDH) level, poor PS, and/or symptomatic CNS metastases, a short course of target therapy (sandwich regimen) allowed disease control prior to ICI treatment.[15] It found a 3 year OS of 54% (95% confidence interval [CI], 41–67) for targeted therapy as initial therapy, 62% (95% CI, 48–76) for ICI as initial therapy, and 60% (95% CI, 58–72) for the sandwich regimen.

PATIENTS WITH CENTRAL NERVOUS SYSTEM INVOLVEMENT

Melanoma brain metastasis (MBM) is of particularly poor prognosis and occurs in approximately 50% of patients with metastatic melanoma.[16,17] Historically, median OS following diagnosis of MBM was 3 to 13 months.[16–18] The remarkable advances in the systemic therapy of metastatic melanoma have now improved the clinical outcome of MBM. Durable responses were observed with ICI in patients with asymptomatic MBM.[18–20] In the phase 2 trial CheckMate 204, half of the asymptomatic patients with MBM (n = 54; 53·5% [43·3–63·5]) who were treated with nivolumab plus ipilimumab achieved intracranial clinical response.[18] After 3 years of follow-up, the median duration of response was not reached, with the majority of responses (29 [58%] of 50 patients) lasting more than 2 years and most first responses occurring early in treatment (median 2·8 months interquartile range [IQR 1·3–4·1]).[18] The rate of durable responses remained stable after 3 years of follow-up in patients with asymptomatic brain metastases, with 85% of ongoing intracranial responses.[18,21] Of note, more than 50% of patients who had a durable response had unirradiated brain metastases. The median PFS and OS was not reached, with 3 year intracranial PFS of 54·1% and an OS of 71·9%.[18,21] The combination of ipilimumab and nivolumab showed a low efficacy in patients with symptomatic brain metastases, with an objective response rates (ORR) of 16·7% in patients with stable brain metastases. In patients with stable symptomatic MBM, the ORR was modest (16·7%); however, symptomatic patients who achieved a response maintained durable disease control.[18]

These findings were consistent with those reported in the phase 2 trial ABC and the phase 3 trial NIBIT-M2.[19,20] They demonstrate the durable clinical efficacy of ipilimumab plus nivolumab in the control of melanoma brain metastases, and the similar intracranial and extracranial tumor control.[19,20]

The combination of BRAF/MEK inhibitors provide up to 58% of intracranial response rates, as seen in the COMBI-MB trial that evaluated dabrafenib and trametinib in MBM.[22] However, the durability of responses (DOR) induced by BRAF/MEK inhibitors seems to be even shorter than in extracranial disease. The median DOR was only of 6.5 months which is less than for extracranial disease for targeted therapies.[22]

Combination treatment using immune anti-PD1 antibodies plus targeted therapies has been shown to be effective in patients with MBM, but with an increased toxicity rate.[23] In the TRICOTEL trial, the triplet combination of atezolizumab plus vemurafenib plus cobimetinib provided intracranial activity in patients with BRAF V600-mutated melanoma with MBM. Intracranial ORR was 42% (95% CI 29–54) in the BRAF V600-mutation-positive cohort.[23] However, treatment-related grade 3 or worse AEs occurred in 41 (68%) of 60 patients who received atezolizumab plus vemurafenib plus cobimetinib in the BRAF V600 mutation-positive cohort, the most common of which were lipase increased (15 [25%] of 60 patients) and blood creatine phosphokinase increased (11 [18%]).[23]

The impact of whole-brain radiation therapy (WBRT) on MBM is likely to be limited, which is not surprisingly given the DNA repair capacity of melanoma cells and the relative resistance to radiation.[24] WBRT is reserved for recurrence after stereotactic radiosurgery (SRS), a large number of metastases, or leptomeningeal disease.[25] SRS may effectively lead to local control of established brain metastases, but its use is limited to oligometastatic MBM.[25]

ADJUVANT TREATMENTS FOR STAGE II AND III MELANOMA

Patients with stage IIB, IIC (melanoma with a Breslow thickness >2 mm with ulceration or >4 mm) and stage III (regional skin or lymphatic involvement) melanoma have traditionally been treated with surgery, but they are still at a high risk of relapse. The 5 year melanoma-specific survival rates for patients with stage IIB/C and stage III melanoma range from 82% to 87% and 32% to 93%, respectively.[26]

In 2010, adjuvant ipilimumab 10 mg/kg every 3 weeks was approved for stage III melanoma. It showed a 25% decrease in the risk of recurrence and distant metastasis, and a nearly 30% decrease in the risk of death compared to placebo.[27,28] However, the treatment resulted in severe immune-related AEs in 54% and death in 1% of treated patients. A few years later, 1 year treatment with nivolumab and pembrolizumab were evaluated in the adjuvant setting.

Nivolumab 3 mg/kg every 2 weeks for 1 year demonstrated a 35% decrease in the risk of recurrence compared to ipilimumab and had a lower rate of AEs.[29,30] Treatment-related grade 3 or 4 AEs were reported in 14.4% of the patients in the nivolumab group and in 45.9% of those in the ipilimumab group.[29] Pembrolizumab showed a 40% reduction in the risk of recurrence and an increase in distant metastasis-free survival (DMFS) versus placebo in patients with stage III melanoma versus placebo.[31,32]

In patients with stage IIB/IIC melanoma, adjuvant pembrolizumab and nivolumab given for one year provided a significant reduction in the risk of relapse or death with HR of 0.42 and 0.61 versus placebo respectively.[33,34] Both nivolumab and pembrolizumab are now approved for adjuvant treatments for stage IIB and IIC melanoma. Several physicians now skip the sentinel node surgery for patients with stage IIB or IIC and directly prescribe adjuvant anti-PD1 treatment for one year.

Moreover, for patients with stage III BRAF-V600 mutant melanoma, 1 year of adjuvant treatment with the combination of the BRAF inhibitor dabrafenib and the MEK inhibitor trametinib resulted in a 53% lower risk of relapse. Combination therapy also resulted in higher rates of OS, DMFS, and recurrence-free survival (RFS), with clinically meaningful lower risks of 43%, 49%, and 53%, respectively.[35]

This benefit versus placebo is similar to the one obtained with pembrolizumab versus placebo. Although AEs are frequent with targeted therapy, they are not durable whereas some of the AEs associated with anti-PD1 such as endocrine alteration are usually permanent. The choice of adjuvant treatment of resected stage III melanoma between targeted therapy and anti-PD1 is therefore an important question to be discussed on a case-by-case basis with the patient. Overall, prescribing an adjuvant systemic therapy always implies to carefully consider the balance between the treatment's AEs and its potential benefit. Indeed, an adjuvant treatment treats a risk, and for subpopulations of patients with a low risk of relapse, such as those with minimal tumor load in the sentinel node or with stage IIB and IIC melanoma, who have a 10 year survival rate superior to 75%, the indication of an adjuvant treatment can be debated.

COMBINATION OF IMMUNE CHECKPOINT INHIBITORS WITH RNA VACCINE

A highly innovative strategy combining a tumor-specific RNA vaccine with pembrolizumab has recently shown very promising results in macroscopic stage III resected patients versus pembrolizumab alone. The phase 2b trial KEYNOTE-942 evaluated mRNA-4157 plus pembrolizumab versus pembrolizumab monotherapy in patients with resected, high-risk, stage IIIB–IV cutaneous melanoma.[36] The results showed a positive and clinically meaningful outcome in the randomized setting for an individualized neoantigen therapy approach. RFS was longer with the combination versus pembrolizumab monotherapy (HR for recurrence or death, $0 \cdot 561$ [95% CI $0 \cdot 309–1 \cdot 017$]), with lower recurrence or death event rate (22% vs 40%); 18 month RFS was 79% (95% CI $69 \cdot 0–85 \cdot 6$) versus 62% ($46 \cdot 9–74 \cdot 3$).[36]

SYSTEMIC IMMUNOTHERAPY BEFORE SURGERY IN RESECTABLE DISEASE: NEOADJUVANT TREATMENT

With the success of ICI in both the adjuvant and metastatic settings, a neoadjuvant approach has emerged in patients with macroscopic stage III melanoma.

The rationale for neoadjuvant immunotherapy stems from preclinical and clinical trials that demonstrated an enhanced systemic antitumor immune response with neoadjuvant immunotherapy compared with adjuvant treatment. The ability to generate tumor-specific CD8 T cells is hence increased, resulting in an improved clinical outcome for neoadjuvant-treated versus adjuvant-treated patients.[37–40] The evaluation of pathologic response (PR) after neoadjuvant settings provides a strong personalized predictive biomarker of RFS and OS in patients with early-stage disease.[38]

Hence, over the past 5 years, a paradigm shift into a neoadjuvant approach was observed through several clinical trials.[41,42]

The Optimal Adjuvant Combination Scheme of Ipilimumab and Nivolumab in Melanoma Patients (OpACIN) pilot study demonstrated translational and clinical evidence of improved outcomes when ICI was administered neoadjuvantly rather than adjuvantly.[43] This led to the (OpACIN)-neo trial, which tested 3 different neoadjuvant ipilimumab and nivolumab dosing schedule to take into account the potential risk of treatment-related AEs. The regimen consisting in ipilimumab 1 mg/kg dose and nivolumab at 3 mg/kg every 3 weeks for 2 cycles was identified as the preferable regimen for a preserved PR rate (defined as the percentage of patients with <50% residual viable tumor in the resection specimen) and the lowest incidence of grade 3 to 4 AEs (PR rate: 77% and grade 3 or 4 AE: 20%). The estimated 5 year RFS and OS rates for the neoadjuvant arm were 70% and 90% versus 60% and 70% for the adjuvant arm.[43]

Following the OpACIN trial, the PRADO trial tested whether adjuvant therapy could be omitted in case of major PR.[44] Therapeutic lymph node dissection (TLND) and adjuvant therapy were omitted in patients with a major PR. Patients with a partial PR underwent TLND only, whereas those with a pathologic non-response underwent TLND and adjuvant systemic therapy. The 2 year RFS and DMFS were 93% and 98% in patients with a major PR, 64% and 64% in those with a partial PR, and 71% and 76% in those with a pathologic non-response.[44] These results suggest that adjuvant therapy can be omitted in patients with a major PR, but may be important in those with a pathologic non-response, as patients with major PR showed better RFS than non-responders in the OpaCIN-neo trial, where no adjuvant therapy was given (71% vs 36%), and even a better outcome than partial-responders in the PRADO trial, where adjuvant therapy was also omitted.[43,44]

The combination of nivolumab and relatlimab was evaluated in the neoadjuvant setting in patients with resectable clinical stage III or oligometastatic stage IV melanoma.[7,45] Patients received 2 cycles of neoadjuvant nivolumab and relatlimab at fixed doses of 480 mg and 160 mg, respectively, every 4 weeks, followed by surgical resection, and then 10 doses of adjuvant nivolumab–relatlimab combination. 57% of patients included in the trial had a pathologic complete response (pCR). PR rate was 70%. No grade 3 or 4 AEs were observed in the neoadjuvant setting. The 2 year RFS was 92% for patients who had any PR, and 55% for patients who did not have a PR ($P=.005$).[45]

The Southwest Oncology Group S1801 trial compared adjuvant and neoadjuvant pembrolizumab among patients with clinical stage III or oligometastatic, resectable stage IV melanoma. Patients were randomized to either undergo surgery followed by 18 doses of pembrolizumab 200 mg every 3 weeks, or receive 3 doses of neoadjuvant pembrolizumab followed by surgery, then 15 doses of adjuvant pembrolizumab. Patients were required to undergo planned surgical resection and TLND regardless of response to neoadjuvant therapy; and no de-escalation of surgery occurred. Event-free survivalEFS at 2 years was 72% (95% CI 64–80) in the neoadjuvant–adjuvant group and 49% (95% CI 41–59) in the adjuvant-only group. Treatment-related AE rates were similar among both treatment arms. Around 21% of neoadjuvant participants with submitted pathology reports achieved a pCR.[40]

The Morpheus-Melanoma trial (NCT05116202) is currently underway to evaluate efficacy, safety, and pharmacokinetics of different combinations simultaneously that may enhance antitumor activity, including inhibitors of LAG-3, TIGIT, and PD-1. The simultaneous evaluation of several combinations in the Morpheus-Melanoma trial is a promising approach to accelerate the development of novel neoadjuvant.

The NADINA trial is also currently underway to evaluate 2 cycles of neoadjuvant nivolumab (3 mg/kg) combined with ipilimumab (1 mg/kg) versus standard adjuvant nivolumab in biopsy-proven resectable clinical stage III melanoma (NCT04949113).

PREDICTIVE BIOMARKERS

Many efforts are directed at predicting the treatment outcome of patients based on tumor or microenvironmental biomarkers.

Several prognostic and/or predictive biomarkers have been identified among which PDL-1 expression, LDH, S100B protein, circulating tumor DNA (ctDNA), tumor mutation burden, transcriptomic inflammatory or interferon gamma signatures and circulating tumor cells (CTCs).

Among thse markers, only LDH is routinely used in clinical practice.

More recently, technological evolutions have made it possible to detect more precise tumor elements.

Notably, ctDNA monotoring is associated with the clinical course of the disease and can predict relapses a few months before relpases seen on CT-scan. Various techniques can be used with various sensitivities. The personnalized and tumor-informed methods seem to be the most reliable.[46]

Multiple studies found that the presence of a high TMB, especially if these mutations are found in all tumor cells (clonal TMB), are associated with ICI treatment benefit.[47] This is explained by the higher potential for neoantigens production by tumor with high TMB. Other reported parameters associated with ICI response include an inflamed/IFN-gamma transcriptomic signature and the presence of CD8 + T cells B cells, tertiary lymphoid structures and specialized vessels named high endothelial venules in tumor microenvironment.[48,49] However, none of these results can be used in the clinic today and practical predictive biomarkers to guide treatment strategies are still lacking.[50]

POSSIBILITY TO STOP TREATMENT IN CASE OF COMPLETE RESPONSE

Data from clinical trials have shown that ICI had durable antitumor activity in patients with advanced melanoma.[51,52] The most recent update of anti-PD-1 monotherapy is provided by the analysis of the long-term efficacy of pembrolizumab at 7 years in the phase 3 trial KEYNOTE-006.[51] Among the overall population, 93 patients who received pembrolizumab (16.7%) had CR, 191 (34.4%) had partial response (PR), and 184 (33.1%) had SD. The patients with CR or PR had an improved OS and PFS when compared with patients who had SD.[51] After more than 7 years of follow-up, pembrolizumab continued to demonstrate improved OS compared with ipilimumab. The median OS in the overall population (n = 834) was prolonged with pembrolizumab versus ipilimumab (HR, 0.70; 95% CI, 0.58–0.83), with 7 year OS of 37.8% and 25.3%, respectively. Recent data emerged from the follow-up of patients in the KEYNOTE-006 who received pembrolizumab for 2 years, with at least stable disease (SD) upon discontinuation.[51,52] Long-term data from these patients indicate that up to 76% of patients who had CR or PR had ongoing disease control after 5 years of follow-up.[23] Interestingly, 8 (8%) patients with a previous PR upon discontinuation converted to CR after cessation of pembrolizumab.[23] Patients who completed 2 years of pembrolizumab with SD relapsed earlier than did those with CR or PR.[51,52] Tumor relapse occurred in 27 of the 103 patients (26%) who initially completed the 2 years of pembrolizumab, with a median time to progression of 33·3 months (IQR 26·0 months—not available) from the end of pembrolizumab.[52] Among these patients, 16 received a second course of pembrolizumab.[22] Among them, 7 patients had achieved initially CR as a best overall response, 7 had PR, and 2 had SD. The median time to progression was 33·3 months (IQR 26·0 months—not available) from the end of first-course pembrolizumab. The lymph nodes were the most frequent site of disease at relaspse.[51] Second-course pembrolizumab provided additional clinical benefit in some patients. Hence, patients with a best overall response of CR or PR to first-course pembrolizumab tended to have a better response to second-course pembrolizumab than patients who had SD.[22] The ORR to second-course pembrolizumab was 56% (95% CI, 30% to 80%), with 4 patients (25%) achieving CR, 5 (31%) PR, 5 (31%) SD, and 2 (13%) PD. The median duration of second-course pembrolizumab was 9·0 months (IQR 4·2–10·6).[51]

Despite these promising long-term remissions in a group of patients, many questions remain unanswered and many efforts are made to address them in the near future. Further trials are needed to establish the optimal duration of ICI treatment and to define potential predictive biomarkers to discontinue ICI.

SUMMARY AND PERSPECTIVES

Melanoma prognosis has been radically improved with the advent of ICI particularly anti-PD1 that can be used as monotherapy or combined either anti-CTLA-4 or anti-LAG-3, constituting the most effective anti-melanoma therapies, leading to durable remission and hopefully a cure for some patients.

However, there is no standard effective treatment for patients with primary or secondary resistance to ICI. Obtaining a clinical benefit in patients who fail ICI treatment is thus a major objective in the current therapeutic landscape, with several clinical trial from phase I to III targeting this population. Tumor-infiltrating lymphocytes were evaluated in a phase II single arm trial and demonstrated a 31.4% ORR.[53] These results led to the authorization of lifileucel in the United States in March 2023 (TILs developed by Iovance). However, this adoptive immunotherapy can only be prescribed to highly selected patients and is currently available only in highly specialized centers.

An ongoing phase III is evaluating the immune mobilizing monoclonal TCR against a gp100 peptide presented in the HLA 0201, tebentafusp, combined with anti-PD1 versus physician' choice in this population of patient (NCT06112314).

In the coming years, other critical goals for will be to optimize ICI base therapies by developing robust biomarkers to guide treatment choices, predict efficacy and toxicity, and adjust the dose and duration of treatment in patients with low-risk diseases.

CLINICS CARE POINTS

- The choice of first-line treatment is based on multiple factors including BRAF status, metastasis location, symptoms, comorbidities and in particular autoimmune diseases.
- Nivolumab plus ipilimumab may be considered as a first-line therapy in patients with CNS metastases and in asymptomatic BRAF-mutant melanoma.
- Nivolumab plus relatlimab could be considered in patients with BRAF wild-type melanoma lacking CNS metastases or those not felt to be able to tolerate nivolumab plus ipilimumab due to comorbidities.

DISCLOSURE

C. Boutros has received travel fees from Pierre Fabre, Amgen and MSD, and has received compensation from MSD for participation in conferences, and from BMS for participation to advisory boards. H. Herrscher reports fees from Mudipharma, Mylan Medical, Ipsen an Jansen and honoraria from Astrazeneca and Novartis. C. Robert reports consultancy for BMS, Roche, Novartis, Pierre Fabre, MSD, Sanofi, AstraZeneca, and Merck and Sunpharma.

REFERENCES

1. Robert C, Thomas L, Bondarenko I, et al. Ipilimumab plus dacarbazine for previously untreated metastatic melanoma. N Engl J Med 2011;364(26):2517–26.
2. Boutros C, Tarhini A, Routier E, et al. Safety profiles of anti-CTLA-4 and anti-PD-1 antibodies alone and in combination. Nat Rev Clin Oncol 2016;13(8):473–86.

3. Robert C, Long GV, Brady B, et al. Nivolumab in previously untreated melanoma without BRAF mutation. N Engl J Med 2015;372(4):320–30.
4. Robert C, Schachter J, Long GV, et al. Pembrolizumab versus ipilimumab in advanced melanoma. N Engl J Med 2015;372(26):2521–32.
5. Wolchok JD, Chiarion-Sileni V, Gonzalez R, et al. Long-term outcomes with nivolumab plus ipilimumab or nivolumab alone versus ipilimumab in patients with advanced melanoma. J Clin Oncol 2022;40(2):127–37.
6. Robert C. LAG-3 and PD-1 blockade raises the bar for melanoma. Nat Cancer 2021;2(12):1251–3.
7. Tawbi HA, Schadendorf D, Lipson EJ, et al. Relatlimab and nivolumab versus nivolumab in untreated advanced melanoma. N Engl J Med 2022;386(1):24–34.
8. Sidaway P. LAG3 inhibition improves outcomes. Nat Rev Clin Oncol 2022; 19(3):149.
9. Dummer R, Long GV, Robert C, et al. Randomized phase III trial evaluating spartalizumab plus dabrafenib and trametinib for BRAF V600-mutant unresectable or metastatic melanoma. J Clin Oncol 2022;40(13):1428–38.
10. Gutzmer R, Stroyakovskiy D, Gogas H, et al. Atezolizumab, vemurafenib, and cobimetinib as first-line treatment for unresectable advanced BRAF^{V600} mutation-positive melanoma (IMspire150): primary analysis of the randomised, double-blind, placebo-controlled, phase 3 trial [published correction appears in Lancet. 2020 Aug 15;396(10249):466]. Lancet 2020;395(10240):1835–44.
11. Regan MM, Mantia CM, Werner L, et al. Treatment-free survival over extended follow-up of patients with advanced melanoma treated with immune checkpoint inhibitors in CheckMate 067. J Immunother Cancer 2021;9(11):e003743.
12. Switzer B, Piperno-Neumann S, Lyon J, et al. Evolving management of stage IV melanoma. Am Soc Clin Oncol Educ Book 2023;43:e397478.
13. Sondak VK, Atkins MB, Messersmith H, et al. Systemic therapy for melanoma: ASCO guideline update Q and A. JCO Oncol Pract 2024;20(2):173–7.
14. Atkins MB, Lee SJ, Chmielowski B, et al. Combination dabrafenib and trametinib versus combination nivolumab and ipilimumab for patients with advanced BRAF-mutant melanoma: the DREAMseq trial-ECOG-ACRIN EA6134. J Clin Oncol 2023;41(2):186–97.
15. Ascierto PA, Mandalà M, Ferrucci PF, et al. Sequencing of ipilimumab plus nivolumab and encorafenib plus binimetinib for untreated BRAF-mutated metastatic melanoma (SECOMBIT): a randomized, three-arm, open-label phase II trial. J Clin Oncol 2023;41(2):212–21.
16. Internò V, Sergi MC, Metta ME, et al. Melanoma brain metastases: a retrospective analysis of prognostic factors and efficacy of multimodal therapies. Cancers (Basel) 2023;15(5):1542. Published 2023 Feb 28.
17. Sperduto PW, Mesko S, Li J, et al. Survival in patients with brain metastases: summary report on the updated diagnosis-specific graded prognostic assessment and definition of the eligibility quotient. J Clin Oncol 2020;38(32):3773–84.
18. Tawbi HA, Forsyth PA, Hodi FS, et al. Long-term outcomes of patients with active melanoma brain metastases treated with combination nivolumab plus ipilimumab (CheckMate 204): final results of an open-label, multicentre, phase 2 study. Lancet Oncol 2021;22(12):1692–704.
19. Long G.V., Atkinson V., Lo S., et al., Five-year overall survival from the anti-PD1 brain collaboration (ABC Study): Randomized phase 2 study of nivolumab (nivo) or nivo+ ipilimumab (ipi) in patients (pts) with melanoma brain metastases (mets). J Clin Oncol, 39 (15_suppl). https://doi.org/10.1200/JCO.2021.39.15_suppl.9508.

20. Di Giacomo AM, Chiarion-Sileni V, Del Vecchio M, et al. Primary Analysis and 4-Year Follow-Up of the Phase III NIBIT-M2 Trial in Melanoma Patients With Brain Metastases. Clin Cancer Res 2021;27(17):4737–45.

21. Boutros C, Belkadi-Sadou D, Marchand A, et al. Cured or Not? Long-term Outcomes of Immunotherapy Responders. Focus on Melanoma. Curr Oncol Rep 2023;25(9):989–96.

22. Davies MA, Saiag P, Robert C, et al. Dabrafenib plus trametinib in patients with BRAF^{V600}-mutant melanoma brain metastases (COMBI-MB): a multicentre, multi-cohort, open-label, phase 2 trial. Lancet Oncol 2017;18(7):863–73.

23. Dummer R, Queirolo P, Gerard Duhard P, et al. Atezolizumab, vemurafenib, and cobimetinib in patients with melanoma with CNS metastases (TRICOTEL): a multi-centre, open-label, single-arm, phase 2 study. Lancet Oncol 2023;24(12): e461–71.

24. Pak BJ, Lee J, Thai BL, et al. Radiation resistance of human melanoma analysed by retroviral insertional mutagenesis reveals a possible role for dopachrome tautomerase. Oncogene 2004;23(1):30–8.

25. Tawbi HA, Boutros C, Kok D, et al. New Era in the Management of Melanoma Brain Metastases. Am Soc Clin Oncol Educ Book 2018;38:741–50.

26. Miller R, Walker S, Shui I, et al. Epidemiology and survival outcomes in stages II and III cutaneous melanoma: a systematic review. Melanoma Manag 2020;7(1): MMT39. Published 2020 Mar 19.

27. Eggermont AM, Chiarion-Sileni V, Grob JJ, et al. Adjuvant ipilimumab versus placebo after complete resection of high-risk stage III melanoma (EORTC 18071): a randomised, double-blind, phase 3 trial [published correction appears in Lancet Oncol. 2015 Jun;16(6):e262] [published correction appears in Lancet Oncol. 2016 Jun;17 (6):e223]. Lancet Oncol 2015;16(5):522–30.

28. Eggermont AMM, Chiarion-Sileni V, Grob JJ, et al. Adjuvant ipilimumab versus placebo after complete resection of stage III melanoma: long-term follow-up results of the European Organisation for Research and Treatment of Cancer 18071 double-blind phase 3 randomised trial. Eur J Cancer 2019;119:1–10.

29. Weber J, Mandala M, Del Vecchio M, et al. Adjuvant Nivolumab versus Ipilimumab in Resected Stage III or IV Melanoma. N Engl J Med 2017 09;377(19):1824–35.

30. Ascierto PA, Del Vecchio M, Mandalá M, et al. Adjuvant nivolumab versus ipilimumab in resected stage IIIB-C and stage IV melanoma (CheckMate 238): 4-year results from a multicentre, double-blind, randomised, controlled, phase 3 trial [published correction appears in Lancet Oncol. 2021 Oct;22(10):e428]. Lancet Oncol 2020;21(11):1465–77.

31. Eggermont AMM, Blank CU, Mandala M, et al. Adjuvant Pembrolizumab versus Placebo in Resected Stage III Melanoma. N Engl J Med 2018;378(19):1789–801.

32. Eggermont AMM, Blank CU, Mandala M, et al. Longer Follow-Up Confirms Recurrence-Free Survival Benefit of Adjuvant Pembrolizumab in High-Risk Stage III Melanoma: Updated Results From the EORTC 1325-MG/KEYNOTE-054 Trial. J Clin Oncol 2020;38(33):3925–36.

33. Luke JJ, Ascierto PA, Carlino MS, et al. KEYNOTE-716: Phase III study of adjuvant pembrolizumab versus placebo in resected high-risk stage II melanoma. Future Oncol 2020;16(3):4429–38.

34. Luke JJ, Ascierto PA, Khattak MA, et al. Adjuvant Pembrolizumab Shows Efficacy in High-Risk Stage II Melanoma in Adults and Children Older Than 12 - The ASCO Post [Internet]. [cited 2022 Mar 26]. Available at: https://ascopost.com/issues/october-10-2021/adjuvant-pembrolizumab-shows-efficacy-in-high-risk-stage-ii-melanoma-in-adults-and-children-older-than-12.

35. Long GV, Hauschild A, Santinami M, et al. Adjuvant Dabrafenib plus Trametinib in Stage III BRAF-Mutated Melanoma. N Engl J Med 2017;377(19):1813–23.
36. Weber JS, Carlino MS, Khattak A, et al. Individualised neoantigen therapy mRNA-4157 (V940) plus pembrolizumab versus pembrolizumab monotherapy in resected melanoma (KEYNOTE-942): a randomised, phase 2b study. Lancet 2024;403(10427):632–44.
37. Witt RG, Erstad DJ, Wargo JA. Neoadjuvant therapy for melanoma: rationale for neoadjuvant therapy and pivotal clinical trials. Ther Adv Med Oncol 2022;14. https://doi.org/10.1177/17588359221083052. 17588359221083052. Published 2022 Mar 2.
38. Hieken TJ, Kreidieh F, Aedo-Lopez V, et al. Neoadjuvant Immunotherapy in Melanoma: The Paradigm Shift. Am Soc Clin Oncol Educ Book 2023;43:e390614.
39. Lucas MW, Lijnsvelt J, Pulleman S, et al. The NADINA trial: A multicenter, randomised, phase 3 trial comparing the efficacy of neoadjuvant ipilimumab plus nivolumab with standard adjuvant nivolumab in macroscopic resectable stage III melanoma. J Clin Oncol 2022;40(suppl 16). abstr TPS9605).
40. Patel SP, Othus M, Chen Y, et al. Neoadjuvant-Adjuvant or Adjuvant-Only Pembrolizumab in Advanced Melanoma. N Engl J Med 2023;388(9):813–23.
41. Tetzlaff MT, Adhikari C, Lo S, et al. Histopathological features of complete pathological response predict recurrence-free survival following neoadjuvant targeted therapy for metastatic melanoma. Ann Oncol 2020;31(11):1569–79.
42. Tetzlaff MT, Messina JL, Stein JE, et al. Pathological assessment of resection specimens after neoadjuvant therapy for metastatic melanoma. Ann Oncol 2018;29(8):1861–8.
43. Versluis JM, Menzies AM, Sikorska K, et al. Survival update of neoadjuvant ipilimumab plus nivolumab in macroscopic stage III melanoma in the OpACIN and OpACIN-neo trials. Ann Oncol 2023;34(4):420–30.
44. Reijers ILM, Menzies AM, van Akkooi ACJ, et al. Personalized response-directed surgery and adjuvant therapy after neoadjuvant ipilimumab and nivolumab in high-risk stage III melanoma: the PRADO trial. Nat Med 2022;28(6):1178–88.
45. Amaria RN, Postow M, Burton EM, et al. Neoadjuvant relatlimab and nivolumab in resectable melanoma [published correction appears in Nature. 2023 Mar;615(7953):E23]. Nature 2022;611(7934):155–60.
46. Eroglu Z, Krinshpun S, Kalashnikova E, et al. Circulating tumor DNA-based molecular residual disease detection for treatment monitoring in advanced melanoma patients. Cancer 2023;129(11):1723–34.
47. Litchfield K, Reading JL, Puttick C, et al. Meta-analysis of tumor- and T cell-intrinsic mechanisms of sensitization to checkpoint inhibition. Cell 2021;184(3):596–614.e14.
48. Helmink BA, Reddy SM, Gao J, et al. B cells and tertiary lymphoid structures promote immunotherapy response. Nature 2020;577(7791):549–55.
49. Asrir A, Tardiveau C, Coudert J, et al. Tumor-associated high endothelial venules mediate lymphocyte entry into tumors and predict response to PD-1 plus CTLA-4 combination immunotherapy. Cancer Cell 2022;40(3):318–34.e9.
50. Robert C, Gautheret D. Multi-omics prediction in melanoma immunotherapy: A new brick in the wall. Cancer Cell 2022;40(1):14–6.
51. Robert C, Carlino MS, McNeil C, et al. Seven-Year Follow-Up of the Phase III KEYNOTE-006 Study: Pembrolizumab Versus Ipilimumab in Advanced Melanoma. J Clin Oncol 2023;41(24):3998–4003.
52. Robert C, Ribas A, Schachter J, et al. Pembrolizumab versus ipilimumab in advanced melanoma (KEYNOTE-006): post-hoc 5-year results from an open-

label, multicentre, randomised, controlled, phase 3 study. Lancet Oncol 2019; 20(9):1239–51.

53. Chesney J, Lewis KD, Kluger H, et al. Efficacy and safety of lifileucel, a one-time autologous tumor-infiltrating lymphocyte (TIL) cell therapy, in patients with advanced melanoma after progression on immune checkpoint inhibitors and targeted therapies: pooled analysis of consecutive cohorts of the C-144-01 study. J Immunother Cancer 2022;10(12):e005755.

Cancer Therapy-induced Dermatotoxicity as a Window to Understanding Skin Immunity

Yanek Jiménez-Andrade, PhD, Jessica L. Flesher, PhD, Jin Mo Park, PhD*

KEYWORDS

- Rash • Pruritis • Depigmentation • T cell • Macrophage • Epidermis • Nerve

KEY POINTS

- Therapy-induced dermatotoxicity reveals mechanisms governing skin immunity.
- Immune checkpoint inhibitors unleash T cell responses and trigger cytokine-driven dermatitis.
- Various cancer therapies alter skin neuroimmune interactions and cause itch.
- Epidermal growth factor receptor/MEK inhibitors disrupt the epidermal barrier and promote skin infection.

INTRODUCTION

The advent of targeted molecular therapy and immunotherapy in clinical oncology heralded explosive growth of data from the clinic that would shed new light on basic biology and accelerate research progress in molecular medicine. Conventional cancer therapies, which rely on nonspecific cytotoxic chemicals and radiation, generated limited insight into complex molecular pathways operating in cells and tissues and producing physiologic and pathologic outputs. Human biology could be approached and understood only through extrapolating data from preclinical model systems where sophisticated genetic tools for functional analysis were available. These limitations impeded the exploration of exactly how molecules and cells function in human tissues and the generation of mechanistic insights directly relevant to human health and disease. Unlike conventional oncology drugs, small-molecule inhibitors of signaling enzymes and monoclonal antibodies blocking ligand–receptor interactions—the main

Cutaneous Biology Research Center, Massachusetts General Hospital and Harvard Medical School, 149 Thirteenth Street, Charlestown, MA 02129, USA
* Corresponding author.
E-mail address: jmpark@mgh.harvard.edu

Hematol Oncol Clin N Am 38 (2024) 1011–1025
https://doi.org/10.1016/j.hoc.2024.05.002
0889-8588/24/© 2024 Elsevier Inc. All rights reserved.

staples of targeted molecular therapy and immunotherapy—exert their pharmacologic effects by creating a highly specific loss-of-function or gain-of-function state in vivo, akin to gene knockout and transgene expression in mice. Not only do the intended pharmacologic actions of these advanced therapeutics provide meaningful insights but their unintended adverse effects, if on-target, also reveal precious information regarding the physiologic role of the targeted molecules in the tissues where toxicity is observed.

The skin is a large organ that serves as the interface between the body and the environment. It protects against physical and chemical threats and microbial pathogens. This essential function depends on the interplay between the epidermal barrier structure and the immune system. Epidermal barrier dysfunction or impaired immunity leads to diverse forms of skin pathology. Cancer therapies are designed to suppress tumor growth or enhance antitumor immunity, but many (almost all) of those developed to date also interfere with molecular processes crucial for epithelial or immune homeostasis in the skin, producing on-target dermatotoxicity. In this review, we examine various forms of dermatotoxicity occurring in such scenarios, portray newly emerging mechanistic insights coming from their analysis, and present an updated conceptual framework of how skin immunity operates. This knowledge will also help devise novel clinical strategies for the detection, prevention, and treatment of therapy-induced dermatotoxicity in patients with cancer. For detailed information on the epidemiology, clinicopathological features, and management of cancer therapy-induced dermatotoxicity, we refer readers to comprehensive expert reviews focused on these subjects.[1–4]

THREE TELLING CASES IN CANCER THERAPY-INDUCED DERMATOTOXICITY
Cutaneous Adverse Events Caused by Immune Checkpoint Inhibitor Therapy

Cytotoxic T lymphocyte-associated protein-4 (CTLA-4), programmed cell death protein-1 (PD-1), and other immune checkpoint molecules play a crucial role in the control of adaptive immunity, restraining T cell activation in lymphoid and nonlymphoid tissues. CTLA-4 is expressed on antigen-encountered T cells and intercepts costimulatory signals from antigen-presenting cells, thereby limiting antigen-specific T cell priming.[5] PD-1 is highly expressed in T cells undergoing chronic antigen stimulation in peripheral tissues and interacts with its ligands, programmed cell death ligand-1 (PD-L1) and PD-L2, to induce a dysfunctional T cell state.[6] Monoclonal antibodies blocking CTLA-4, PD-1, and PD-L1 are major immune checkpoint inhibitors (ICIs) used in the treatment of a growing number of cancer types. In addition, new ICIs, including a lymphocyte-activated gene-3 (LAG-3) inhibitor, have become available for clinical use or are under development, expanding the arsenal of cancer immunotherapy.[7]

Immune-related adverse events (irAEs) occur in a substantial population of patients receiving all known regimens of ICI monotherapy and combination therapy. IrAEs are diverse in etiology and affect a variety of organs.[8] Being barrier tissues with continuous exposure to environmental immune stimuli and large immune cell pools in residence and transit, the skin and intestinal mucosa are the 2 most common sites where ICI-induced immunopathology is manifested. Cutaneous irAEs (cirAEs) are the most frequent type of ICI toxicity, and they develop early relative to other types of irAEs.[3] cirAE development has been consistently shown to correlate with patient response to ICI and improved survival.[9–11] ICI-induced dermatotoxicity ranges from pruritus and rash to leukoderma and alopecia and, albeit rare, also includes severe forms such as Stevens–Johnson syndrome and toxic epidermal necrolysis. Skin rashes in ICI-treated patients are heterogeneous in clinicopathological characteristics and categorized into distinct forms of dermatitis, including maculopapular, lichenoid, psoriasiform, eczematous, and bullous eruptions. Despite this broad spectrum of manifestations, ICI-induced cutaneous adversities likely share some mechanistic elements ultimately traceable to aberrant T cell activation, given that ICIs are designed to unleash T cell responses and activate T cell effector mechanisms. We revisit ICI-induced cirAEs and discuss their underlying mechanisms in upcoming sections of this review.

Cutaneous Adverse Events Caused by Macrophage-targeting Cancer Therapy

Macrophages exist in multiple subtypes and serve subtype-specific functions related to immunity and tissue maintenance. Tumor-associated macrophages (TAMs) contribute to both tumor growth and antitumor immunity depending on their functional state and interactions with other components of the tumor microenvironment. A variety of macrophage-targeted therapies have been developed and are tested for their efficacy against certain types of cancer. These therapies target molecular pathways essential for macrophage survival, recruitment, phagocytic activity, functional polarization, and interplay with adaptive immunity.[12] Macrophage-targeting agents are often combined with ICIs and other pharmacologic agents in clinical settings, making it difficult to discern macrophage-specific study outcomes. Some agents developed for macrophage-targeted therapy exert their effects on nonmacrophage targets as well. A few clinical trials, however, investigated therapeutics specifically targeting macrophages and examined their performance as monotherapy, revealing therapeutic and toxic effects most likely attributable to macrophage biology.

Colony stimulating factor-1 receptor (CSF1R), the receptor for macrophage-colony stimulating factor, transduces signals essential for macrophage development and survival. Intriguingly, preclinical studies found that CSF1R inhibition produces antitumor effects mainly by shifting TAM phenotype to an antitumor state rather than achieving complete TAM depletion.[13,14] The early promise of CSF1R inhibitors has led to numerous clinical trials on a variety of tumor types, but these studies, which evaluated CSF1R inhibition as monotherapy or its combination with ICI or CD40 agonist treatment, have shown only marginal improvements in patient response.[15–21] Another macrophage-targeting strategy that has entered clinical trials seeks to promote macrophage phagocytosis through the disruption of the CD47–signal regulatory protein α (SIRPα) axis.[22–24] Preclinical studies have shown that a range of CD47–SIRPα signaling inhibitors can promote cancer cell clearance by phagocytosis and enhance tumor immunogenicity in mice.[25–27] Macrophage-targeted therapies have been shown to cause a wide range of adverse effects including those associated with the skin. Pruritus, edema, and xerosis (dry skin) are common adverse events among patients with cancer treated with antibody or small-molecule inhibitors of CSF1R[15,18,19,21] and engineered CD47-blocking proteins.[24] These skin manifestations may be secondary to cutaneous or systemic inflammatory responses. Alternatively, perturbation of macrophage function may contribute directly to changes in sensory nerve activity and epidermal and vascular permeability in the skin.

Cutaneous Adverse Events Caused by Epidermal Growth Factor Receptor/MEK Inhibitor Therapy

The RAS-RAF-MEK-ERK pathway is activated by epidermal growth factor receptor (EGFR) and other growth factor receptors and transduces intracellular signals for cell proliferation during tissue development and regeneration. This growth factor signaling cascade is constitutively activated by mutations in a wide range of cancer types and becomes a prime target for intervention. In addition to functioning as oncogenic drivers in cancer cells, EGFR and MEK appear to serve functions essential for skin barrier integrity and antimicrobial defense. Patients with cancer treated with EGFR and MEK inhibitors display similar and closely related cutaneous toxicities in the first week of treatment initiation, including papulopustular rash in the trunk and face, pruritus, xerosis, folliculitis, and paronychia.[28,29] Both antibody and small-molecule inhibitors of EGFR cause these adverse events, suggesting on-target dermatotoxicity. EGFR inhibitor-induced dermatotoxicity is dose-dependent and correlates with treatment effectiveness.[28,29] Treatment with EGFR and MEK inhibitors results in drastic changes in the skin immune landscape and altered gene expression, which could be attributed to and downstream of skin barrier dysfunction and microbial stimulation. We discuss in detail the mechanisms linking EGFR/MEK-dependent epidermal barrier function to skin immune homeostasis in the subsequent section of this review.

MECHANISMS DRIVING CANCER THERAPY-INDUCED DERMATOTOXICITY
Pathogenic T cell States Resulting from Impaired Immune Tolerance

Developing T and B lymphocytes bearing receptors specific for self-antigens are clonally eliminated in a process referred to as central tolerance. Small fractions of self-reactive lymphocytes that have escaped this purge and exited generative lymphoid organs are subjected to additional control in peripheral tissues, which induces a state of unresponsiveness to antigen stimulation and attenuated effector function. CTLA-4 and PD-1 play a role in peripheral tolerance, mediating cell-autonomous as well as regulatory T cell-dependent mechanisms suppressing T cell activation. These immune checkpoint functions are essential for preventing autoimmunity and uncontrolled immune responses to foreign antigens from innocuous sources. ICIs enhance T cell priming against tumor antigens and steer tumor-infiltrating T cells (TILs) toward a state of augmented antitumor effector function, yet they also appear to break peripheral T cell tolerance and disrupt immune homeostasis, permitting self-destructive inflammatory responses (**Fig. 1**).

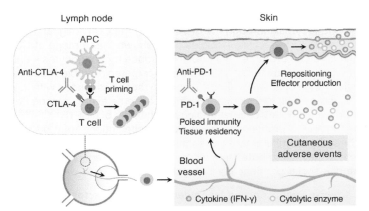

Fig. 1. Immune checkpoint inhibition unleashes T cell responses and drives T cell-mediated and cytokine-mediated dermatotoxicity. CTLA-4 inhibition enhances antigen-specific T cell priming, whereas PD-1 inhibition repositions T cells for antigen access and unlocks their effector potential. CTLA-4 and PD-1 inhibitor treatment causes cutaneous adverse events by mobilizing T cells reactive to self-antigens and commensal bacterial antigens.

Multiplex immunofluorescence imaging and spatial transcriptomics analysis have been performed of skin lesions resulting from ICI treatment (mostly PD-1 inhibitor monotherapy); this study revealed increased CD4 and CD8 T cell abundance in maculopapular, lichenoid, and bullous lesions and detected gene expression signatures of tissue-resident T cell memory (CD103, CD69) and interferon γ (IFN-γ)/tumor necrosis factor (TNF) signaling (IFN-γ, interleukin [IL]-15, TNF, chemokine [C-X-C] ligand-9/10/11 [CXCL9/10/11]) as immune features common to the 3 clinical types of dermatotoxicity.[30] These findings are, in part, consistent with what was observed in patients with ICI colitis: the single-cell transcriptomics analysis performed in 2 independent studies captured IFN-γ-producing and cytolytic enzyme-producing colonic CD8 T cells as the most prominently expanded T cell cluster during ICI-induced inflammation and provided evidence suggesting tissue-resident memory T cells as the precursor of these pathogenic effector T cells.[31,32] Taken together, these data from ICI dermatitis and colitis call attention to the need for deeper research into T cells committed to tissue residency and IFN-γ-dependent effector function as a major responder to ICI treatment in barrier organs and a driver of irAEs.

Immune checkpoint molecules appear to hold antigen-experienced T cells in check and allow them to silently coexist with their cognate antigens in peripheral tissues, a condition rendered precarious by ICIs. This idea was tested in a study that used mice in which transgenic expression of an experimental antigen was induced in adult skin and subsequently led to the mobilization of antigen-specific CD8 T cells.[33] The mouse line used in this study was designed to exert multiple layers of genetic and pharmacologic control over the transgene such that its expression would be switched on in skin areas exposed to a topically administered chemical inducer while its leaky expression in the thymus (hence central tolerance to the antigen expressed from the transgene) would be prevented. The experimental antigen, mainly detected in the epidermis upon induction, elicited skin infiltration of CD8 T cells but did not cause overt skin pathology; these T cells expressed checkpoint inhibitor molecules but did not actively produce cytokines. This local antigen expression precipitated lichenoid dermatitis, however, when combined with administration of anti-PD-1 antibody; in this pathologic condition, antigen-specific T cells, which mostly remained in the dermal area in the absence of ICI treatment, penetrated across the dermoepidermal junction, accessed antigen-expressing epidermal cells, and underwent differentiation into fully mature effector cells producing IFN-γ, TNF, and cytolytic enzymes.[33] These findings shed light on how immune checkpoint molecules keep T cells inactive upon antigen encounter in peripheral tissues and point to the T cell states and effector pathways mediating irAEs in barrier tissues. Pathogenic T cells driving cirAEs likely react to self-antigens produced from skin cells or skin microbiota-derived antigens. The source of cirAE-associated antigens as well as the type of immunity directed to them are critical determinants of the specific form of the resulting pathology.

Antigens Shared between Cancer Cells and Normal Skin Structures

The immune response to neoantigens, which arise from cancer-specific DNA, RNA, and protein alterations, is the mechanistic underpinning of ICI therapy, but the occurrence of vitiligo-like depigmentation (VLD) in ICI-treated patients with melanoma hints at an additional contribution of antigens common to melanoma cells and normal melanocytes (**Fig. 2**). Vitiligo is a group of autoimmune disorders where melanocytes are targeted for destruction by cytotoxic T cells. The prevailing mechanism for vitiligo posits a sequence of events that begins with innate immune sensing of stressed melanocytes, proceeds through the formation and skin infiltration of melanocyte-reactive CD8 T cells producing IFN-γ, and ends with T cell killing of melanocytes.[34] This

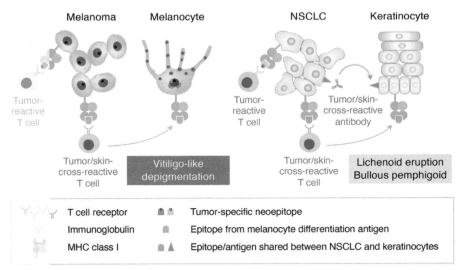

Fig. 2. T cells and antibodies recognizing antigens shared between cancer cells and normal skin cells drive autoimmune-mediated cutaneous adverse events. Melanoma and NSCLC may elicit autoreactive T cells and autoantibodies that attack melanocytes and keratinocytes.

pathogenic process is amplified by IFN-γ-stimulated keratinocytes, which produce the chemokines CXCL9/10 and thereby recruit additional T cells,[35,36] and sustained by tissue-resident memory T cells, which depend on IL-15 for persistence in lesional skin.[37] T cells recognizing melanocyte differentiation antigens (MDAs)—pigmentation-related proteins expressed in highly differentiated melanocytes such as Melan-A (also known as MART-1), tyrosinase, and gp100—have been detected in patients with vitiligo[38,39] as well as in patients with melanoma who responded to ICI therapy.[40,41] Studies have identified T cell receptor (TCR) clonotypes shared between patient-matched melanoma and VLD lesions.[42,43] Research performed in mouse models has shown that melanoma immunotherapy, when effectively controlling tumors through neoantigen-directed immune responses, leads to an increase in MDA-specific TILs and memory T cells, immune-mediated depigmentation, and protection against newly engrafted MDA-expressing tumors with a low neoantigen load,[41,44,45] suggesting a widened repertoire of antigens associated with T cell immunity. This epitope spreading may be attributable to either de novo formation of MDA-specific T cells or a drastic expansion of their pools from pre-existing precursors. In addition to MDAs, immune attack of melanocytes in ICI-treated patients may involve other self-antigens expressed across multiple tissues given that VLD has been reported to develop in patients with nonmelanoma cancer.[46–48]

Non-small cell lung cancer (NSCLC) and normal skin exhibit a substantial degree of overlap in their transcriptomes with many predicted T cell antigens coexpressed in both tissues (see **Fig. 2**). An analysis of ICI-treated patients with NSCLC revealed that some of these shared antigens, including keratin-6, keratin-14, desmocollin-3, maspin (also known as serpin-B5), and LL37 (also known as cathelicidin), were associated with cirAE incidence; some TCR clonotypes of peripheral blood T cells reactive to these antigens were also detected among the TILs and lesional skin T cells of these patients.[49] A study performed under a similar design of sampling and analysis found that other proteins common to NSCLC tumors and normal skin, such as BP180 (also known as the α1 chain of collagen-7), served as B-cell antigens: titers of serum immunoglobulin (Ig)-G specific for BP180 were associated with the rate of cirAEs and predictive of ICI response and prolonged survival.[50] Of note, although autoantibodies against BP180 are best known as a pathogenic factor of bullous pemphigoid with their ability to promote skin blister formation well established, the form of dermatotoxicity with which BP180-specific IgG titers showed a correlation in this study was lichenoid dermatitis. This finding does not necessarily indicate a causal role for BP180-specific IgG in the formation of lichenoid lesions; this autoantibody may arise as a byproduct of immune dysregulation in ICI-treated NSCLC patients, yet still it has the potential to serve as a predictive marker for cirAE development.

Aberrant Neuroimmune Interactions and Sensitized Pruritic Neural Circuits

Pruritus is common among patients with cancer treated with ICIs, CSF1R inhibitors, CD47 blockers, and EGFR/MEK inhibitors. The mechanisms by which these therapeutics induce itch have yet to be understood. Itch is mediated by a subset of unmyelinated C-fibers in the skin. These pruriceptive nerves relay signals to the spinal cord and brain to evoke itch and trigger scratching.[51] Immune cell-derived and keratinocyte-derived cytokines, derivatives of amino acids and arachidonic acids, neuropeptides, and proteases activate or sensitize pruriceptive nerves, thereby functioning as endogenous pruritogens (**Fig. 3**).

Skin biopsies and serum from patients with ICI-induced eczematous rash and bullous pemphigoid often exhibit histologic and molecular features associated with pruritus, such as eosinophilia[52,53] and elevated production of IgE[52] and IL-4/IL-13[54,55]; high percentages of these patients respond to omalizumab and dupilumab, antibodies neutralizing IgE and blocking IL-4Rα, respectively, showing a significant improvement in pruritis and rash.[52,53,55,56] IL-4 Rα, a chain of the receptor that binds

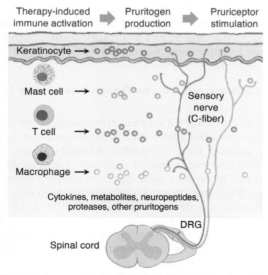

Fig. 3. Cancer therapy activates neuroimmune signaling and stimulates pruritic neural circuits. Keratinocytes and immune cells produce various endogenous pruritogens and stimulate pruriceptive sensory neurons, a subset of DRG neurons relaying itch signals to the central nervous system.

to both IL-4 and IL-13, is expressed in a multitude of cell types and serves signaling functions related to barrier tissue inflammation and allergic reactions. Intriguingly, IL-4Rα is also highly expressed in the subtypes of sensory neurons crucial for itch and has been shown to mediate IL-4/IL-13-dependent sensitization of skin nerves to various pruritogens.[57] There are other cytokines known to exert direct action on sensory neurons and trigger or sensitize to itch, the most notable of which are thymic stromal lymphopoietin,[58] IL-31,[59] and oncostatin-M.[60] Multiplex cytokine profiling has captured IL-31 in elevated amounts in the skin of ICI-treated patients with pruritus.[61] Whether IL-31 and other pruritogenic cytokines are produced in amounts sufficient to induce itch in cirAE settings remains to be rigorously studied.

Sensory neurons innervating the skin have been reported to express PD-1 and PD-L1; studies of neuronal PD-1 and PD-L1 signaling in mice have shown its ability to modulate the excitability of nociceptive and pruriceptive neurons and inhibit pain and itch.[62–67] These studies yielded results that were incongruous with one another in mechanistic details but raised the interesting possibility that ICIs might cause pruritus by acting directly on sensory neurons and disinhibiting pruriception rather than through mechanisms secondary to inflammation and mediated by neuroactive cytokines produced from nonneuronal cells.

Pruritus is common and often the most frequent type of adverse event among patients with cancer treated with macrophage-targeting agents, including CSF1R inhibitors[15,18,19,21] and CD47 antagonists.[24] The dorsal root ganglion (DRG) contains the somata of pruriceptors and other sensory neurons innervating the skin as well as immune cells including macrophages. Subsets of DRG-resident and skin-resident macrophages patrol neuronal somata and nerve fibers for surveillance and contribute to their regeneration after tissue injury.[68,69] Furthermore, these macrophages have been shown to modulate neuronal gene expression and metabolism to set the threshold for and terminate sensory stimulation[70,71] as well as produce IL-31 and other pruritogens.[72–74] CSF1R inhibitors, CD47 blockers, and other macrophage-targeting agents may cause pruritus by depleting or functionally disrupting macrophages in the DRG and skin. A better understanding of the nature of these sensory anomalies requires studies that delve deeper into the mechanisms governing macrophage–neuron interactions and macrophage-dependent maintenance and functional modulation of pruriceptive neurons.

Epithelial Barrier Dysfunction and Immune Dysregulation Linked to Skin and Gut Bacteria

Acneiform eruptions and bacterial superinfection frequently occur in patients with cancer treated with EGFR and MEK inhibitors.[28,29] *Staphylococcus aureus* is one of the bacteria frequently isolated from EGFR/MEK inhibitor-induced skin lesions.[75–77] Studies that generated and characterized mice with keratinocyte-restricted EGFR gene ablation found that these mice exhibited increased epidermal permeability (as extrapolated from a higher rate of transepidermal water loss) and a signature of skin gene expression indicative of a defective skin barrier.[77,78] Skin barrier dysfunction in mice lacking epidermal EGFR expression was accompanied by the influx of mast cells, macrophages, eosinophils, neutrophils, and T cells in lesional skin (**Fig. 4**); among these immune cell types, macrophage function and mast cell degranulation were found to contribute to skin pathology, as macrophage depletion and inhibition of histamine signaling with pharmacologic agents suppressed abnormal epidermal differentiation and T cell infiltration in skin lesions, respectively.[78,79] The outgrowth of bacteria in the skin of EGFR/MEK inhibitor-treated patients with cancer likely activates microbial sensor-dependent innate immune signaling. Bacterial stimuli and EGFR/MEK inhibition

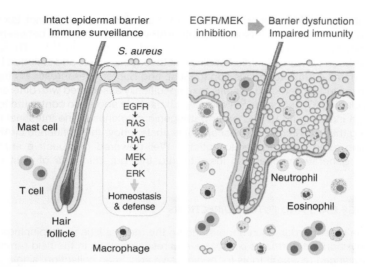

Fig. 4. EGFR/MEK inhibitors disrupts the skin barrier function and impairs antibacterial defense. Intracellular signaling downstream of EGFR is essential for skin homeostasis and immune defense. Inhibition of this signaling results in barrier dysfunction, hair follicle infection, and immunopathology. *Staphylococcus aureus* is the common etiologic agent associated with EGFR/MEK inhibitor-induced cutaneous adverse events.

have indeed been shown to act together to reshape keratinocyte gene expression, induce epithelial cytokines such as IL-36γ, and promote cutaneous neutrophilia.[80]

Commensal bacteria in healthy human skin perform functions beneficial to the host, such as controlling pathogenic microbial growth and training the skin immune system. T cells primed to respond to commensal bacterial antigens or innate-like T cells hard-wired to sense microbial metabolites are recruited to barrier tissues inhabited by the antigen/metabolite-producing microbes, yet these T cells persist there without triggering inflammation and pathology, a state referred to as homeostatic immunity.[81] Immune checkpoint molecules are thought to play an essential role in keeping commensal-specific T cells locked in a poised state for activation and cytokine production and preventing their activation in the steady-state skin with an intact epidermal barrier. This idea was supported by a study that investigated mice whose skin was colonized with *Staphylococcus epidermidis*, a commensal inhabiting the human skin. *S epidermidis*-colonized mice did not display perceptible skin pathology but developed severe dermatitis when administered anti-CTLA-4 antibody, which by itself did not induce inflammation.[82] Skin disease resulting from *S epidermidis* colonization in the absence of CTLA-4 function was driven by both CD4 and CD8 T cells and depended on IL-17A but not IFN-γ. Similar commensal-CTLA-4 inhibitor cooperation has been observed in mice harboring the gut microbiota from wild-caught mice; these mice developed colitis in a manner dependent on IFN-γ-producing CD4 T cells but not CD8 T cells or IL-17 A/F-producing T cells.[83] These findings show that ICIs can break T cell tolerance in barrier tissues and unleash inflammatory responses driven by T cells specific to self-antigens or antigens derived from innocuous commensals.

The gut microbiota, the largest microbial community in the human body, exerts local and systemic influences on physiology and pathology by interacting with the immune and neuroendocrine systems. Gut microbiota composition affects not only response to ICIs but also irAE incidence. Studies have captured several distinct taxa of the baseline gut microbiota as associated with irAEs although there is between-cohort and interstudy heterogeneity in the data and conclusions.[84–87] These irAE-associated bacteria were identified at different taxonomic levels and included Lachno-spiraceae (family), *Streptococcus* spp (genus), and *Bacteroides intestinalis* (species). One of these studies detected specific taxa specifically associated with different types of irAEs including ICI dermatitis.[87] Whereas gut bacteria appear to contribute to ICI co-litis through inducing IL-1β and other pathogenic cytokines in the intestinal mucosa and altering the local immune landscape, it is unclear how they influence cirAE development and exert other systemic actions. Well-powered prospective studies are needed to generate mechanistic insights into this gut–skin axis of host–microbe interactions.

KNOWLEDGE GAPS AND FUTURE DIRECTIONS

Despite the recent progress in understanding the mechanistic underpinnings of cancer therapy-induced dermatotoxicity, several research gaps in the field remain to be closed. Advanced research tools for noninvasive specimen collection, single-cell molecular profiling, and spatial imaging should be leveraged to analyze skin lesions from patients developing cirAEs. Comprehensive and unbiased data from such analyses will uncover as-yet-unidentified molecular processes causally linked to cirAE mechanisms. Preclinical models that closely resemble pruritus, rash, VLD, and other manifestations of dermatotoxicity in humans will propel research into the underlying molecular mechanisms and help discover targets for the management of cutaneous adverse events. Severe dermatotoxicity often results in therapy interruption and discontinuation, preventing otherwise promising cancer therapeutics from realizing their full potential. Effective treatments tailored to individual forms of dermatotoxicity will improve toxicity management and maximize patient benefit. Another important question in the areas of targeted molecular therapy and immunotherapy is whether clinical strategies could be devised to suppress the toxicity of therapeutic agents while preserving their efficacy. A preclinical study showed that although anti-CTLA-4 therapy promoted both antitumor immune responses and intestinal inflammatory damage in mice, the latter (ICI colitis) depended on Ig Fcγ receptor signaling, whereas this signaling function is dispensable for the former (tumor eradication); anti-CTLA-4 nano-bodies, which lacked an Fc domain, could circumvent intestinal toxicity without sacrificing their antitumor effects.[83] The management of cirAEs, and irAEs in general, in ICI-treated patients requires such strategies for dissociating antitumor immunity and treatment toxicity.

The use of targeted molecular therapy and immunotherapy for cancer treatment will continue to grow. Their armamentarium is expanding with new small-molecule therapeutics and biologics entering the clinical space. This progress will certainly push cancer treatment forward; it will also generate massive amounts of data that deepen our understanding of human biology and enable the development of more powerful technologies for improved patient care.

DISCLOSURE

J.L. Flesher is supported by NIH, United States T32AR007098 (Dermatology Training Grant). J.M. Park is supported by NIH R01AI177414, has a consulting role with Chong Kun Dang Pharmaceutical, and has received research funding from Pfizer, United States and Evommune.

REFERENCES

1. Lacouture ME. Mechanisms of cutaneous toxicities to EGFR inhibitors. Nat Rev Cancer 2006;6:803–12.
2. Lacouture M, Sibaud V. Toxic side effects of targeted therapies and immunotherapies affecting the skin, oral mucosa, hair, and nails. Am J Clin Dermatol 2018; 19:31–9.
3. Geisler AN, Phillips GS, Barrios DM, et al. Immune checkpoint inhibitor-related dermatologic adverse events. J Am Acad Dermatol 2020;83:1255–68.
4. Allais BS, Fay CJ, Kim DY, et al. Cutaneous immune-related adverse events from immune checkpoint inhibitor therapy: Moving beyond "maculopapular rash". Immunol Rev 2023;318:22–36.
5. Sharma P, Siddiqui BA, Anandhan S, et al. The next decade of immune checkpoint therapy. Cancer Discov 2021;11:838–57.
6. Sharpe AH, Pauken KE. The diverse functions of the PD1 inhibitory pathway. Nat Rev Immunol 2018;18:153–67.
7. Sharma P, Goswami S, Raychaudhuri D, et al. Immune checkpoint therapy-current perspectives and future directions. Cell 2023;186:1652–69.
8. Dougan M, Luoma AM, Dougan SK, et al. Understanding and treating the inflammatory adverse events of cancer immunotherapy. Cell 2021;184:1575–88.
9. Teulings HE, Limpens J, Jansen SN, et al. Vitiligo-like depigmentation in patients with stage III-IV melanoma receiving immunotherapy and its association with survival: a systematic review and meta-analysis. J Clin Oncol 2015;33:773–81.
10. Min Lee CK, Li S, Tran DC, et al. Characterization of dermatitis after PD-1/PD-L1 inhibitor therapy and association with multiple oncologic outcomes: A retrospective case-control study. J Am Acad Dermatol 2018;79:1047–52.
11. Zhang S, Tang K, Wan G, et al. Cutaneous immune-related adverse events are associated with longer overall survival in advanced cancer patients on immune checkpoint inhibitors: A multi-institutional cohort study. J Am Acad Dermatol 2023;88:1024–32.
12. Mantovani A, Allavena P, Marchesi F, et al. Macrophages as tools and targets in cancer therapy. Nat Rev Drug Discov 2022;21:799–820.
13. Pyonteck SM, Akkari L, Schuhmacher AJ, et al. CSF-1R inhibition alters macrophage polarization and blocks glioma progression. Nat Med 2013;19:1264–72.
14. Zhu Y, Knolhoff BL, Meyer MA, et al. CSF1/CSF1R blockade reprograms tumor-infiltrating macrophages and improves response to T-cell checkpoint immunotherapy in pancreatic cancer models. Cancer Res 2014;74:5057–69.
15. Cassier PA, Italiano A, Gomez-Roca CA, et al. CSF1R inhibition with emactuzumab in locally advanced diffuse-type tenosynovial giant cell tumours of the soft tissue: a dose-escalation and dose-expansion phase 1 study. Lancet Oncol 2015;16:949–56.
16. Wiehagen KR, Girgis NM, Yamada DH, et al. Combination of CD40 Agonism and CSF-1R blockade reconditions tumor-associated macrophages and drives potent antitumor immunity. Cancer Immunol Res 2017;5:1109–21.
17. Hoves S, Ooi CH, Wolter C, et al. Rapid activation of tumor-associated macrophages boosts preexisting tumor immunity. J Exp Med 2018;215:859–76.
18. Gomez-Roca CA, Italiano A, Le Tourneau C, et al. Phase I study of emactuzumab single agent or in combination with paclitaxel in patients with advanced/metastatic solid tumors reveals depletion of immunosuppressive M2-like macrophages. Ann Oncol 2019;30:1381–92.

19. Cassier PA, Italiano A, Gomez-Roca C, et al. Long-term clinical activity, safety and patient-reported quality of life for emactuzumab-treated patients with diffuse-type tenosynovial giant-cell tumour. Eur J Cancer 2020;141:162–70.

20. Gomez-Roca C, Cassier P, Zamarin D, et al. Anti-CSF-1R emactuzumab in combination with anti-PD-L1 atezolizumab in advanced solid tumor patients naïve or experienced for immune checkpoint blockade. J Immunother Cancer 2022;10: e004076.

21. Johnson M, Dudek AZ, Sukari A, et al. ARRY-382 in combination with pembrolizumab in patients with advanced solid tumors: results from a phase 1b/2 study. Clin Cancer Res 2022;28:2517–26.

22. Johnson LDS, Banerjee S, Kruglov O, et al. Targeting CD47 in Sézary syndrome with SIRPαFc. Blood Adv 2019;3:1145–53.

23. Ansell SM, Maris MB, Lesokhin AM, et al. Phase I Study of the CD47 Blocker TTI-621 in Patients with Relapsed or Refractory Hematologic Malignancies. Clin Cancer Res 2021;27:2190–9.

24. Lakhani NJ, Chow LQM, Gainor JF, et al. Evorpacept alone and in combination with pembrolizumab or trastuzumab in patients with advanced solid tumours (ASPEN-01): a first-in-human, open-label, multicentre, phase 1 dose-escalation and dose-expansion study. Lancet Oncol 2021;22:1740–51.

25. Willingham SB, Volkmer JP, Gentles AJ, et al. The CD47-signal regulatory protein alpha (SIRPa) interaction is a therapeutic target for human solid tumors. Proc Natl Acad Sci U S A 2012;109:6662–7.

26. Sockolosky JT, Dougan M, Ingram JR, et al. Durable antitumor responses to CD47 blockade require adaptive immune stimulation. Proc Natl Acad Sci U S A 2016;113:E2646–54.

27. Weiskopf K, Jahchan NS, Schnorr PJ, et al. CD47-blocking immunotherapies stimulate macrophage-mediated destruction of small-cell lung cancer. J Clin Invest 2016;126:2610–20.

28. Macdonald JB, Macdonald B, Golitz LE, et al. Cutaneous adverse effects of targeted therapies: Part I: Inhibitors of the cellular membrane. J Am Acad Dermatol 2015;72:203–18.

29. Macdonald JB, Macdonald B, Golitz LE, et al. Cutaneous adverse effects of targeted therapies: Part II: Inhibitors of intracellular molecular signaling pathways. J Am Acad Dermatol 2015;72:221–36.

30. Reschke R, Shapiro JW, Yu J, et al. Checkpoint blockade-induced dermatitis and colitis are dominated by tissue-resident memory T Cells and Th1/Tc1 Cytokines. Cancer Immunol Res 2022;10:1167–74.

31. Luoma AM, Suo S, Williams HL, et al. Molecular pathways of colon inflammation induced by cancer immunotherapy. Cell 2020;182:655–71.

32. Sasson SC, Slevin SM, Cheung VTF, et al. Interferon-Gamma-Producing CD8+ Tissue Resident Memory T Cells Are a Targetable Hallmark of Immune Checkpoint Inhibitor-Colitis. Gastroenterology 2021;161:1229–44.

33. Damo M, Hornick NI, Venkat A, et al. PD-1 maintains CD8 T cell tolerance towards cutaneous neoantigens. Nature 2023;619:151–9.

34. Frisoli ML, Essien K, Harris JE. Vitiligo: Mechanisms of Pathogenesis and Treatment. Annu Rev Immunol 2020;38:621–48.

35. Rashighi M, Agarwal P, Richmond JM, et al. CXCL10 is critical for the progression and maintenance of depigmentation in a mouse model of vitiligo. Sci Transl Med 2014;6:223ra23.

36. Richmond JM, Bangari DS, Essien KI, et al. Keratinocyte-Derived Chemokines Orchestrate T-Cell Positioning in the Epidermis during Vitiligo and May Serve as Biomarkers of Disease. J Invest Dermatol 2017;137:350–8.

37. Richmond JM, Strassner JP, Zapata L Jr, et al. Antibody blockade of IL-15 signaling has the potential to durably reverse vitiligo. Sci Transl Med 2018;10:eaam7710.

38. Ogg GS, Rod Dunbar P, Romero P, et al. High frequency of skin-homing melanocyte-specific cytotoxic T lymphocytes in autoimmune vitiligo. J Exp Med 1998; 188:1203–8.

39. Palermo B, Campanelli R, Garbelli S, et al. Specific cytotoxic T lymphocyte responses against Melan-A/MART1, tyrosinase and gp100 in vitiligo by the use of major histocompatibility complex/peptide tetramers: the role of cellular immunity in the etiopathogenesis of vitiligo. J Invest Dermatol 2001;117:326–32.

40. Klein O, Ebert LM, Nicholaou T, et al. Melan-A-specific cytotoxic T cells are associated with tumor regression and autoimmunity following treatment with anti-CTLA-4. Clin Cancer Res 2009;15:2507–13.

41. Lo JA, Kawakubo M, Juneja VR, et al. Epitope spreading toward wild-type melanocyte-lineage antigens rescues suboptimal immune checkpoint blockade responses. Sci Transl Med 2021;13:eabd8636.

42. Becker JC, Guldberg P, Zeuthen J, et al. Accumulation of identical T cells in melanoma and vitiligo-like leukoderma. J Invest Dermatol 1999;113:1033–8.

43. Carbone ML, Capone A, Guercio M, et al. Insight into immune profile associated with vitiligo onset and anti-tumoral response in melanoma patients receiving anti-PD-1 immunotherapy. Front Immunol 2023;14:1197630.

44. Zhang P, Côté AL, de Vries VC, et al. Induction of postsurgical tumor immunity and T-cell memory by a poorly immunogenic tumor. Cancer Res 2007;67:6468–76.

45. Byrne KT, Côté AL, Zhang P, et al. Autoimmune melanocyte destruction is required for robust CD8+ memory T cell responses to mouse melanoma. J Clin Invest 2011;121:1797–809.

46. Yin ES, Totonchy MB, Leventhal JS. Nivolumab-associated vitiligo-like depigmentation in a patient with acute myeloid leukemia: A novel finding. JAAD Case Rep 2017;3:90–2.

47. Kosche C, Mohindra N, Choi JN. Vitiligo in a patient undergoing nivolumab treatment for non-small cell lung cancer. JAAD Case Rep 2018;4:1042–4.

48. Liu RC, Consuegra G, Chou S, et al. Vitiligo-like depigmentation in oncology patients treated with immunotherapies for nonmelanoma metastatic cancers. Clin Exp Dermatol 2019;44:643–6.

49. Berner F, Bomze D, Diem S, et al. Association of Checkpoint Inhibitor-Induced Toxic Effects With Shared Cancer and Tissue Antigens in Non-Small Cell Lung Cancer. JAMA Oncol 2019;5:1043–7.

50. Hasan Ali O, Bomze D, Ring SS, et al. BP180-specific IgG is associated with skin adverse events, therapy response, and overall survival in non-small cell lung cancer patients treated with checkpoint inhibitors. J Am Acad Dermatol 2020;82: 854–61.

51. Cevikbas F, Lerner EA. Physiology and Pathophysiology of Itch. Physiol Rev 2020;100:945–82.

52. Phillips GS, Wu J, Hellmann MD, et al. Treatment Outcomes of Immune-Related Cutaneous Adverse Events. J Clin Oncol 2019;37:2746–58.

53. Barrios DM, Phillips GS, Geisler AN, et al. IgE blockade with omalizumab reduces pruritus related to immune checkpoint inhibitors and anti-HER2 therapies. Ann Oncol 2021;32:736–45.

54. Lim SY, Lee JH, Gide TN, et al. Circulating Cytokines Predict Immune-Related Toxicity in Melanoma Patients Receiving Anti-PD-1-Based Immunotherapy. Clin Cancer Res 2019;25:1557–63.

55. Shipman WD, Singh K, Cohen JM, et al. Immune checkpoint inhibitor-induced bullous pemphigoid is characterized by interleukin (IL)-4 and IL-13 expression and responds to dupilumab treatment. Br J Dermatol 2023;189:339–41.

56. Kuo AM, Gu S, Stoll J, et al. Management of immune-related cutaneous adverse events with dupilumab. J Immunother Cancer 2023;11:e007324.

57. Oetjen LK, Mack MR, Feng J, et al. Sensory Neurons Co-opt Classical Immune Signaling Pathways to Mediate Chronic Itch. Cell 2017;171:217–28.

58. Wilson SR, Thé L, Batia LM, et al. The epithelial cell-derived atopic dermatitis cytokine TSLP activates neurons to induce itch. Cell 2013;155:285–95.

59. Cevikbas F, Wang X, Akiyama T, et al. A sensory neuron-expressed IL-31 receptor mediates T helper cell-dependent itch: Involvement of TRPV1 and TRPA1. J Allergy Clin Immunol 2014;133:448–60.

60. Tseng PY, Hoon MA. Oncostatin M can sensitize sensory neurons in inflammatory pruritus. Sci Transl Med 2021;13:eabe3037.

61. Wang E, Lyubchenko T, Goleva E, et al. Checkpoint inhibition induced pruritus during cancer therapy is associated with skin IL-31 and CCL22 expression. J Allergy Clin Invest 2022;149:ab173.

62. Chen G, Kim YH, Li H, et al. PD-L1 inhibits acute and chronic pain by suppressing nociceptive neuron activity via PD-1. Nat Neurosci 2017;20:917–26.

63. Liu BL, Cao QL, Zhao X, et al. Inhibition of TRPV1 by SHP-1 in nociceptive primary sensory neurons is critical in PD-L1 analgesia. JCI Insight 2020;5:e137386.

64. Zhao L, Luo H, Ma Y, et al. An analgesic peptide H-20 attenuates chronic pain via the PD-1 pathway with few adverse effects. Proc Natl Acad Sci U S A 2022;119. e2204114119.

65. Meerschaert KA, Edwards BS, Epouhe AY, et al. Neuronally expressed PDL1, not PD1, suppresses acute nociception. Brain Behav Immun 2022;106:233–46.

66. Wanderley CWS, Maganin AGM, Adjafre B, et al. PD-1/PD-L1 Inhibition Enhances Chemotherapy-Induced Neuropathic Pain by Suppressing Neuroimmune Antinociceptive Signaling. Cancer Immunol Res 2022;10:1299–308.

67. Xu ZH, Zhang JC, Chen K, et al. Mechanisms of the PD-1/PD-L1 pathway in itch: From acute itch model establishment to the role in chronic itch in mouse. Eur J Pharmacol 2023;960:176128.

68. Kolter J, Feuerstein R, Zeis P, et al. A Subset of Skin Macrophages Contributes to the Surveillance and Regeneration of Local Nerves. Immunity 2019;50:1482–97.

69. Feng R, Muraleedharan SV, Mokalled MH, et al. Self-renewing macrophages in dorsal root ganglia contribute to promote nerve regeneration. Proc Natl Acad Sci U S A 2023;120. e2215906120.

70. van der Vlist M, Raoof R, Willemen HLDM, et al. Macrophages transfer mitochondria to sensory neurons to resolve inflammatory pain. Neuron 2022;110:613–26.

71. Tanaka T, Okuda H, Isonishi A, et al. Dermal macrophages set pain sensitivity by modulating the amount of tissue NGF through an SNX25-Nrf2 pathway. Nat Immunol 2023;24:439–51.

72. Luo J, Feng J, Yu G, et al. Transient receptor potential vanilloid 4-expressing macrophages and keratinocytes contribute differentially to allergic and nonallergic chronic itch. J Allergy Clin Immunol 2018;141:608–19.

73. Hashimoto T, Kursewicz CD, Fayne RA, et al. Mechanisms of Itch in Stasis Dermatitis: Significant Role of IL-31 from Macrophages. J Invest Dermatol 2020;140: 850–9.

74. Hashimoto T, Yokozeki H, Karasuyama H, et al. IL-31-generating network in atopic dermatitis comprising macrophages, basophils, thymic stromal lympho-poietin, and periostin. J Allergy Clin Immunol 2023;151:737–46.
75. Grenader T, Gipps M, Goldberg A. Staphylococcus aureus bacteremia second-ary to severe erlotinib skin toxicity. Clin Lung Cancer 2008;9:59–60.
76. Balagula Y, Barth Huston K, Busam KJ, et al. Dermatologic side effects associ-ated with the MEK 1/2 inhibitor selumetinib (AZD6244, ARRY-142886). Invest New Drugs 2011;29:1114–21.
77. Lichtenberger BM, Gerber PA, Holcmann M, et al. Epidermal EGFR controls cuta-neous host defense and prevents inflammation. Sci Transl Med 2013;5:199ra111.
78. Klufa J, Bauer T, Hanson B, et al. Hair eruption initiates and commensal skin mi-crobiota aggravate adverse events of anti-EGFR therapy. Sci Transl Med 2019; 11:eaax2693.
79. Mascia F, Lam G, Keith C, et al. Genetic ablation of epidermal EGFR reveals the dynamic origin of adverse effects of anti-EGFR therapy. Sci Transl Med 2013;5: 199ra110.
80. Satoh TK, Mellett M, Meier-Schiesser B, et al. IL-36γ drives skin toxicity induced by EGFR/MEK inhibition and commensal Cutibacterium acnes. J Clin Invest 2020;130:1417–30.
81. Belkaid Y, Harrison OJ. Homeostatic Immunity and the Microbiota. Immunity 2017;46:562–76.
82. Hu ZI, Link VM, Lima-Junior DS, et al. Immune checkpoint inhibitors unleash path-ogenic immune responses against the microbiota. Proc Natl Acad Sci U S A 2022;119. e2200348119.
83. Lo BC, Kryczek I, Yu J, et al. Microbiota-dependent activation of CD4+ T cells in-duces CTLA-4 blockade-associated colitis via Fcγ receptors. Science 2024;383: 62–70.
84. Chaput N, Lepage P, Coutzac C, et al. Baseline gut microbiota predicts clinical response and colitis in metastatic melanoma patients treated with ipilimumab. Ann Oncol 2017;28:1368–79.
85. Dubin K, Callahan MK, Ren B, et al. Intestinal microbiome analyses identify mel-anoma patients at risk for checkpoint-blockade-induced colitis. Nat Commun 2016;7:10391.
86. Andrews MC, Duong CPM, Gopalakrishnan V, et al. Gut microbiota signatures are associated with toxicity to combined CTLA-4 and PD-1 blockade. Nat Med 2021; 27:1432–41.
87. McCulloch JA, Davar D, Rodrigues RR, et al. Intestinal microbiota signatures of clinical response and immune-related adverse events in melanoma patients treated with anti-PD-1. Nat Med 2022;28:545–56.

Melanoma Brain Metastasis
Biology and Therapeutic Advances

Merve Hasanov, MD[a],*, Yusuf Acikgoz, MD[b],
Michael A. Davies, MD, PhD[c]

KEYWORDS

- Melanoma brain metastasis • Immunotherapy • Targeted therapy

KEY POINTS

- Melanoma brain metastasis (MBM) is a common and deadly complication of advanced melanoma.
- Outcomes in MBM patients have improved with the development of more effective systemic therapies and radiation, but outcomes remain poor for patients with symptomatic MBMs or leptomeningeal disease.
- The identification of unique molecular and immune characteristics of MBMs provides new insights into their pathogenesis and therapeutic resistance and suggests new therapeutic opportunities.

INTRODUCTION

Melanoma, the deadliest of the common skin cancers, has the highest propensity to metastasize to the brain among solid tumors. Approximately 11% to 17% of early-stage melanoma[1,2] and up to 60% of stage IV melanoma patients develop brain metastasis.[3] Risk factors for melanoma brain metastasis (MBM) include patient sex, age, American Joint Committee on Cancer stage, primary tumor site, Breslow thickness, and primary tumor mitotic rate.[1,2,4] While MBMs can cause multiple symptoms (including headaches, seizures, or neurologic changes), many melanoma patients are

Funding statement: Dr M.A. Davies acknowledges grant funding support from the Dr. Miriam and Sheldon G. Adelson Medical Research Foundation (FP17016), the NIH/NCI (5P50CA221703–05), the American Cancer Society (134148-MRAT-19–168–01), and the Melanoma Research Alliance (#687055)
[a] Division of Medical Oncology, Department of Internal Medicine, The Ohio State University Comprehensive Cancer Center, Suite 1335, Lincoln Tower, 1800 Cannon Drive, Columbus, OH, 43210, USA; [b] Division of Medical Oncology, Department of Internal Medicine, The Ohio State University Comprehensive Cancer Center, 13th floor, Lincoln Tower, 1800 Cannon Drive, Columbus, OH, 43210, USA; [c] Division of Cancer Medicine, Department of Melanoma Medical Oncology, The University of Texas MD Anderson Cancer Center, 1515 Holcombe Boulevard, Unit 0430, Houston, TX 77030, USA
* Corresponding author. Suite 1335 Lincoln Tower, 1800 Cannon Drive, Columbus, OH 43210.
E-mail address: merve.hasanov@osumc.edu

Hematol Oncol Clin N Am 38 (2024) 1027–1043
https://doi.org/10.1016/j.hoc.2024.05.008
hemonc.theclinics.com
0889-8588/24/© 2024 Elsevier Inc. All rights reserved.

diagnosed with asymptomatic tumors because of regular central nervous system (CNS) radiographic surveillance.[3,5]

In the past, the prognosis of MBM patients was grim, with a median overall survival (OS) of 4 to 6 months.[6] However, recent studies support that median OS is now 1 to 1.5 years, likely because of improved local stereotactic radiosurgery (SRS) and systemic (immune and targeted therapies) treatment options.[5,7,8] Despite these advances, responses to these treatments in MBMs are often not as robust and durable as in extracranial metastases (ECMs). Recent research suggests that this may be due, at least in part, to the unique molecular and immune features of MBMs. Interestingly, some of these distinctive features also confer unique vulnerabilities and therapeutic opportunities.

THERAPEUTIC ADVANCES IN MELANOMA BRAIN METASTASIS
Immunotherapies

High-dose interleukin-2 was the first immunotherapy approved for stage IV melanoma. However, this treatment was suboptimal for MBM patients because of its toxicity profile and low efficacy, with intracranial response rates (ICRR) of 6% in previously untreated MBMs.[9] There have been several immune checkpoint inhibitors (ICIs) approved as single agents and in combinations over the past decade for patients with stage IV melanoma. The registrational studies of all these agents excluded patients with new or progressing MBMs. However, post-approval studies have demonstrated their safety, activity, and limitations in patients with MBMs (Table 1).

The first prospective clinical trial of an ICI for MBM patients was a 2-arm phase II trial of ipilimumab, an anti-CTLA-4 antibody approved for stage II melanoma patients in 2011.[10] The study included 2 cohorts of patients: cohort A patients (n = 51) had asymptomatic MBMs and cohort B patients (n = 21) had symptomatic MBMs on a stable steroid dose. Patients received 4 doses of high-dose ipilimumab (HD-Ipi; 10 mg/kg) every 3 weeks; patients with clinical benefit could then receive maintenance HD-Ipi every 12 weeks. The ICRR per immune-related response criteria was 16% and 5% in cohorts A and B, respectively. The intracranial progression-free survival (iPFS) was 1.9 months and 1.2 months, respectively. A randomized phase III trial for asymptomatic MBM, comparing HD-Ipi (n = 65) to Food and Drug Administration (FDA)-approved dose ipilimumab (Ipi; 3 mg/kg, n = 62), resulted in similar median OS of 7.0 and 5.7 months, respectively. This was a larger study than the initial ipilimumab study and showed that HD-Ipi achieved greater OS benefit in patients with MBMs (HR 0.71) than in patients without MBMs (HR 0.92). Although the rate of toxicities was relatively high, there were no new or unexpected toxicities of ipilimumab observed in the MBM patients.[11,12] Additionally, the analysis of the Italian Early Access Program of Ipi reported a global objective response rate (ORR) of 11% with a median OS of 4.3 months in patients with MBM.[20] Several studies have also reported promising outcomes for radiotherapy with Ipi. A prospective cohort study of patients receiving SRS reported improved OS in patients who received Ipi (median 21.3 months) versus those who did not (4.9 months).[21] Other retrospective studies have also reported promising outcomes.[22,23]

Single-agent pembrolizumab and nivolumab are ICIs that inhibit programmed cell death protein 1 (PD-1). Clinical trials in patients without MBMs showed that each agent improved ORR, PFS, and OS with decreased toxicity compared with Ipi.[24–27] Pembrolizumab was evaluated in a post-approval phase II trial in patients with asymptomatic MBMs (or asymptomatic brain metastases from non-small-cell lung cancer). Among the 23 MBM patients, the ICRR was 26%, and the median PFS and OS were 2 and 17 months, respectively.[13,28] Single-agent nivolumab was evaluated in MBM patients

Table 1
Key immunotherapy trials in melanoma brain metastasis management

Clinical Trial and Drug/ Characteristics	Ipilimumab NCT00623766		Ipilimumab NCT01515189		Pembrolizumab NCT02085070	Nivolumab ± Ipilimumab NCT02374242 (ABC Trial)			Nivolumab + Ipilimumab NCT02320058 (Checkmate-204)		Ipilimumab + Nivolumab, Ipilimumab + Fotemustine, Fotemustine (NIBIT-M2)		
Treatment Arms	HD-Ipi (n = 51)	HD-Ipi (n = 21)	HD-Ipi (n = 65)	Ipi (n = 62)	Pembrolizumab (n = 23)	Nivo + Ipi (n = 36)	Nivo (n = 27)	Nivo (n = 16)	Nivo + Ipi then Nivo (n = 101 + 18)		Ipi + Nivo (n = 27)	Ipi + Fote (n = 26)	Fote (n = 23)
Study Description	Phase II Open label		Phase III, Randomized, Double-blinded		Phase II	Phase II, Randomized, Open label			Phase II, Open label		Phase III		
Characteristics													
Prior Systemic Tx	78%	71%	56%	57%	70%	23%	24%	75%	17%	22%	None	None	None
Prior Local MBM Tx	41%	48%	-	-	78%	None	None	Some	9%	17%	26%	19%	17%
Symptomatic MBM	None	100%	None	None	None	None	None	63%	None	100%	None	None	None
ECOG	0-1	0-1	0-1	0-1	0-1	0-2	0-1	0-2	0-1	0-2	0-1	0-1	0-1
Median Follow-up (mo)	-		14.5	11.2	11.6	14	17	31	34.3	7.5	67		
Response Rate (%)													
Extracranial	14%	5%	-	-	30%	57%	29%	25%	49%	22%	44%	23%	0%
Intracranial	16%	5%	-	-	26%	46%	20%	6%	54%	17%	44%	19%	0%
Median PFS (mo)													
Extracranial	2.6	1.3	-	-	2	13.8	2.6	2.6	NR	1.2	-	-	-
Intracranial	1.9	1.2	-	-		NR	2.5	2.3	NR	2.2	8.7	3.3	3.0
Median OS (mo)	7	3.7	7.0	5.7	17	NR	18.5	5.1	NR	8.7	29.2	8.2	8.5
Citation	Margolin et al,[10] 2012		Ascierto et al,[11] 2020; Ascierto et al,[12] 2017		Kluger et al,[13] 2019	Long et al,[14] 2018			Tawbi et al,[15] 2018; Tawbi et al,[16] 2021; Tawbi et al,[17] 2021		Di Giacomo et al,[18] 2021; Di Giacomo et al,[19] 2024		

Abbreviations: Fote, Fotemustine; HD-Ipi, High dose ipilimumab (10 mg/kg); Ipi, ipilimumab (3 mg/kg); mo, month; Nivo, nivolumab; NR, not reached; Tx, Treatment.

in the Australian anti-PD-1 brain collaboration (ABC) study. Nivolumab had an ICRR of 20% in patients with asymptomatic and untreated MBMs (n = 27), but only 6% in patients with MBMs that were symptomatic or that had failed previous local therapies (n = 16).[14] Although those trials should be interpreted cautiously because of the heterogeneous nature of trials, the ICRR of ICI monotherapy is consistently around 20% to 25% in patients with asymptomatic MBMs and virtually all such responses appear to be durable (>2 years).

The combination of nivolumab and ipilimumab has demonstrated much more promising efficacy in patients with MBMs than was observed with monotherapy. In the phase II Checkmate 204 trial, patients were treated with ipilimumab 3 mg per kg every 3 weeks for 4 doses with concurrent nivolumab 1 mg per kg every 3 weeks; patients with clinical benefit without unacceptable toxicity then continued treatment with single-agent nivolumab 3 mg per kg every 2 weeks until disease progression or for a maximum of 24 months.[15] In patients with asymptomatic MBMs (n = 101), the ICRR response rate was 54%, with long-term follow-up demonstrating that 84% of those responses were ongoing at 3 years from treatment initiation. The median iPFS, duration of response (DOR), and OS were not yet reached at a median follow-up of 34 months. Based on these promising results, the Checkmate 204 trial was amended to include a cohort of patients (n = 18) with symptomatic MBMs, including patients on up to 4 mg per day of dexamethasone. Those patients had a lower ICRR of 17%, but the responses that did occur were durable.[16,17] In the ABC trial, patients (n = 36) with asymptomatic MBMs treated with the same ipilimumab + nivolumab regimen had an ICRR of 46%; the ICRR was 56% in the patients not previously treated with targeted therapy.[14] In a phase III trial (NIBIT-M2) comparing the efficacy of nivolumab plus ipilimumab, ipilimumab plus fotemustine, and fotemustine alone in asymptomatic MBM patients,[18,19] the ICRRs were 44.4%, 19.2%, and 0%, respectively. The median OS was also significantly longer in the nivolumab plus ipilimumab arm compared with the other regimens (29.2 vs 8.2 vs 8.5 months).[18,19] Similar to single-agent ICIs, no new or unexpected toxicities were reported with ipilimumab + nivolumab in MBM patients. However, the rate of toxicities was higher than was observed with monotherapies. Another ICI combination, nivolumab + relatlimab, was approved for stage IV melanoma patients based on a phase III trial that excluded patients with untreated MBMs.[29] A phase II trial will assess the safety and efficacy of this combination in patients with asymptomatic MBMs (NCT05704647).

Targeted Therapy

Several non-randomized trials have evaluated FDA-approved single-agent BRAF inhibitors (BRAFi) and FDA-approved BRAFi plus MEK inhibitor (MEKi) combination regimens in post-approval studies in patients with MBM with a BRAF V600 mutation (**Table 2**). Similar to trials in patients with ECMs, initial trials evaluated single-agent BRAFi. The phase II BREAK-MB trial evaluated single-agent dabrafenib in 2 distinct cohorts of patients with asymptomatic MBMs: cohort A patients (n = 89) had treatment-naïve MBMs, while those in cohort B (n = 83) had progressed after prior brain-directed treatment (craniotomy or radiation).[30] The ICRRs were 39% and 31%; the median iPFS were 3.8 and 3.8 months; and the median OS were 7.7 and 7.3 months in Cohorts A and B, respectively. Vemurafenib was also assessed in a 2-cohort study (Cohort A, previously untreated, n = 90; Cohort B, previously treated, n = 56) of patients with asymptomatic BRAF-mutant MBMs.[31] The ICRRs were 18% and 18%; the median iPFS were 3.7 months and 4.0 months; and the median OS were 8.9 and 9.6 months in cohorts A and B, respectively.[31] A single-arm study that assessed the safety and efficacy of vemurafenib in patients with symptomatic MBMs demonstrated an ICRR of 16% along with a

Table 2
Key targeted therapy trials in melanoma brain metastasis management

Clinical Trial and Drug/ Characteristics	Dabrafenib NCT01266967 (BREAK-MB)	Vemurafenib	Vemurafenib NCT01253564	Dabrafenib + Trametinib NCT02039947 (COMBI-MB)	Atezolizumab + Vemurafenib + Cobimetinib NCT03625141 (TRICOTEL)	
Treatment Arms	Dabrafenib (Cohort A n = 89, B n = 83)	Vemurafenib (Cohort 1 n = 90, Cohort 2 n = 56)	Vemurafenib (n = 24)	Dabrafenib + Trametinib (Cohorts A n = 76, B n = 16, C n = 16, D n = 17)	Atezo + Vem + Cobi BRAF V600 mut (n = 65)	Atezo + Cobi BRAF V600 WT (n = 15)
Study description	Phase II, Open label	Phase II	Open label Pilot study	Phase II, Open label	Phase II, Open label	
Characteristics	>26% / >42%	20% / 39%	83%	22% / 31% / 19% / 41%	11%	7%
Prior Systemic Tx	None / 100%	None / 100%	Some	None / 100% / Some / Some	-	-
Prior Local MBM Tx	None / None	- / Some	100%	None / None / None / 100%	40%	47%
Symptomatic MBM ECOG	0–1 / 0–1	0–1 / 0–1	0–2	0–2 / 0–1 / 0–1 / 0–2	0–2	0–2
Median follow-up (mo.)	>4	9.6	8.5	20 / 9.5 / 11	9.7	6.2
Response Rate (%) Extracranial	38% / 31%	33% / 18%	62%	55% / 44% / 44% / 41%	57%	-
Intracranial	39% / 31%	23% / 18%	16%	58% / 56% / 56% / 59%	42%	27%
Median PFS (mo.) Extracranial	3.8 / 3.9	- / 4.0	3.9	5.6 / 7.2 / 4.2 / 5.5	9.4	-
Intracranial	3.8 / 3.9	3.7 / 4.0	3.9	-	5.3	2.2
Median OS (mo.)	7.7 / 7.3	8.9 / 9.6	5.3	10.8 / 24.3 / 10.2 / 11.5	13.7	
Citation	Long et al,[30] 2012	McArthur et al,[31] 2017	Dummer et al,[33] 2014	Davies et al,[34] 2017	Dummer et al,[35] 2023	

Abbreviations: Atezo, atezolizumab; Cobi, Cobimetinib; Tx, treatment; Vem, Vemurafenib.

median PFS of 3.9 and a median OS of 5.3 months.[32,33] Similar to the immunotherapy trials, no new or unexpected toxicities were reported with BRAFi in MBM patients.

The phase II COMBI-MB trial was the first study to evaluate BRAFi and MEKi combination in MBM patients, with dabrafenib plus trametinib.[34] The trial included a total of 125 patients who received the same treatment but were analyzed in 4 cohorts: cohort A (n = 76) had *BRAF* V600 E mutation, asymptomatic MBM, and no prior local brain therapy; cohort B (n = 16) had *BRAF* V600 E mutation, asymptomatic MBM, with prior local brain therapy; cohort C (n = 16) had a *BRAF* V600D/K/R mutation, asymptomatic MBM, with or without prior local brain therapy; and cohort D (n = 17) had a *BRAF* V600D/E/K/R mutation with or without prior local brain therapy, and had symptomatic MBM. The ICRR were 58%, 56%, 44%, and 59%, respectively. The median PFS/OS were 5.6/10.8 months, 7.2/24.3 months, 4.2/10.2 months, and 5.5/11.5, respectively. Notably, the median intracranial DOR ranged from 4.5 to 8.3 months, which was shorter than the extracranial DOR, and approximately 50% of the patients experienced progression of MBMs while their ECMs were still controlled.[34] A subsequent multivariable analysis demonstrated that patients on steroids at baseline had lower ICRR and shorter iPFS than patients who did not require steroids, reminiscent of the results of clinical trials of ICIs for MBM patients.[36]

To enhance the intracranial activity of BRAFi and ICI, the TRICOTEL trial evaluated the safety and efficacy of atezolizumab (anti-PD-L1 ICI) combined with vemurafenib (a BRAFi) and cobimetinib (a MEKi) for patients with BRAF-mutant, previously untreated MBM.[35] The trial included 65 patients, 26 (40%) of whom had symptomatic MBMs (including 11 receiving steroids). For the full cohort, the ICRR was 42%, the median DOR was 7.4 months, and the median iPFS was 5.3 months. In a post-hoc analysis, the ICRR was 35% and 46% and the median iPFS was 4.5 and 5.5 months in the symptomatic and asymptomatic MBM patients, respectively. The combination of atezolizumab and cobimetinib was also evaluated in a small (n = 15) cohort of BRAF wild-type (WT) MBM patients. The trial was stopped early because of other trial results; the ICRR was 27% and the median iPFS was 2.2 months.

Chemotherapy

ICIs and targeted therapies have replaced chemotherapy in the frontline treatment of MBM patients. Before these agents, evaluations focused on chemotherapies that penetrate the blood brain barrier (BBB). Trials of fotemustine[37] and temozolomide[38,39] reported an ICRR of approximately5% for each agent.

Local Treatments: Surgery and Radiation

Several of the MBM patients present with concurrent extracranial disease. The development of effective systemic therapies for MBMs provides a promising approach to address both entities. However, local therapies continue to play an important role in the management of patients with MBM.

Radiation therapy for patients with MBMs previously consisted predominantly of whole-brain radiotherapy (WBRT). However, WBRT has generally had minimal impact on survival in MBM patients, and long-term survivors can experience detrimental effects on neurocognitive function from this treatment.[40,41] Focal radiotherapy with SRS allows for the delivery of higher doses of radiation to brain tumors with reduced damage to surrounding healthy brain tissue and, thus, less impact on neurocognition. In a phase III trial, WBRT combined with SRS extended median OS to 6.5 versus 4.9 months for WBRT alone in patients with a single brain metastasis (*P* = .0393) and improved 6-month Karnofsky performance status to 43% versus 27% with the WBRT alone group (*P* = .03).[42] In a prospective study, patients undergoing SRS plus WBRT exhibited a higher decline in learning and memory function at 4 months (52% mean posterior probability of decline vs 24% for SRS alone). The mortality rate at 4 months was higher in the SRS plus WBRT group (29%) versus the SRS alone group (13%). However, 1-year CNS-recurrence-free survival was 73% and 27% (P = .0003) for patients who received SRS plus WBRT and SRS alone, respectively.[43]

SRS, beneficial for tumors less than 3 cm or near critical brain areas, has proven effective in patients with up to 10 lesions.[44–46] Studies report similar median OS (10.8 vs 8.5 months) and local control rates (95% vs 97%) at 6 months between patients with lesser than or equal to 4 and those with greater than or equal to 5 brain metastases receiving SRS, respectively.[47–49] Specifically, an MBM-focused retrospective study of SRS indicated a local control rate of 87% and 68% at 6 months and 12 months, respectively,[47] with another study reporting 90% local control, including 11% tumor disappearance post-SRS.[49] The role of adjuvant WBRT following SRS or surgery to prevent further metastases has also been examined. A phase III trial comparing adjuvant WBRT with observation post-SRS/surgery showed no significant difference in distant intracranial control at 12 months or in median OS, although a lower local failure rate was noted in the WBRT group (52% vs 58%).[50] The efficacy of adjuvant SRS to the surgical cavity has also been explored, with phase III trials reporting local control rates of approximately 70% to 90%.[51,52]

Both clinical and preclinical studies suggest that ICI immunotherapy may synergize with radiation, including the induction of responses in non-radiated lesions.[53,54] A comparison to a retrospective patient cohort suggested that giving SRS within 30 days of ipilimumab may result in improved local control and OS in MBM patients.[55] This observation was supported by a meta-analysis of retrospective data from 534 patients that reported 1-year OS of 65% and 52%, and local control rates of 89% and 68% in patients with concurrent (SRS + ICI) and non-concurrent therapy, respectively.[56] While these studies are very promising, questions remain about the potential risk of increased radiation necrosis with such combination approaches and toxicity that can cause symptoms similar to progressive disease.[55–58] Ultimately, prospective clinical trial data (from, for example, NCT03340129) will help to define the relative risks and benefits of such combinatorial approaches.

Similar to WBRT, the use of surgical resection of MBMs has decreased over time with the development of effective, less invasive treatments. However, surgery is still frequently used in clinical scenarios where such treatments are unlikely to be effective (for example, in large symptomatic lesions larger than 3 cm), for lesions that have progressed after radiation and systemic therapy, or in cases where tissue is needed to establish a diagnosis. However, a retrospective study of 355 MBM patients highlighted the potential benefit of integrating surgery (or SRS) with systemic treatment to enhance OS.[59] Another single-institution retrospective study of 142 MBM patients treated with ICI immunotherapy reported improved OS (median 22.7 months) in patients that underwent resection of larger tumors followed by ICI compared with treatment with ICI alone (median 10.8 months) or ICI followed by surgery (median 9.4 months).[60] Together, the results suggest the continued need for multidisciplinary evaluation and research for patients with MBMs.

DISTINCT IMMUNE AND MOLECULAR FEATURES OF MELANOMA BRAIN METASTASES
Immune Microenvironment of Melanoma Brain Metastasis

The brain has historically been regarded as a site of immunologic privilege because of the BBB and reduced expression of major histocompatibility complex molecules.[61–63]

However, this assumption has been challenged and reevaluated due to many recent studies demonstrating the potential for the development of distinct immune responses that diverge from those in ECMs.[64–67] The assumption has also been challenged by the clinical efficacy of ICI immunotherapy for MBMs.

Single-cell/nucleus RNA-sequencing (snRNA-seq) of 22 MBMs and 10 ECMs delineated the contrasting immunologic landscapes of these tumors.[64] MBMs featured increased dysfunctional CD8 + T cells and macrophages with a pro-tumorigenic phenotype compared with ECMs. Macrophages in MBMs exhibited reduced expression of antigen presentation genes (HLA types, B2M, and CD74) and matrix proteases, coupled with elevated expression of CD163, TLR2, MERTK, AXL, and IL2RA.[64] Other studies similarly observed the lowest density of CD3 + T cells and CD68+ macrophages around melanoma cells and the lowest number of tumor-infiltrating lymphocytes in MBMs compared with other ECM sites.[66,68]

Further characterization of T cells has identified a heightened abundance of TOX+CD8+ T cells (exhausted T cells) and CXCL13+ CD4 + T follicular helper (TFH)-like cells in MBMs compared with ECMs.[64,69] The TOX+CD8+ T cells, characterized by dynamic proliferation and anti-tumor activities, and CXCL13+ CD4 + TFH-like cells, which are crucial in tumor antigen recognition and enhancing the response to anti-PD-1 therapy, underscore the complexity of the T cell milieu in MBMs. Furthermore, T cells in MBMs displayed reduced expression of exhaustion markers such as PD1, LAG3, TIGIT, and TIM-3 relative to ECMs.[64]

Plasma cell aggregates have been reported to be more prominent in MBMs than in ECMs, albeit spatially restricted, suggesting intratumoral B cell to plasma cell differentiation, potentially indicative of a response to immune checkpoint blockade.[64,70] Integrated snRNA-seq and spatial transcriptomic analyses unveiled a spatially restricted cancer cell expression of type I interferon responses despite extensive antigen presentation, alluding to potential immune evasion zones, especially in areas lacking an effective T cell response.[64]

Metabolic Features and Dependencies of Melanoma Brain Metastasis

The brain is characterized by its high glucose oxidation rates, which are necessary to meet the energy demands of neurons.[71] It is also a lipid-rich organ, with about half its composition being lipids, predominantly polyunsaturated fatty acids, regulated largely by astrocytes.[72] Moreover, the brain's interstitial and cerebrospinal fluids are relatively nutrient-poor, especially in amino acids, compared with plasma.[73,74] Cancer cells, including melanoma, rewire their metabolic pathways in this unique setting.

RNAseq of patient-matched MBMs and ECMs showed that MBMs are enriched in the oxidative phosphorylation (OXPHOS) pathway.[75,76] This metabolic shift has important clinical implications, as OXPHOS has been linked to resistance to mitogen-activated protein kinase (MAPK) pathway inhibitors and anti-PD-1 immunotherapy.[77–80] Notably, patients with MBMs have inferior outcomes with both approved BRAFi and MEKi and with single-agent anti-PD1, compared with melanoma patients with ECMs only.[14,28,34] Consistent with those results, another study showed that MBMs with the highest levels of OXPHOS were associated with decreased post-craniotomy survival. Interestingly, this metabolic change resulted in a new vulnerability, as MBMs were more sensitive to IACS-010759, a potent OXPHOS inhibitor, than primary tumors or lung metastases in mouse models.[76] High-OXPHOS MBMs also demonstrated an augmented glutamine metabolic pathway and sensitivity to CB839, a specific glutaminase inhibitor. High-OXPHOS MBMs were characterized by a transcriptional profile indicative of suppressed immune activation, which was reversed by metformin inhibiting OXPHOS in preclinical models.[75]

In exploiting the brain's lipid-rich environment, melanoma cells utilize the proliferator-activated receptor (PPAR) pathway.[81] PPARs, which are fatty acid-activated transcription factors, facilitate the utilization of fatty acids such as arachidonic acid and mead acid supplied by neighboring astrocytes.[82] This interaction activates PPARγ signaling in cancer cells, stimulating their growth. Research indicates that blocking the PPAR pathway can slow the progression of MBMs.[81]

The brain environment is characterized by low amino acid levels.[83–85] To survive, investigators showed that brain metastases increase the synthesis of nonessential amino acids such as serine, glycine, and aspartate by diverting glycolytic intermediates into serine and glycine synthesis pathways. This adaptation was achieved by upregulation of 3-phosphoglycerate dehydrogenase (PHGDH).[85] Similar to OXPHOS, PHGDH inhibition prevented or slowed the growth of brain metastases, including MBM, in preclinical models without impacting ECMs.[85]

Molecular Changes in Melanoma Brain Metastasis

Studies have revealed differences in oncogenic signaling pathways in MBMs that may contribute to their pathogenesis and may serve as therapeutic targets.

The MAPK pathway is activated in the overwhelming majority of the cutaneous melanomas, and it is critical to their growth and survival. The pathway is frequently activated genetically, most commonly by activating mutation in *BRAF* or *NRAS*, or by loss-of-function mutations in *NF1*.[86–89] Mutations that result in the expression of BRAF V600 E (~70%) and V600 K (~20%) account for over 90% of V600 mutations in this disease, and they cause constitutive hyperactivation of MAPK signaling.[90,91] Approximately 20% of cutaneous melanomas feature *NRAS* mutations, predominantly affecting Q61. Mutations in *NRAS* are generally mutually exclusive of BRAF V600 mutations.[92] Loss-of-function mutations in *NF1*, a negative regulator of RAS, are identified in 15% of all melanomas, and up to 46% of cutaneous melanomas with WT *BRAF* and *NRAS*.[86,89,93] BRAF and NRAS mutation statuses show high (>95%) concordance between MBMs and ECMs/primary tumors, respectively.[76,94,95] Several studies have reported that *BRAF* mutations are associated with an increased risk of developing MBMs.[96,97]

Several studies have implicated the activation of the PI3K/AKT pathway in the development and pathogenesis of MBMs. Proteomic characterization of the PI3K-AKT pathway in melanoma cell lines and clinical samples showed that constitutive pathway activation consistently correlated with loss of function or expression of the tumor suppressor PTEN, a lipid phosphatase that counteracts PI3K. Interestingly, while there was no global difference in PI3K-AKT pathway activation between melanoma regional and distant metastases, significantly higher pathway activity and more frequent loss of PTEN were observed in MBMs than in metastases to any other site.[98] Subsequently, 2 independent studies showed that patient-matched MBMs and ECMs from individual patients consistently demonstrated higher activation of the PI3K-AKT pathway in the brain tumors (but no difference in MAPK pathway activation).[95,99] Further supporting a role for this pathway in MBMs, analysis of the status of *BRAF, NRAS,* and PTEN in stage III melanomas showed that loss of PTEN was associated with a higher risk of developing MBMs, but not metastases to other organ sites.[100] In parallel to these clinical studies, experiments in a murine model of melanoma featuring a BRAF V600 E mutation and loss of CDKN2A showed that concurrent activation of the PI3K-AKT pathway resulted in spontaneous MBM development.[101] Finally, independent studies showed that targeting the PI3K-AKT pathway inhibited the growth of MBMs, particularly when combined with approved MAPK inhibitors, in preclinical models.[95,102]

LEPTOMENINGEAL DISEASE

Leptomeningeal disease (LMD) is defined by the spread of tumor cells to the lining (meninges) of the brain or spinal cord. Multiple clinical studies have demonstrated that the presence of LMD is associated with markedly worse prognosis in MBM patients, even in contemporary therapies,[5,6] which has not meaningfully improved over the last decade (median OS $\leq$3 months).[103,104] One key challenge for melanoma patients with LMD is their continued exclusion from clinical trials, including in most studies for patients with MBMs.[10–13,15–19,30,31,33–35] However, a recent phase I trial of combined intrathecal (IT) and systemic administration of nivolumab successfully accrued 48 patients ahead of schedule, supporting the feasibility of trials for melanoma patients with LMD.[105,106] In this trial, the 6- and 12-month OS rates were 44% and 26%, even though virtually all patients had progressed on systemically administered anti-PD-1 therapy; further, there were no toxicities attributable to IT treatment. Additional trials are needed, as currently available systemic therapies have limited activity.[104,107–109] Interestingly, pilot studies suggest that the immune microenvironment of LMD may differ from that of MBMs and primary tumors,[110] and that the tumors may have unique molecular features and dependencies.[111]

SUMMARY

There has been progress on multiple fronts for MBMs. However, there remain many unmet needs, including effective therapies for patients who fail to respond to current immunotherapies, have symptomatic MBMs, and who have LMD. Fortunately, recent clinical experiences have demonstrated the feasibility of clinical trials for MBM patients, which hopefully will accelerate progress. There is also a strong rationale and opportunity to explore combining different treatment modalities instead of simply comparing them to each other.

In parallel, basic and translational research studies have provided new insights into the pathogenesis of MBMs. These studies provide growing evidence that MBMs can harbor unique features that may contribute to the aggressive nature of these tumors but that may also result in new vulnerabilities that can be exploited for potential new treatments. Such features have also been detected in brain metastases in other tumor types, supporting the potential impact of continued MBM research. These findings also support the need for similar studies of other clinically significant metastatic sites.

CLINICS CARE POINTS

- Combination immunotherapy with Ipilimumab + Nivolumab achieves high rates of durable responses in patients with asymptomatic MBMs.
- Targeted therapy with BRAF + MEK inhibitors achieves high response rates in BRAF-mutant MBMs but with a shorter duration of response than in ECMs.
- SRS is very effective at controlling small MBMs with less neurotoxicity than WBRT.
- Retrospective studies support the rationale to evaluate combinations of radiation and systemic therapies in prospective clinical trials.

ACKNOWLEDGMENTS

The authors would like to thank Angela Dahlberg, editor in the Division of Medical Oncology at The Ohio State University, for editing and proofreading this manuscript.

DISCLOSURE

M. Hasanov and Y. Acikgoz do not report any conflicts of interest. M.A. Davies is supported by the Dr Miriam and Sheldon G. Adelson Medical Research Foundation, United States, the AIM at Melanoma Foundation, , United States, the NIH, United States/NCI (P50CA221703), the American Cancer Society and the Melanoma Research Alliance, Cancer Fighters of Houston, the Anne and John Mendelsohn Chair for Cancer Research, and philanthropic contributions to the Melanoma Moon Shots Program of MD Anderson. M.A. Davies has been a consultant to Roche/Genentech, Array, Pfizer, Novartis, BMS, GSK, Sanofi-Aventis, Vaccinex, Apexigen, Eisai, Iovance, Merck, and ABM Therapeutics, and has been the PI of research grants to MD Anderson by Roche/Genentech, GSK, Sanofi-Aventis, Merck, Myriad, Oncothyreon, Pfizer, ABM Therapeutics, and LEAD Pharma.

REFERENCES

1. Haydu LE, Lo SN, McQuade JL, et al. Cumulative incidence and predictors of CNS metastasis for patients with american joint committee on cancer 8th edition stage III melanoma. J Clin Oncol 2020;38(13):1429–41.
2. Hasanov M, Milton DR, Lo SN, et al. External validation and nomogram for risk factors of CNS metastasis in patients with clinically localized melanoma. J Clin Oncol 2023;41(16_suppl):2012.
3. Zakrzewski J, Geraghty LN, Rose AE, et al. Clinical variables and primary tumor characteristics predictive of the development of melanoma brain metastases and post-brain metastases survival. Cancer 2011;117(8):1711–20.
4. Hasanov M, Milton DR, Patel SP, et al. Incidence, timing, and predictors of CNS metastasis in patients (Pts) with clinically localized cutaneous melanoma (CM). J Clin Oncol 2021;39(15_suppl):9580.
5. Hasanov M, Milton DR, Davies AB, et al. Changes in outcomes and factors associated with survival in melanoma patients with brain metastases. Neuro Oncol 2023;25(7):1310–20.
6. Davies MA, Liu P, McIntyre S, et al. Prognostic factors for survival in melanoma patients with brain metastases. Cancer 2011;117(8):1687–96.
7. Vosoughi E, Lee JM, Miller JR, et al. Survival and clinical outcomes of patients with melanoma brain metastasis in the era of checkpoint inhibitors and targeted therapies. BMC Cancer 2018;18(1):490.
8. Bander ED, Yuan M, Carnevale JA, et al. Melanoma brain metastasis presentation, treatment, and outcomes in the age of targeted and immunotherapies. Cancer 2021;127(12):2062–73.
9. Guirguis LM, Yang JC, White DE, et al. Safety and efficacy of high-dose interleukin-2 therapy in patients with brain metastases. J Immunother 2002;25(1):82–7.
10. Margolin K, Ernstoff MS, Hamid O, et al. Ipilimumab in patients with melanoma and brain metastases: an open-label, phase 2 trial. Lancet Oncol 2012;13(5):459–65.
11. Ascierto PA, Del Vecchio M, Mackiewicz A, et al. Overall survival at 5 years of follow-up in a phase III trial comparing ipilimumab 10 mg/kg with 3 mg/kg in patients with advanced melanoma. J Immunother Cancer 2020;8(1). https://doi.org/10.1136/jitc-2019-000391.
12. Ascierto PA, Del Vecchio M, Robert C, et al. Ipilimumab 10 mg/kg versus ipilimumab 3 mg/kg in patients with unresectable or metastatic melanoma: a randomised, double-blind, multicentre, phase 3 trial. Lancet Oncol 2017;18(5):611–22.

13. Kluger HM, Chiang V, Mahajan A, et al. Long-term survival of patients with melanoma with active brain metastases treated with pembrolizumab on a phase II trial. J Clin Oncol 2019;37(1):52–60.

14. Long GV, Atkinson V, Lo S, et al. Combination nivolumab and ipilimumab or nivolumab alone in melanoma brain metastases: a multicentre randomised phase 2 study. Lancet Oncol 2018;19(5):672–81.

15. Tawbi HA, Forsyth PA, Algazi A, et al. Combined nivolumab and ipilimumab in melanoma metastatic to the brain. N Engl J Med 2018;379(8):722–30.

16. Tawbi HA, Forsyth PA, Hodi FS, et al. Long-term outcomes of patients with active melanoma brain metastases treated with combination nivolumab plus ipilimumab (CheckMate 204): final results of an open-label, multicentre, phase 2 study. Lancet Oncol 2021;22(12):1692–704.

17. Tawbi HA, Forsyth PA, Hodi FS, et al. Safety and efficacy of the combination of nivolumab plus ipilimumab in patients with melanoma and asymptomatic or symptomatic brain metastases (CheckMate 204). Neuro Oncol 2021;23(11): 1961–73.

18. Di Giacomo AM, Chiarion-Sileni V, Del Vecchio M, et al. Primary analysis and 4-year follow-up of the phase III NIBIT-M2 trial in melanoma patients with brain metastases. Clin Cancer Res 2021;27(17):4737–45.

19. Di Giacomo AM, Chiarion-Sileni V, Del Vecchio M, et al. Nivolumab plus ipilimumab in melanoma patients with asymptomatic brain metastases: 7-year outcomes and quality of life from the multicenter phase III NIBIT-M2 trial. Eur J Cancer 2024;199:113531.

20. Queirolo P, Spagnolo F, Ascierto PA, et al. Efficacy and safety of ipilimumab in patients with advanced melanoma and brain metastases. J Neuro Oncol 2014; 118(1):109–16.

21. Knisely JP, Yu JB, Flanigan J, et al. Radiosurgery for melanoma brain metastases in the ipilimumab era and the possibility of longer survival. J Neurosurg 2012;117(2):227–33.

22. Silk AW, Bassetti MF, West BT, et al. Ipilimumab and radiation therapy for melanoma brain metastases. Cancer Med 2013;2(6):899–906.

23. Tazi K, Hathaway A, Chiuzan C, et al. Survival of melanoma patients with brain metastases treated with ipilimumab and stereotactic radiosurgery. Cancer Med 2015;4(1):1–6.

24. Robert C, Schachter J, Long GV, et al. Pembrolizumab versus ipilimumab in advanced melanoma. N Engl J Med 2015;372(26):2521–32.

25. Robert C, Ribas A, Schachter J, et al. Pembrolizumab versus ipilimumab in advanced melanoma (KEYNOTE-006): post-hoc 5-year results from an open-label, multicentre, randomised, controlled, phase 3 study. Lancet Oncol 2019; 20(9):1239–51.

26. Larkin J, Chiarion-Sileni V, Gonzalez R, et al. Combined nivolumab and ipilimumab or monotherapy in untreated melanoma. N Engl J Med 2015;373(1):23–34.

27. Wolchok JD, Chiarion-Sileni V, Gonzalez R, et al. Long-term outcomes with nivolumab plus ipilimumab or nivolumab alone versus ipilimumab in patients with advanced melanoma. J Clin Oncol 2022;40(2):127–37.

28. Goldberg SB, Gettinger SN, Mahajan A, et al. Pembrolizumab for patients with melanoma or non-small-cell lung cancer and untreated brain metastases: early analysis of a non-randomised, open-label, phase 2 trial. Lancet Oncol 2016; 17(7):976–83.

29. Tawbi HA, Schadendorf D, Lipson EJ, et al. Relatlimab and Nivolumab versus Nivolumab in Untreated Advanced Melanoma. N Engl J Med 2022;386(1):24–34.

30. Long GV, Trefzer U, Davies MA, et al. Dabrafenib in patients with Val600Glu or Val600Lys BRAF-mutant melanoma metastatic to the brain (BREAK-MB): a multi-centre, open-label, phase 2 trial. Lancet Oncol 2012;13(11):1087–95.

31. McArthur GA, Maio M, Arance A, et al. Vemurafenib in metastatic melanoma patients with brain metastases: an open-label, single-arm, phase 2, multicentre study. Ann Oncol 2017;28(3):634–41.

32. Blank CU, Larkin J, Arance AM, et al. Open-label, multicentre safety study of vemurafenib in 3219 patients with BRAF(V600) mutation-positive metastatic melanoma: 2-year follow-up data and long-term responders' analysis. Eur J Cancer 2017;79:176–84.

33. Dummer R, Goldinger SM, Turtschi CP, et al. Vemurafenib in patients with BRAF(V600) mutation-positive melanoma with symptomatic brain metastases: final results of an open-label pilot study. Eur J Cancer 2014;50(3):611–21.

34. Davies MA, Saiag P, Robert C, et al. Dabrafenib plus trametinib in patients with BRAF(V600)-mutant melanoma brain metastases (COMBI-MB): a multicentre, multicohort, open-label, phase 2 trial. Lancet Oncol 2017;18(7):863–73.

35. Dummer R, Queirolo P, Gerard Duhard P, et al. Atezolizumab, vemurafenib, and cobimetinib in patients with melanoma with CNS metastases (TRICOTEL): a multicentre, open-label, single-arm, phase 2 study. Lancet Oncol 2023;24(12):e461–71.

36. Wilmott JS, Tawbi H, Engh JA, et al. Clinical features associated with outcomes and biomarker analysis of dabrafenib plus trametinib treatment in patients with BRAF-mutant melanoma brain metastases. Clin Cancer Res 2023;29(3):521–31.

37. Jacquillat C, Khayat D, Banzet P, et al. Final report of the French multicenter phase II study of the nitrosourea fotemustine in 153 evaluable patients with disseminated malignant melanoma including patients with cerebral metastases. Cancer 1990;66(9):1873–8.

38. Schadendorf D, Hauschild A, Ugurel S, et al. Dose-intensified bi-weekly temozolomide in patients with asymptomatic brain metastases from malignant melanoma: a phase II DeCOG/ADO study. Ann Oncol 2006;17(10):1592–7.

39. Agarwala SS, Kirkwood JM, Gore M, et al. Temozolomide for the treatment of brain metastases associated with metastatic melanoma: a phase II study. J Clin Oncol 2004;22(11):2101–7.

40. de la Fuente M, Beal K, Carvajal R, et al. Whole-brain radiotherapy in patients with brain metastases from melanoma. CNS Oncol 2014;3(6):401–6.

41. Morris SL, Low SH, A'Hern RP, et al. A prognostic index that predicts outcome following palliative whole brain radiotherapy for patients with metastatic malignant melanoma. Br J Cancer 2004;91(5):829–33.

42. Andrews DW, Scott CB, Sperduto PW, et al. Whole brain radiation therapy with or without stereotactic radiosurgery boost for patients with one to three brain metastases: phase III results of the RTOG 9508 randomised trial. Lancet 2004;363(9422):1665–72.

43. Chang EL, Wefel JS, Hess KR, et al. Neurocognition in patients with brain metastases treated with radiosurgery or radiosurgery plus whole-brain irradiation: a randomised controlled trial. Lancet Oncol 2009;10(11):1037–44.

44. Rava P, Leonard K, Sioshansi S, et al. Survival among patients with 10 or more brain metastases treated with stereotactic radiosurgery. J Neurosurg 2013;119(2):457–62.

45. Salvetti DJ, Nagaraja TG, McNeill IT, et al. Gamma Knife surgery for the treatment of 5 to 15 metastases to the brain: clinical article. J Neurosurg 2013;118(6):1250–7.

46. Yamamoto M, Serizawa T, Shuto T, et al. Stereotactic radiosurgery for patients with multiple brain metastases (JLGK0901): a multi-institutional prospective observational study. Lancet Oncol 2014;15(4):387–95.

47. Bernard ME, Wegner RE, Reineman K, et al. Linear accelerator based stereotactic radiosurgery for melanoma brain metastases. J Cancer Res Therapeut 2012;8(2):215–21.

48. Knoll MA, Oermann EK, Yang AI, et al. Survival of patients with multiple intracranial metastases treated with stereotactic radiosurgery: does the number of tumors matter? Am J Clin Oncol 2018;41(5):425–31.

49. Mori Y, Kondziolka D, Flickinger JC, et al. Stereotactic radiosurgery for cerebral metastatic melanoma: factors affecting local disease control and survival. Int J Radiat Oncol Biol Phys 1998;42(3):581–9.

50. Hong AM, Fogarty GB, Dolven-Jacobsen K, et al. Adjuvant whole-brain radiation therapy compared with observation after local treatment of melanoma brain metastases: a multicenter, randomized phase III trial. J Clin Oncol 2019;37(33): 3132–41.

51. Brown PD, Ballman KV, Cerhan JH, et al. Postoperative stereotactic radiosurgery compared with whole brain radiotherapy for resected metastatic brain disease (NCCTG N107C/CEC.3): a multicentre, randomised, controlled, phase 3 trial. Lancet Oncol 2017;18(8):1049–60.

52. Mahajan A, Ahmed S, McAleer MF, et al. Post-operative stereotactic radiosurgery versus observation for completely resected brain metastases: a single-centre, randomised, controlled, phase 3 trial. Lancet Oncol 2017;18(8):1040–8.

53. Finkelstein SE, Timmerman R, McBride WH, et al. The confluence of stereotactic ablative radiotherapy and tumor immunology. Clin Dev Immunol 2011;2011: 439752.

54. Postow MA, Callahan MK, Barker CA, et al. Immunologic correlates of the abscopal effect in a patient with melanoma. N Engl J Med 2012;366(10):925–31.

55. Skrepnik T, Sundararajan S, Cui H, et al. Improved time to disease progression in the brain in patients with melanoma brain metastases treated with concurrent delivery of radiosurgery and ipilimumab. OncoImmunology 2017;6(3):e1283461.

56. Lehrer EJ, Peterson J, Brown PD, et al. Treatment of brain metastases with stereotactic radiosurgery and immune checkpoint inhibitors: An international meta-analysis of individual patient data. Radiother Oncol 2019;130:104–12.

57. Patel KR, Shoukat S, Oliver DE, et al. Ipilimumab and stereotactic radiosurgery versus stereotactic radiosurgery alone for newly diagnosed melanoma brain metastases. Am J Clin Oncol 2017;40(5):444–50.

58. Colaco RJ, Martin P, Kluger HM, et al. Does immunotherapy increase the rate of radiation necrosis after radiosurgical treatment of brain metastases? J Neurosurg 2016;125(1):17–23.

59. Tio M, Wang X, Carlino MS, et al. Survival and prognostic factors for patients with melanoma brain metastases in the era of modern systemic therapy. Pigment Cell Melanoma Res 2018;31(4):509–15.

60. Alvarez-Breckenridge C, Giobbie-Hurder A, Gill CM, et al. Upfront surgical resection of melanoma brain metastases provides a bridge toward immunotherapy-mediated systemic control. Oncol 2019;24(5):671–9.

61. Quail DF, Joyce JA. The microenvironmental landscape of brain tumors. Cancer Cell 2017;31(3):326–41.

62. Shrikant P, Benveniste EN. The central nervous system as an immunocompetent organ: role of glial cells in antigen presentation. J Immunol 1996;157(5):1819–22.

63. Nimmerjahn A, Kirchhoff F, Helmchen F. Resting microglial cells are highly dynamic surveillants of brain parenchyma in vivo. Science 2005;308(5726): 1314–8.

64. Biermann J, Melms JC, Amin AD, et al. Dissecting the treatment-naive ecosystem of human melanoma brain metastasis. Cell 2022;185(14):2591–2608 e30.

65. Boire A, Brastianos PK, Garzia L, et al. Brain metastasis. Nat Rev Cancer 2020; 20(1):4–11.

66. Conway JW, Rawson RV, Lo S, et al. Unveiling the tumor immune microenvironment of organ-specific melanoma metastatic sites. J Immunother Cancer 2022; 10(9). https://doi.org/10.1136/jitc-2022-004884.

67. Arvanitis CD, Ferraro GB, Jain RK. The blood-brain barrier and blood-tumour barrier in brain tumours and metastases. Nat Rev Cancer 2020;20(1):26–41.

68. Weiss SA, Zito C, Tran T, et al. Melanoma brain metastases have lower T-cell content and microvessel density compared to matched extracranial metastases. J Neuro Oncol 2021;152(1):15–25.

69. Cohen M, Giladi A, Barboy O, et al. The interaction of CD4(+) helper T cells with dendritic cells shapes the tumor microenvironment and immune checkpoint blockade response. Nat Cancer 2022;3(3):303–17.

70. Patil NS, Nabet BY, Muller S, et al. Intratumoral plasma cells predict outcomes to PD-L1 blockade in non-small cell lung cancer. Cancer Cell 2022;40(3): 289–300 e4.

71. Garcia-Espinosa MA, Rodrigues TB, Sierra A, et al. Cerebral glucose metabolism and the glutamine cycle as detected by in vivo and in vitro 13C NMR spectroscopy. Neurochem Int 2004;45(2–3):297–303.

72. Katz R, Hamilton JA, Pownall HJ, et al. Brain uptake and utilization of fatty acids, lipids & lipoproteins: recommendations for future research. J Mol Neurosci 2007;33(1):146–50.

73. Jones CM, Smith M, Henderson MJ. Reference data for cerebrospinal fluid and the utility of amino acid measurement for the diagnosis of inborn errors of metabolism. Ann Clin Biochem 2006;43(Pt 1):63–6.

74. Rainesalo S, Keranen T, Palmio J, et al. Plasma and cerebrospinal fluid amino acids in epileptic patients. Neurochem Res 2004;29(1):319–24.

75. Fischer GM, Guerrieri RA, Hu Q, et al. Clinical, molecular, metabolic, and immune features associated with oxidative phosphorylation in melanoma brain metastases. Neurooncol Adv 2021;3(1):vdaa177.

76. Fischer GM, Jalali A, Kircher DA, et al. Molecular Profiling Reveals Unique Immune and Metabolic Features of Melanoma Brain Metastases. Cancer Discov 2019;9(5):628–45.

77. Gopal YN, Rizos H, Chen G, et al. Inhibition of mTORC1/2 overcomes resistance to MAPK pathway inhibitors mediated by PGC1alpha and oxidative phosphorylation in melanoma. Cancer Res 2014;74(23):7037–47.

78. Haq R, Shoag J, Andreu-Perez P, et al. Oncogenic BRAF regulates oxidative metabolism via PGC1alpha and MITF. Cancer Cell 2013;23(3):302–15.

79. Najjar YG, Menk AV, Sander C, et al. Tumor cell oxidative metabolism as a barrier to PD-1 blockade immunotherapy in melanoma. JCI Insight 2019;4(5). https://doi.org/10.1172/jci.insight.124989.

80. Scharping NE, Menk AV, Whetstone RD, et al. Efficacy of PD-1 blockade is potentiated by metformin-induced reduction of tumor hypoxia. Cancer Immunol Res 2017;5(1):9–16.

81. Zou Y, Watters A, Cheng N, et al. Polyunsaturated fatty acids from astrocytes activate ppargamma signaling in cancer cells to promote brain metastasis. Cancer Discov 2019;9(12):1720–35.

82. Pfrieger FW, Ungerer N. Cholesterol metabolism in neurons and astrocytes. Prog Lipid Res 2011;50(4):357–71.

83. Dolgodilina E, Imobersteg S, Laczko E, et al. Brain interstitial fluid glutamine homeostasis is controlled by blood-brain barrier SLC7A5/LAT1 amino acid transporter. J Cerebr Blood Flow Metabol 2016;36(11):1929–41.

84. Maggs DG, Jacob R, Rife F, et al. Interstitial fluid concentrations of glycerol, glucose, and amino acids in human quadricep muscle and adipose tissue. Evidence for significant lipolysis in skeletal muscle. J Clin Invest 1995;96(1):370–7.

85. Ngo B, Kim E, Osorio-Vasquez V, et al. Limited environmental serine and glycine confer brain metastasis sensitivity to PHGDH inhibition. Cancer Discov 2020; 10(9):1352–73.

86. Cancer Genome Atlas N. Genomic classification of cutaneous melanoma. Cell 2015;161(7):1681–96.

87. Fedorenko IV, Paraiso KH, Smalley KS. Acquired and intrinsic BRAF inhibitor resistance in BRAF V600E mutant melanoma. Biochem Pharmacol 2011;82(3): 201–9.

88. Fedorenko IV, Gibney GT, Smalley KS. NRAS mutant melanoma: biological behavior and future strategies for therapeutic management. Oncogene 2013; 32(25):3009–18.

89. Krauthammer M, Kong Y, Bacchiocchi A, et al. Exome sequencing identifies recurrent mutations in NF1 and RASopathy genes in sun-exposed melanomas. Nat Genet 2015;47(9):996–1002.

90. McQuade J, Davies MA. Converting biology into clinical benefit: lessons learned from BRAF inhibitors. Melanoma Manag 2015;2(3):241–54.

91. Davies H, Bignell GR, Cox C, et al. Mutations of the BRAF gene in human cancer. Nature 2002;417(6892):949–54.

92. Jakob JA, Bassett RL Jr, Ng CS, et al. NRAS mutation status is an independent prognostic factor in metastatic melanoma. Cancer 2012;118(16):4014–23.

93. Colombino M, Capone M, Lissia A, et al. BRAF/NRAS mutation frequencies among primary tumors and metastases in patients with melanoma. J Clin Oncol 2012;30(20):2522–9.

94. Varaljai R, Horn S, Sucker A, et al. Integrative genomic analyses of patient-matched intracranial and extracranial metastases reveal a novel brain-specific landscape of genetic variants in driver genes of malignant melanoma. Cancers (Basel) 2021;13(4). https://doi.org/10.3390/cancers13040731.

95. Chen G, Chakravarti N, Aardalen K, et al. Molecular profiling of patient-matched brain and extracranial melanoma metastases implicates the PI3K pathway as a therapeutic target. Clin Cancer Res 2014;20(21):5537–46.

96. Maxwell R, Garzon-Muvdi T, Lipson EJ, et al. BRAF-V600 mutational status affects recurrence patterns of melanoma brain metastasis. Int J Cancer 2017; 140(12):2716–27.

97. Wang Y, Lian B, Si L, et al. Cumulative incidence and risk factors of brain metastasis for acral and mucosal melanoma patients with stages I-III. Eur J Cancer 2022;175:196–203.

98. Davies MA, Stemke-Hale K, Lin E, et al. Integrated Molecular and Clinical Analysis of AKT Activation in Metastatic Melanoma. Clin Cancer Res 2009;15(24): 7538–46.

99. Niessner H, Forschner A, Klumpp B, et al. Targeting hyperactivation of the AKT survival pathway to overcome therapy resistance of melanoma brain metastases. Cancer Med 2013;2(1):76–85.

100. Bucheit AD, Chen G, Siroy A, et al. Complete loss of PTEN protein expression correlates with shorter time to brain metastasis and survival in stage IIIB/C melanoma patients with BRAFV600 mutations. Clin Cancer Res 2014;20(21):5527–36.

101. Cho JH, Robinson JP, Arave RA, et al. AKT1 activation promotes development of melanoma metastases. Cell Rep 2015;13(5):898–905.

102. Niessner H, Schmitz J, Tabatabai G, et al. PI3K pathway inhibition achieves potent antitumor activity in melanoma brain metastases in vitro and in vivo. Clin Cancer Res 2016;22(23):5818–28.

103. Cohen JV, Tawbi H, Margolin KA, et al. Melanoma central nervous system metastases: current approaches, challenges, and opportunities. Pigment Cell Melanoma Res 2016;29(6):627–42.

104. Ferguson SD, Bindal S, Bassett RL Jr, et al. Predictors of survival in metastatic melanoma patients with leptomeningeal disease (LMD). J Neuro Oncol 2019; 142(3):499–509.

105. Glitza Oliva IC, Ferguson SD, Bassett R Jr, et al. Concurrent intrathecal and intravenous nivolumab in leptomeningeal disease: phase 1 trial interim results. Nat Med 2023;29(4):898–905.

106. Glitza IC, Phillips S, John I, et al. 10820 - Concurrent intrathecal (IT) and intravenous (IV) nivolumab (N) for melanoma (MM) patients (pts) with leptomeningeal disease (LMD). Annals of Oncology. ESMO 2023.

107. Glitza IC, Ferguson SD, Guha-Thakurta N. Rapid resolution of leptomeningeal disease with targeted therapy in a metastatic melanoma patient. J Neuro Oncol 2017;133(3):663–5.

108. Kim DW, Barcena E, Mehta UN, et al. Prolonged survival of a patient with metastatic leptomeningeal melanoma treated with BRAF inhibition-based therapy: a case report. BMC Cancer 2015;15:400.

109. Lee JM, Mehta UN, Dsouza LH, et al. Long-term stabilization of leptomeningeal disease with whole-brain radiation therapy in a patient with metastatic melanoma treated with vemurafenib: a case report. Melanoma Res 2013;23(2):175–8.

110. Smalley I, Chen Z, Phadke M, et al. Single-cell characterization of the immune microenvironment of melanoma brain and leptomeningeal metastases. Clin Cancer Res 2021;27(14):4109–25.

111. Boire A, Zou Y, Shieh J, et al. Complement component 3 adapts the cerebrospinal fluid for leptomeningeal metastasis. Cell 2017;168(6):1101–1113 e13.

Advances in Vaccines for Melanoma

Can Cui, MD, PhD[a,b], Patrick A. Ott, MD, PhD[b,c,d,e],
Catherine J. Wu, MD[b,c,d,e],*

KEYWORDS

- Melanoma • Neoantigen • Personalized cancer vaccine • Immunotherapy

KEY POINTS

- Melanoma serves as a critical platform for the development of immunotherapy, including cancer vaccines.
- Advances in sequencing technologies and computational algorithms have enabled rapid and cost-effective discovery of neoantigens.
- Clinical trials in melanoma have validated the feasibility, safety, immunogenicity of personal neoantigen vaccines, and have shown promising efficacy findings in combination with checkpoint blockade immunotherapy.

MELANOMA HAS BEEN INEXTRICABLY INTERTWINED WITH ADVANCES IN CANCER IMMUNOTHERAPY, INCLUDING VACCINES

The modern era of cancer immunotherapy was arguably launched by the discovery of cytokines, particularly the T-cell growth factor now known as interleukin-2 (IL)-2 by Morgan in 1976.[1] Tumor regression seen in subsets of patients treated with high-dose IL-2 or adoptive transfer of tumor-infiltrating lymphocytes (TILs) pointed to the potential immune-responsiveness of melanoma early on.[2,3] Melanoma was also identified early as responsive to checkpoint blockade immunotherapy (CBI) with anti-CTLA4[4–6] and anti-PD1 antibodies,[7–12] now a cornerstone of therapy for melanoma and many other solid and hematologic malignancies.

Melanoma has also been a "testing ground" for therapeutic cancer vaccines from the start. There is a long history of identifying and testing tumor-associated antigens (TAAs) as targets of vaccines, yet therapeutic success has been largely elusive, likely explained, at least in part, by immune tolerance and lack of tumor specificity. Recently, vaccines that target tumor-mutation-encoded, highly specific neoantigens, have

[a] Department of Medicine, Massachusetts General Hospital, Boston, MA, USA; [b] Harvard Medical School, Boston, MA, USA; [c] Department of Medical Oncology, Dana-Farber Cancer Institute, Boston, MA, USA; [d] Department of Medicine, Brigham and Women's Hospital, Boston, MA, USA; [e] Broad Institute of MIT and Harvard, Cambridge, MA, USA
* Corresponding author.
E-mail address: catherine_wu@dfci.harvard.edu

Hematol Oncol Clin N Am 38 (2024) 1045–1060
https://doi.org/10.1016/j.hoc.2024.05.009
0889-8588/24/© 2024 Elsevier Inc. All rights reserved, including those for text and data mining, AI training, and similar technologies.

hemonc.theclinics.com

shown the ability to generate robust and durable vaccine-specific immune responses, as well as early signals of vaccine-mediated tumor control, potentially ushering in a new chapter in the development of effective anticancer therapeutics. Because the majority of neoantigens are unique to each individual's tumor, neoantigen vaccines require customization for each patient. Next-generation sequencing (NGS) and in silico epitope prediction algorithms now allow fast and relatively low-cost neoantigen discovery and selection, thus enabling such a personalized vaccine approach. Early clinical trials in melanoma have demonstrated the feasibility, safety, and immunogenicity of personalized neoantigen vaccines, and have demonstrated signals of efficacy in combination with CBI.

THE BASICS OF VACCINOLOGY INFORM NEW DIRECTIONS FOR MELANOMA VACCINE DEVELOPMENT

Vaccination, pioneered by Edward Jenner in the 1790s, laid the foundation for modern immunology and has since became a cornerstone of public health, providing long-lasting immunity against infectious diseases.[13] The application of vaccines has broadened from disease prevention to treatment, due to their ability to generate durable immune responses. The concept of employing an individual's own immune system to treat cancer dates back to the 1890s with Coley's toxin, a mixture of heat-inactivated gram-positive Streptococcus pyogenes and gram-negative Serratia marcescens that was found to mediate tumor regression by enhancing antitumor immune responses.[14] A conceptually similar approach using bacille Calmette-Guerin was studied first in 1950s by Old and colleagues[15] and later explored in multiple cancer types including melanoma.[16–18] Further progress in the development of therapeutic cancer vaccines has revolved around advances in the core pillars of vaccinology—antigen (to be discussed below), adjuvant, and delivery platform. A fundamental question in the field has been how to overcome immune tolerance and engage both the innate and adaptive immune system to elicit antigen-specific T-cell responses capable of mediating tumor regression.

Several key elements have emerged as critical for achieving a successful immunotherapy-induced T-cell response: (1) the delivery of antigens in high quantities and of high quality; (2) the efficient capture, processing, and presentation of tumor antigens by professional antigen-presenting cells (APCs) such as dendritic cells (DCs), fueled by proinflammatory milieu; (3) the optimal activation of CD4 and CD8 T cells; (4) the infiltration of T cells into the tumor microenvironment (TME) and their effective destruction of cancer cells through antigen/MHC-T-cell receptor (TCR) interactions; (5) the maintenance of the immune response and a steady influx of various immune cells, driven by chemokine and cytokine gradients.[19] As shown in **Fig. 1**, antigen-specific T-cell responses involve a series of sequential steps that take place in both secondary lymphoid organs (SLOs; eg, draining lymph nodes, dLNs) and TME. MHC I-restricted and II-restricted antigens are captured and processed by APCs such as DCs and presented by DCs to CD8 and CD4 T cells, respectively, leading to their activation and differentiation. Priming of naïve T cells typically starts in SLOs, yet in certain cases, priming may also occur in tertiary lymphoid structures (TLSs),[20–22] which are organized lymphoid aggregates developed in TMEs resembling SLOs with orchestrated vascular and chemokine networks.[23,24] Upon activation, CD8 T cells undergo a differentiation process, branching into 2 developmental pathways: one eventually resulting in the formation of memory T cells and the other one in the generation of exhausted T (Tex) cells. Tex cells have been conventionally characterized by increased expression of inhibitory coreceptors (eg, PD-1, CTLA4, TIM-3, LAG-3, CD39) and

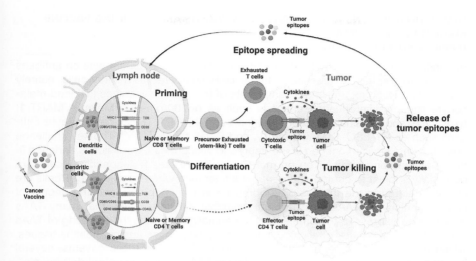

Fig. 1. Model of vaccine-induced T-cell responses. Essential steps for a successful therapeutic response to cancer vaccines: antigen presentation in lymph nodes, T-cell priming, differentiation, migration to the tumor, effective tumor cell killing, and subsequent epitope spreading that further amplifies the immune response. (Figure created with BioRender.com)

decreased production of cytokines (eg, IFN-γ, TNF-α, IL-2).[25] Based on their developmental stage, Tex cells can be further classified into various subsets, including precursor exhausted T cells (T_{PE}), also commonly referred to as TCF1 + stem-like T cells for their stem-cell-like features, and terminally exhausted T cells (T_{TE}).[26] T_{PE} cells have been identified as primary responders to CBI[27–30] and are enriched in dLNs and TLSs, functioning as "reservoirs" or "hubs," where T_{PE} cells can join with CD4 helper T cells, DCs, and B cells to create a tetrad, thereby jointly enhancing antitumor immune responses.[31–36]

An important component of a cancer vaccine is the "immune adjuvant." A vaccine adjuvant is aimed at enhancing immunogenicity and is thus designed to deliver or mimic innate danger signals, that is, pathogen-associated and damage-associated molecular patterns, thereby facilitating the activation of pattern-recognition receptors from APCs. Examples include poly-ICLC, CpG ODN, CMP-001, as well as cotherapies with CD40 or fms-like tyrosine kinase 3 ligand (FLT3L) agonists to target DCs and to presumably facilitate DC–T-cell interactions.[19,37]

Therapeutic cancer vaccines are aimed at optimal priming and activation of antigen-specific responses by ensuring the delivery and loading of a large quantity of high-quality antigen targets to DCs in dLNs. This leads to priming of T cells and shapes their future developmental trajectories.[38] Subsequent to priming, activated antigen-specific T cells migrate to and infiltrate tumors as well as surrounding stroma, where they can recognize and kill tumor cells, a process that can lead to release of additional tumor antigens. This can, in turn, lead to a secondary wave of immunity, termed epitope spreading (**Fig. 1**). Notably, this phenomenon has been observed across various studies testing personalized cancer vaccines, and has associated with improved patient outcomes.[39–43] The detection of epitope spreading has been interpreted to indicate on-target tumor cytotoxicity and rejuvenation of the de novo T-cell response against cancer.

TUMOR NEOANTIGENS AND ALTERNATIVE ANTIGENS ARE PROMISING VACCINE TARGETS IN MELANOMA
Tumor-associated Antigens

Historically, the focus of therapeutic cancer vaccine development was on antigens that are preferentially expressed in tumor cells compared to healthy cells, namely TAAs.[44] In melanoma, these antigen targets of therapeutic vaccines included melanocyte lineage/differentiation antigens such as gp100/pmel17, Melan A/MART-1, tyrosinase, and tyrosinase-related proteins 1 and 2 (TRP1, TRP2); cancer-testis antigens such as NY-ESO-1, MAGE family, and BAGE family.[19,45,46] The key challenge posed by this class of antigen is the degree to which their expression is enriched in tumor tissues and minimal on normal tissue. Therefore, TAA-specific T cells are potentially subject to central and peripheral tolerance where high-affinity T cells are clonally deleted in the thymus or suppressed in the periphery, and the degree of immunogenicity of TAAs can be highly variable. Of note, given that many TAAs may be also expressed to some extent in nonmalignant cells, the targeting of TAAs carries the possible risk of eliciting self-reactive responses against healthy tissues, which may lead to autoimmune-related toxicity.[47] Despite these caveats, several recent studies have focused on the targeting of TAAs using new potent delivery platforms, given their well-established expression profiles. A phase 1 multicenter, dose-escalation trial (NCT02410733) testing FixVac (BNT111), which target 4 melanoma TAAs (NY-ESO-1, MAGE-A3, tyrosinase, and TPTE), with delivery through a mRNA lipoplex vaccine platform, demonstrated promising early results: in 17 patients treated with FixVac and anti-PD1 combination therapy, six achieved partial response (PR) and two reached stable disease (SD), with the majority of PR and SD exhibiting sustained disease control.[48] Encouraged by these promising phase 1 findings, the investigators proceeded to initiate randomized phase 2 trials in melanoma (NCT04526899), and expanded this strategy in other solid tumors, including prostate cancer (NCT04382898), HPV16-positive head and neck cancer (NCT04534205), and non-small cell lung cancer (NCT05142189). TAAs have also been the therapeutic target of Tebentafusp (KIMMTRAK), a bispecific protein comprising a soluble gp-100 targeting TCR fused to an CD3 effector; this agent demonstrated prolonged overall survival and progression-free survival (PFS) in adult HLA-A*02:01-positive patients with uveal melanoma,[49,50] and was recently approved by the Food and Drug Administration for use in the metastatic setting.

Tumor-specific Antigens

Unlike TAAs, tumor-specific antigens (TSAs) are novel epitopes encoded exclusively by tumor cells and arise either from somatic mutations (neoantigens) or from viral oncoproteins. Neoantigen-specific T-cell responses were identified in human melanoma patients before the era of NGS.[51–55] However, over the past decade, advancements in sequencing technologies have transformed our ability to quickly and cost-effectively identify tumor mutations, thus–for the first time–enabling the consistent discovery of immunogenic neoantigens as targets of cancer vaccines.[56] Canonical genomic alteration-derived neoantigens included single-nucleotide variants, single insertions, or deletions of nucleotides (indels) and fusion genes. Previous studies have shown that a high non-synonymous mutational load, indicative of canonical neoantigens, was associated with survival benefit and improved outcomes of cancer patients treated with CBI.[57–62] A typical melanoma has 100s to 1,000s of such mutations, namely "passenger mutations," providing a rich spectrum of targetable neoantigens. In contrast, a smaller number of neoantigens are encoded by oncogenic "driver mutations" that are shared across different individuals. These shared neoantigens, derived from driver mutations, are conceptually appealing because they offer the potential for "off the shelf" vaccine and are critical for tumor development, typically exhibiting stable expression within tumor clones.[38,44] However, computational models have suggested that shared driver mutations are not only rare but also relatively poorly presented by MHC-I and MHC-II to become immunogenic.[63–65] The systematic, unbiased discovery of neoantigens has revealed that the vast majority are "private" neoantigens encoded by "passenger mutations," which are unique to each individual's tumors. These findings have motivated the ongoing efforts to test custom-made personalized vaccines.

While a correlation between CBI response and tumor mutational burden has been observed in melanoma, this association is less pronounced in cancer types with low mutational burden including cancers responsive to CBI.[66–69] Emerging evidence for the role of non-canonical neoantigen sources in this context may explain the apparent discrepancy. These originate from noncoding genomic regions, or from non-canonical transcriptional, translational, or posttranslational aberrations.[70–73] Approaches to the identification of such alterations have included the use of ribosome profiling (Ribo-seq) and MHC-I immunopeptidome mass spectrometry (MS) analyses, through which novel or unannotated open reading frames (ORFs) have been identified as sources of neoantigens, arising from 5′ and 3′ untranslated regions (5′ uORF, 5′ overlap uORF, 3′ dORF, 3′ overlap dORF), long noncoding RNAs (lncRNAs), and pseudogenes.[74,75] Proteogenomic studies have further uncovered other resources of neoantigens such as alternative splicing aberrations[76,77] with tumor-specific exon–exon junctions ("neojunctions"),[78] intron retention,[79,80] "exitron,"[81] splice-site-creating mutations[82]; alternative translational products [83–86] or posttranslational modifications.[87] Such studies promise to provide new avenues for TSA targeting across a broad array of cancers, even beyond melanoma.

It is important to note that only a small proportion of neoantigens, around 1% to 2%, are naturally capable of inducing spontaneous host T-cell responses.[88–90] A better understanding of the characteristics that drive presentation and ultimately lead to immunogenicity of neoantigens is of high priority in the field. The process of cross-presentation of HLA-I restricted epitopes by professional APCs involves a series of steps including epitope acquisition, proteasomal cleavage, and loading onto the polymorphic HLA alleles. Consequently, variables such as expression abundance, HLA-binding affinity and stability, and the degree of similarity between the mutated and wild-type sequences are critical to guide neoantigen selection. Rapid development of NGS-based approaches in the past years, coupled with computational prediction algorithms, has markedly expedited the systematic identification and prioritization of neoantigen targets. Historically, widely used prediction algorithms such as NetMHCpan,[91] MHCflurry,[92] MixMHCpred,[93,94] EDGE,[95] have been trained on binding affinity and/or MS-sequenced eluted peptide databases. A substantial challenge in the advancement of machine learning-based HLA prediction has been the generation of large-scale, high-quality datasets that adequately account for HLA allele bias. In this context, the neural network model trained on MS-derived HLA peptidome dataset from mono-allelic cell lines, HLAthena, has demonstrated improved performance.[96–98] Furthermore, the development of practical computational toolkits such as pVACtools[99] has allowed for the streamlined process of neoantigen prediction and prioritization, with enhanced accessibility and efficiency. To date, there remains a major need for further improvement in predicting epitope immunogenicity, primarily due to the lack of standardized protocols for sequencing, mutation calling, neoantigen prediction, and immunogenicity assessments. Efforts are underway to address these issues through consortium-led efforts.[100]

CLINICAL TRIALS TESTING PERSONALIZED NEOANTIGEN VACCINES IN MELANOMA PATIENTS DEMONSTRATE FEASIBILITY, IMMUNOGENICITY, AND EARLY SIGNALS OF EFFICACY

Generations of vaccine formulations have been tested in melanoma, including peptides, nucleic acids (such as DNA or mRNAs), viral vectors, and DCs. The last 15 years have seen substantial progress in the development and application of innovative vaccine delivery platforms, including synthetic long peptide (SLP) and mRNA vaccines encapsulated with lipid nanoparticles (LNPs). Over the past decade, personalized cancer vaccines have been studied in a series of clinical trials, establishing their feasibility, safety, and immunogenicity (summarized in **Table 1** and **Fig. 2**). Efforts have been also aimed at reducing their "needle-to-needle" manufacturing time spanning from biopsy to vaccination. For example, the Moderna mRNA–LNP vaccine pipeline currently requires approximately 6 weeks from sample collection to product delivery, but a stated goal has been to reduce this time to 30 days.[101]

Initial First in Man Trials Testing Personalized Neoantigen-specific Vaccines

Synthetic long peptide vaccines

In the early 2010s, SLPs as a vaccine platform generated notable interest in the field due to their ability to be directly processed and presented by HLA molecules on professional APCs such as DCs. Based on this evidence, NeoVax, one of the first personalized neoantigen vaccines tested in human patients, was developed utilizing 15 to 30 mer peptides, incorporating up to 20 peptides per patient, and formulated with poly-ICLC, an agonist of Toll-like receptor 3 and melanoma differentiation-associated protein 5. In the first in man phase 1 trial (NCT01970358), immune responses and clinical outcomes of 8 patients with surgically resectable stage IIIB to IV melanoma receiving NeoVax were comprehensively and longitudinally analyzed with immunologic assays, whole-exome sequencing and bulk and single cell RNA/TCR profiling.[39,102–104] Two of these 8 patients developed stage IV disease (lung metastases) following their last vaccination and later achieved complete radiographic responses (CRs) after subsequent anti-PD1 treatment with pembrolizumab. De novo neoantigen-specific CD4 and CD8 T-cell responses were identified weeks after vaccination, with over 30% displaying polyfunctionality (characterized by production of IFNγ, TNFα, and IL-2).[102] In addition to the strong T-cell responses generated promptly after vaccination, a follow-up study revealed that vaccine-specific T-cell responses persisted for several years and exhibited a "memory-like" phenotype on transcriptomic profiling. T-cell receptor clonality analysis demonstrated that vaccine-induced T-cell clones diversified over time.[39] Notably, this study, along with an expanded phase 1b study testing the SLP-based vaccine (NEO-PV-01), in combination with PD-1 blockade in melanoma, non-small cell lung cancer, and bladder cancer (NCT02897765), demonstrated epitope spreading that is, detection of nonvaccine TAA-specific or neoantigen-specific T cells early after vaccination.[39,40] In the latter trial, epitope spreading was also associated with prolonged PFS, consistent with previous reports.[40–43]

RNA vaccines

A proof-of-concept clinical trial testing a personalized mRNA vaccine targeting neoantigens in patients with stage III or stage IV melanoma was reported simultaneously with the NeoVax study described above in the 2010s (NCT02035956).[105] In this study, neoepitope-specific T-cell expansion was detected in several patients after vaccination. Further characterization of these T-cell responses showed central-memory or effector-memory T-cell phenotype as well as polyfunctionality. There was a striking reduction of cumulative metastatic events and improved PFS after vaccinations,

Table 1
Selected trials on personalized neoantigen vaccines in melanoma

Vaccine Name	Company/Institution	Platform	NeoAg Target #	Trial ID	Phase	Status
NeoVax	DFCI	SLP	Up to 20 NeoAgs	NCT01970358	Phase 1	Completed
				NCT03929029	Phase 1	Completed
NEO-PV-01				NCT04930783	Phase 1	Ongoing
				NCT02897765	Phase 1	Completed
EVX-01	Evaxion Biotech	SLP	5–10 NeoAgs	NCT03715985	Phase 1	Completed
				NCT05309421	Phase 2	Ongoing
IVAC mutanome (BNT121)	TRON	mRNA	Up to 10 NeoAgs	NCT02035956	Phase 1	Completed
RO7198457 (BNT122)	BioNTech/Genentech	mRNA	Up to 20 NeoAgs	NCT03289962	Phase 1	Completed
				NCT03815058	Phase 2	Ongoing
mRNA-4157	Moderna/Merck	mRNA	Up to 34 NeoAgs	NCT03313778	Phase 1	Completed
				NCT03897881	Phase 2	Completed
				NCT05933577	Phase 3	Ongoing
VB10.NEO	Nykode/Genentech	DNA	Up to 40 NeoAgs	NCT03548467	Phase 1/2	Completed
EVX-02	Evaxion Biotech	DNA	Up to 13 NeoAgs	NCT04455503	Phase 1/2	Completed

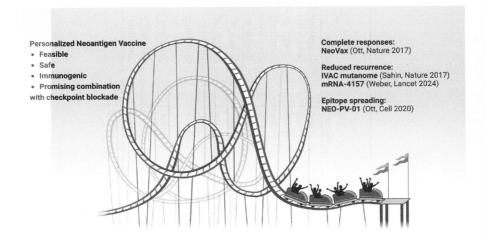

Fig. 2. Trajectory of cancer neoantigen vaccine development. Early clinical trials in melanoma have established that personalized neoantigen vaccines are feasible, safe and highly immunogenic, with promising combination with checkpoint blockade. Reflecting on the past challenges, the field is now entering an exciting new phase of vaccine development. (Figure created with BioRender.com)

providing an early signal of clinical efficacy. RNA-based personalized neoantigen vaccines have been since tested in larger clinical trials including the mRNA-4157 (V940) compound by Moderna/Merck.[106,107] Strikingly, in a randomized, open-label, phase 2 trial (Keynote-942, NCT03897881), patients with surgically resected stage IIIB to IV cutaneous melanoma who received mRNA-4157 plus pembrolizumab had prolonged improved recurrence-free survival (RFS) and distant metastasis-free survival compared to patients receiving pembrolizumab monotherapy.[108] Based on these results, a randomized, double-blind, phase 3 trial of mRNA-4157 has been initiated (NCT05933577). Beyond melanoma, personalized mRNA vaccines have demonstrated a notable association between immunogenicity and clinical outcomes in patients with surgically resected pancreatic ductal adenocarcinoma (PDAC): 16 patients received anti-PD-L1 treatment with atezolizumab followed by RO7198457 (autogene cevumeran) targeting up to 20 neoantigens and mFOLFIRINOX. Eight of 16 patients responded to vaccine and generated de novo neoantigen-specific T-cell responses. These "immune" responders had a prolonged median RFS, compared to nonresponders. Based on the preliminary data in this phase 1 trial where tumor-specific T-cell expansion correlates with delayed recurrence, a randomized, open-label, phase 2 study of autogene cevumeran in resected PDAC has been be initiated (NCT05968326, IMCODE 003).[109]

The Investigational Path Forward

Co-therapies
Given the established role of CBI as a standard of care for high-risk resected as well as advanced melanoma, current trials are exploring the use of neoantigen vaccines in combination with CBI—both in the first-line metastatic and adjuvant settings: NCT03815058 (IMCODE 001), NCT03897881, and NCT05933577. In addition to the reasoning that a melanoma vaccine should be partnered with CBI given it is a key

standard of care therapeutic modality, there is a robust mechanistic rationale for this combinatorial approach. CBI potentiates spontaneous T-cell responses to neoantigens and supports the expansion of T_{PE}/stem-like T cells while therapeutic vaccines can deliver neoantigens in high quantities and of high quality, facilitating de novo priming and activation of T cells. Preclinical studies have also indicated a synergistic effect between CBI and neoantigen vaccines.[29,110] Beyond CBI, there is a large armamentarium of therapies with different mechanistic angles (counteracting the TME, enhanced T-cell activation) that could synergize with a vaccine. Given that CBIs are a "must" ingredient of a combinatorial strategy in melanoma, these agents would need to be added to CBI, rather than substituted. The most effective timing and dosing of these additional agents will be critical for future trial designs.

Clinical setting (neoadjuvant, adjuvant, advanced)
Given the efficacy of neoadjuvant pembrolizumab in patients with resectable stage III or IV melanoma[111] and the prolonged RFS achieved with the combination of pembrolizumab and RNA vaccine in the adjuvant setting,[108] a critical question is how to incorporate a personalized neoantigen vaccine into the neoadjuvant setting. A key challenge here is the lead time of generating a custom-made vaccine. Given the demonstrated excellent outcome associated with a pathologic complete response after neoadjuvant CBI, one approach would be to design a personalized vaccine for all patients starting neoadjuvant therapy, but only manufacture and treat patients whose tumors do not exhibit a major or complete pathologic response post-surgery. While the compelling results achieved in the adjuvant setting[48,108] have led to a general sense in the field that vaccines are most effective in the (neo) adjuvant setting, that is, in patients with surgically resectable or resected melanoma, results are still awaiting from a randomized phase 2 trial comparing autogene cevumeran plus pembrolizumab versus pembrolizumab alone in the first-line metastatic setting. There is also evidence for vaccine mediated antitumor activity in patients with anti-PD-1-resistant melanoma suggesting that vaccination may have a role for patients with advanced melanoma.

Harnessing novel immune assessment tools to better understand and improve vaccine-induced immune and clinical responses
Analyzing the immune responses generated by vaccines and co-therapies, such as CBI, is an essential step to facilitate the optimization of next-generation immunotherapy. Experimental assays including ELISPOT, MHC multimers (eg, tetramers), intracellular cytokine staining were commonly used to analyze T-cell responses induced by cancer vaccines. The emergence of high-throughput single-cell genomics and spatial profiling technologies promises to further refine our analysis of vaccine-induced immune responses, broadening the magnitude and depth of T-cell function data available.[103,104,112,113] Importantly, TCR clonality analyses can provide valuable molecular barcode information to trace dynamic T-cell differentiation along time and space. For instance, in the first NeoVax study, in patients with high-risk melanoma (NCT01970358), longitudinal analyses employing single-cell transcriptomic profiling coupled with single-cell TCR sequencing, provided a comprehensive landscape of T-cell specificity, clonality, phenotype, and functionality in patients pre-vaccination and post-vaccination and after checkpoint blockade, as well as across various anatomic sites. Specifically, shared TCR clones can be traced from T_{PE} cluster (TCF7, CCR7) to T_{TE} cluster (PRF1, GZMB, PD1, HAVCR2, LAG3, CD39),[90,103] suggesting an underlying developmental trajectory consistent with previously reported critical pathways regulating CD8 T-cell differentiation under chronic antigen stimulation.[114-116]

In the case of one patient who achieved CR after vaccine followed by anti-PD1 therapy in this study, tumor-specific TCRs harbored by TILs had more enrichment of T_{PE} cluster, while tumor-specific TCRs in other patients were primarily enriched with T_{TE} cluster (Oliveira and colleagues[103]); these data are in line with the finding that circulating exhausted TCRs were more prominent in patients with disease progression. One hypothesis resulting from these studies is that combined use of a cancer vaccine and checkpoint blockade therapy can efficiently reshuffle the T cell repertoire and promote *de novo* T cell differentiation toward a more stem-like potential, when pre-existing T-cell clones are more exhausted, that is, with diminished functional capacity.

In summation, recent breakthroughs in the field of personalized neoantigen vaccines have opened unprecedented opportunities to expand our knowledge in T-cell biology, neoantigen and MHC characteristics, and their interactions at both molecular and cellular levels. Gaining a deeper understanding of the quantity and quality of these interactions within the therapeutic contexts will inspire the development of next-generation personalized cancer therapies toward the goal of curing more patients with melanoma.

CLINICS CARE POINTS

- Peptide and RNA vaccines for melanoma demonstrated early signals of efficacy
- Ongoing clinical trials are assessing effective co-therapies and optimal clinical settings for personalized neoantigen vaccines

ACKNOWLEDGMENTS

C. J. Wu. is supported by the Lavine Family Foundation. P.A. Ott. is supported by NCI, United States-R01 CA229261; Team Science Award from the Melanoma Research Alliance; the Francis and Adele Kittredge Family Immuno-Oncology and Melanoma Research Fund; the Susan and Bruce Hampton Research Fund; the Fisher Family Fund; the Morgan Family Fund for Melanoma Research.

DISCLOSURE

C.J. Wu. holds equity in BioNTech, receives research funding from Pharmacyclics, United States, and is on the advisory boards of Repertoire and Aethon. P.A. Ott.: Advisory Role: Alexion, Array, Bristol-Myers Squibb, Celldex, CytomX, Genentech, Merck, Neon Therapeutics, Novartis, Pfizer, TRM Oncology, Evaxion, Immunetune, Servier, MyNeo, Phio. Grants to institution: Armo Biosciences, AstraZeneca/MedImmune, Bristol-Myers Squibb, Celldex, CytomX, Genentech, Merck, Neon Therapeutics, Novartis, Pfizer.

REFERENCES

1. Morgan DA, Ruscetti FW, Gallo R. Selective in vitro growth of T lymphocytes from normal human bone marrows. Science 1976;193(4257):1007–8.
2. Rosenberg SA, Lotze MT, Muul LM, et al. Observations on the systemic administration of autologous lymphokine-activated killer cells and recombinant interleukin-2 to patients with metastatic cancer. N Engl J Med 1985;313(23): 1485–92.

3. Rosenberg SA, Packard BS, Aebersold PM, et al. Use of tumor-infiltrating lymphocytes and interleukin-2 in the immunotherapy of patients with metastatic melanoma. a preliminary report. N Engl J Med 1988;319(25):1676–80.
4. Hodi FS, O'Day SJ, McDermott DF, et al. Improved survival with ipilimumab in patients with metastatic melanoma. N Engl J Med 2010;363(8):711–23.
5. Robert C, Thomas L, Bondarenko I, et al. Ipilimumab plus dacarbazine for previously untreated metastatic melanoma. N Engl J Med 2011;364(26):2517–26.
6. Hodi FS, Butler M, Oble DA, et al. Immunologic and clinical effects of antibody blockade of cytotoxic T lymphocyte-associated antigen 4 in previously vaccinated cancer patients. Proc Natl Acad Sci U S A 2008;105(8):3005–10.
7. Larkin J, Chiarion-Sileni V, Gonzalez R, et al. Combined nivolumab and ipilimumab or monotherapy in untreated melanoma. N Engl J Med 2015;373(1):23–34.
8. Topalian SL, Hodi FS, Brahmer JR, et al. Safety, activity, and immune correlates of anti-PD-1 antibody in cancer. N Engl J Med 2012;366(26):2443–54.
9. Wolchok JD, Kluger H, Callahan MK, et al. Nivolumab plus ipilimumab in advanced melanoma. N Engl J Med 2013;369(2):122–33.
10. Robert C, Long GV, Brady B, et al. Nivolumab in previously untreated melanoma without BRAF mutation. N Engl J Med 2015;372(4):320–30.
11. Weber JS, D'Angelo SP, Minor D, et al. Nivolumab versus chemotherapy in patients with advanced melanoma who progressed after anti-CTLA-4 treatment (CheckMate 037): a randomised, controlled, open-label, phase 3 trial. Lancet Oncol 2015;16(4):375–84.
12. Robert C, Schachter J, Long GV, et al. Pembrolizumab versus ipilimumab in advanced melanoma. N Engl J Med 2015;372(26):2521–32.
13. Murphy KM, Weaver C. Janeway's immunobiology. 10th edition. New York, NY: W.W. Norton & Company; 2022.
14. Nauts HC, McLaren JR. Coley toxins — the first century. In: Bicher HI, McLaren JR, Pigliucci GM, editors. Consensus on hyperthermia for the 1990s: clinical practice in cancer treatment. New York, NY: Springer US; 1990. p. 483–500.
15. Old LJ, Clarke DA, Benacerraf B. Effect of bacillus calmette-guerin infection on transplanted tumours in the mouse. Nature 1959;184(Suppl 5):291–2.
16. Morton DL, Eilber FR, Holmes EC, et al. BCG immunotherapy of malignant melanoma: summary of a seven-year experience. Ann Surg 1974;180(4):635–43.
17. Zbar B, Tanaka T. Immunotherapy of cancer: regression of tumors after intralesional injection of living Mycobacterium bovis. Science 1971;172(3980):271–3.
18. Lobo N, Brooks NA, Zlotta AR, et al. 100 years of bacillus calmette-guerin immunotherapy: from cattle to COVID-19. Nat Rev Urol 2021;18(10):611–22.
19. Saxena M, van der Burg SH, Melief CJM, et al. Therapeutic cancer vaccines. Nat Rev Cancer 2021;21(6):360–78.
20. Schumacher TN, Thommen DS. Tertiary lymphoid structures in cancer. Science 2022;375(6576):eabf9419.
21. Schrama D, thor Straten P, Fischer WH, et al. Targeting of lymphotoxin-alpha to the tumor elicits an efficient immune response associated with induction of peripheral lymphoid-like tissue. Immunity 2001;14(2):111–21.
22. Peske JD, Thompson ED, Gemta L, et al. Effector lymphocyte-induced lymph node-like vasculature enables naive T-cell entry into tumours and enhanced anti-tumour immunity. Nat Commun 2015;6:7114.
23. Fridman WH, Meylan M, Pupier G, et al. Tertiary lymphoid structures and B cells: an intratumoral immunity cycle. Immunity 2023;56(10):2254–69.

24. Cui C, Craft J, Joshi NS. T follicular helper cells in cancer, tertiary lymphoid structures, and beyond. Semin Immunol 2023;69:101797.

25. Giles JR, Globig AM, Kaech SM, et al. CD8(+) T cells in the cancer-immunity cycle. Immunity 2023;56(10):2231–53.

26. Gebhardt T, Park SL, Parish IA. Stem-like exhausted and memory CD8(+) T cells in cancer. Nat Rev Cancer 2023;23(11):780–98.

27. Im SJ, Hashimoto M, Gerner MY, et al. Defining CD8+ T cells that provide the proliferative burst after PD-1 therapy. Nature 2016;537(7620):417–21.

28. Miller BC, Sen DR, Al Abosy R, et al. Subsets of exhausted CD8(+) T cells differentially mediate tumor control and respond to checkpoint blockade. Nat Immunol 2019;20(3):326–36.

29. Siddiqui I, Schaeuble K, Chennupati V, et al. Intratumoral Tcf1(+)PD-1(+) CD8(+) T cells with stem-like properties promote tumor control in response to vaccination and checkpoint blockade immunotherapy. Immunity 2019;50(1): 195–211 e10.

30. Kurtulus S, Madi A, Escobar G, et al. Checkpoint blockade immunotherapy induces dynamic changes in PD-1(-)CD8(+) tumor-infiltrating T cells. Immunity 2019;50(1):181–194 e6.

31. Leader AM, Grout JA, Maier BB, et al. Single-cell analysis of human non-small cell lung cancer lesions refines tumor classification and patient stratification. Cancer Cell 2021;39(12):1594–1609 e12.

32. Zhang Y, Chen H, Mo H, et al. Single-cell analyses reveal key immune cell subsets associated with response to PD-L1 blockade in triple-negative breast cancer. Cancer Cell 2021.

33. Zander R, Schauder D, Xin G, et al. CD4(+) T cell help is required for the formation of a cytolytic CD8(+) T cell subset that protects against chronic infection and cancer. Immunity 2019;51(6):1028–1042 e4.

34. Cui C, Wang J, Fagerberg E, et al. Neoantigen-driven B cell and CD4 T follicular helper cell collaboration promotes anti-tumor CD8 T cell responses. Cell 2021; 184(25):6101–6118 e13.

35. Hua Y, Vella G, Rambow F, et al. Cancer immunotherapies transition endothelial cells into HEVs that generate TCF1(+) T lymphocyte niches through a feed-forward loop. Cancer Cell 2022;40(12):1600–1618 e10.

36. Gaglia G, Burger ML, Ritch CC, et al. Lymphocyte networks are dynamic cellular communities in the immunoregulatory landscape of lung adenocarcinoma. Cancer Cell 2023;41(5):871–886 e10.

37. Bhardwaj N, Friedlander PA, Pavlick AC, et al. Flt3 ligand augments immune responses to anti-DEC-205-NY-ESO-1 vaccine through expansion of dendritic cell subsets. Nat Cancer 2020;1(12):1204–17.

38. Lang F, Schrors B, Lower M, et al. Identification of neoantigens for individualized therapeutic cancer vaccines. Nat Rev Drug Discov 2022;21(4):261–82.

39. Hu Z, Leet DE, Allesoe RL, et al. Personal neoantigen vaccines induce persistent memory T cell responses and epitope spreading in patients with melanoma. Nat Med 2021;27(3):515–25.

40. Ott PA, Hu-Lieskovan S, Chmielowski B, et al. A Phase Ib trial of personalized neoantigen therapy plus anti-PD-1 in patients with advanced melanoma, non-small cell lung cancer, or bladder cancer. Cell 2020;183(2):347–362 e24.

41. Corbiere V, Chapiro J, Stroobant V, et al. Antigen spreading contributes to MAGE vaccination-induced regression of melanoma metastases. Cancer Res 2011;71(4):1253–62.

42. Butterfield LH, Ribas A, Dissette VB, et al. Determinant spreading associated with clinical response in dendritic cell-based immunotherapy for malignant melanoma. Clin Cancer Res 2003;9(3):998–1008.

43. Lo JA, Kawakubo M, Juneja VR, et al. Epitope spreading toward wild-type melanocyte-lineage antigens rescues suboptimal immune checkpoint blockade responses. Sci Transl Med 2021;13(581). https://doi.org/10.1126/scitranslmed.abd8636.

44. Shetty K, Ott PA. Personal neoantigen vaccines for the treatment of cancer. Annu Rev Cell Biol 2021;5:259–76.

45. Hodi FS. Well-defined melanoma antigens as progression markers for melanoma: insights into differential expression and host response based on stage. Clin Cancer Res 2006;12(3 Pt 1):673–8.

46. Kalaora S, Nagler A, Wargo JA, et al. Mechanisms of immune activation and regulation: lessons from melanoma. Nat Rev Cancer 2022;22(4):195–207.

47. Blass E, Ott PA. Advances in the development of personalized neoantigen-based therapeutic cancer vaccines. Nat Rev Clin Oncol 2021;18(4):215–29.

48. Sahin U, Oehm P, Derhovanessian E, et al. An RNA vaccine drives immunity in checkpoint-inhibitor-treated melanoma. Nature 2020;585(7823):107–12.

49. Nathan P, Hassel JC, Rutkowski P, et al. Overall survival benefit with tebentafusp in metastatic uveal melanoma. N Engl J Med 2021;385(13):1196–206.

50. Hassel JC, Piperno-Neumann S, Rutkowski P, et al. Three-year overall survival with tebentafusp in metastatic uveal melanoma. N Engl J Med 2023;389(24):2256–66.

51. Wolfel T, Hauer M, Schneider J, et al. A p16INK4a-insensitive CDK4 mutant targeted by cytolytic T lymphocytes in a human melanoma. Science 1995;269(5228):1281–4.

52. Pieper R, Christian RE, Gonzales MI, et al. Biochemical identification of a mutated human melanoma antigen recognized by CD4(+) T cells. J Exp Med 1999;189(5):757–66.

53. Chiari R, Foury F, De Plaen E, et al. Two antigens recognized by autologous cytolytic T lymphocytes on a melanoma result from a single point mutation in an essential housekeeping gene. Cancer Res 1999;59(22):5785–92.

54. Lennerz V, Fatho M, Gentilini C, et al. The response of autologous T cells to a human melanoma is dominated by mutated neoantigens. Proc Natl Acad Sci U S A 2005;102(44):16013–8.

55. Zhou J, Dudley ME, Rosenberg SA, et al. Persistence of multiple tumor-specific T-cell clones is associated with complete tumor regression in a melanoma patient receiving adoptive cell transfer therapy. J Immunother Jan-Feb 2005;28(1):53–62.

56. Gubin MM, Artyomov MN, Mardis ER, et al. Tumor neoantigens: building a framework for personalized cancer immunotherapy. J Clin Invest 2015;125(9):3413–21.

57. Snyder A, Makarov V, Merghoub T, et al. Genetic basis for clinical response to CTLA-4 blockade in melanoma. N Engl J Med 2014;371(23):2189–99.

58. Lauss M, Donia M, Harbst K, et al. Mutational and putative neoantigen load predict clinical benefit of adoptive T cell therapy in melanoma. Nat Commun 2017;8(1):1738.

59. Rizvi NA, Hellmann MD, Snyder A, et al. Cancer immunology. mutational landscape determines sensitivity to PD-1 blockade in non-small cell lung cancer. Science 2015;348(6230):124–8.

60. Yarchoan M, Hopkins A, Jaffee EM. Tumor mutational burden and response rate to PD-1 inhibition. N Engl J Med 2017;377(25):2500–1.

61. Le DT, Durham JN, Smith KN, et al. Mismatch repair deficiency predicts response of solid tumors to PD-1 blockade. Science 2017;357(6349):409–13.

62. Cercek A, Lumish M, Sinopoli J, et al. PD-1 blockade in mismatch repair-deficient, locally advanced rectal cancer. N Engl J Med 2022;386(25):2363–76.

63. Marty R, Kaabinejadian S, Rossell D, et al. MHC-I genotype restricts the oncogenic mutational landscape. Cell 2017;171(6):1272–1283 e15.

64. Marty Pyke R, Thompson WK, Salem RM, et al. Evolutionary pressure against mhc class ii binding cancer mutations. Cell 2018;175(2):416–428 e13.

65. Hoyos D, Zappasodi R, Schulze I, et al. Fundamental immune-oncogenicity trade-offs define driver mutation fitness. Nature 2022;606(7912):172–9.

66. Merchant M, Ranjan A, Pang Y, et al. Tumor mutational burden and immunotherapy in gliomas. Trends Cancer 2021;7(12):1054–8.

67. Turajlic S, Litchfield K, Xu H, et al. Insertion-and-deletion-derived tumour-specific neoantigens and the immunogenic phenotype: a pan-cancer analysis. Lancet Oncol 2017;18(8):1009–21.

68. McDermott DF, Huseni MA, Atkins MB, et al. Clinical activity and molecular correlates of response to atezolizumab alone or in combination with bevacizumab versus sunitinib in renal cell carcinoma. Nat Med 2018;24(6):749–57.

69. Yakirevich E, Patel NR. Tumor mutational burden and immune signatures interplay in renal cell carcinoma. Ann Transl Med 2020;8(6):269.

70. Peri A, Salomon N, Wolf Y, et al. The landscape of T cell antigens for cancer immunotherapy. Nat Cancer 2023;4(7):937–54.

71. Robbins PF, El-Gamil M, Li YF, et al. The intronic region of an incompletely spliced gp100 gene transcript encodes an epitope recognized by melanoma-reactive tumor-infiltrating lymphocytes. J Immunol 1997;159(1):303–8.

72. Wang RF, Johnston SL, Zeng G, et al. A breast and melanoma-shared tumor antigen: T cell responses to antigenic peptides translated from different open reading frames. J Immunol 1998;161(7):3598–606.

73. Gupta RG, Li F, Roszik J, et al. Exploiting tumor neoantigens to target cancer evolution: current challenges and promising therapeutic approaches. Cancer Discov 2021;11(5):1024–39.

74. Ouspenskaia T, Law T, Clauser KR, et al. Unannotated proteins expand the MHC-I-restricted immunopeptidome in cancer. Nat Biotechnol 2022;40(2):209–17.

75. Chong C, Muller M, Pak H, et al. Integrated proteogenomic deep sequencing and analytics accurately identify non-canonical peptides in tumor immunopeptidomes. Nat Commun 2020;11(1):1293.

76. Frankiw L, Baltimore D, Li G. Alternative mRNA splicing in cancer immunotherapy. Nat Rev Immunol 2019;19(11):675–87.

77. Li G, Mahajan S, Ma S, et al. Splicing neoantigen discovery with SNAF reveals shared targets for cancer immunotherapy. Sci Transl Med 2024;16(730):eade2886.

78. Kahles A, Lehmann KV, Toussaint NC, et al. Comprehensive analysis of alternative splicing across tumors from 8,705 patients. Cancer Cell 2018;34(2):211–224 e6.

79. Smart AC, Margolis CA, Pimentel H, et al. Intron retention is a source of neoepitopes in cancer. Nat Biotechnol 2018;36(11):1056–8.

80. Dvinge H, Bradley RK. Widespread intron retention diversifies most cancer transcriptomes. Genome Med 2015;7(1):45.

81. Wang TY, Liu Q, Ren Y, et al. A pan-cancer transcriptome analysis of exitron splicing identifies novel cancer driver genes and neoepitopes. Mol Cell 2021; 81(10):2246–2260 e12.

82. Jayasinghe RG, Cao S, Gao Q, et al. Systematic analysis of splice-site-creating mutations in cancer. Cell Rep 2018;23(1):270–281 e3.

83. Dersh D, Holly J, Yewdell JW. A few good peptides: MHC class I-based cancer immunosurveillance and immunoevasion. Nat Rev Immunol 2021;21(2):116–28.

84. Laumont CM, Vincent K, Hesnard L, et al. Noncoding regions are the main source of targetable tumor-specific antigens. Sci Transl Med 2018;10(470). https://doi.org/10.1126/scitranslmed.aau5516.

85. Starck SR, Tsai JC, Chen K, et al. Translation from the 5' untranslated region shapes the integrated stress response. Science 2016;351(6272):aad3867.

86. Bartok O, Pataskar A, Nagel R, et al. Anti-tumour immunity induces aberrant peptide presentation in melanoma. Nature 2021;590(7845):332–7.

87. Kacen A, Javitt A, Kramer MP, et al. Post-translational modifications reshape the antigenic landscape of the MHC I immunopeptidome in tumors. Nat Biotechnol 2023;41(2):239–51.

88. Parkhurst MR, Robbins PF, Tran E, et al. Unique Neoantigens Arise from Somatic Mutations in Patients with Gastrointestinal Cancers. Cancer Discov 2019;9(8): 1022–35.

89. Leko V, Rosenberg SA. Identifying and targeting human tumor antigens for T cell-based immunotherapy of solid tumors. Cancer Cell 2020;38(4):454–72.

90. Oliveira G, Wu CJ. Dynamics and specificities of T cells in cancer immunotherapy. Nat Rev Cancer 2023;23(5):295–316.

91. Jurtz V, Paul S, Andreatta M, et al. NetMHCpan-4.0: improved peptide-MHC class i interaction predictions integrating eluted ligand and peptide binding affinity data. J Immunol 2017;199(9):3360–8.

92. O'Donnell TJ, Rubinsteyn A, Bonsack M, et al. MHCflurry: open-source class I MHC binding affinity prediction. Cell Syst 2018;7(1):129–132 e4.

93. Bassani-Sternberg M, Chong C, Guillaume P, et al. Deciphering HLA-I motifs across HLA peptidomes improves neo-antigen predictions and identifies allostery regulating HLA specificity. PLoS Comput Biol 2017;13(8):e1005725.

94. Gfeller D, Guillaume P, Michaux J, et al. The length distribution and multiple specificity of naturally presented HLA-I ligands. J Immunol 2018;201(12):3705–16.

95. Bulik-Sullivan B, Busby J, Palmer CD, et al. Deep learning using tumor HLA peptide mass spectrometry datasets improves neoantigen identification. Nat Biotechnol 2018. https://doi.org/10.1038/nbt.4313.

96. Sarkizova S, Klaeger S, Le PM, et al. A large peptidome dataset improves HLA class I epitope prediction across most of the human population. Nat Biotechnol 2020;38(2):199–209.

97. Abelin JG, Keskin DB, Sarkizova S, et al. Mass spectrometry profiling of HLA-associated peptidomes in mono-allelic cells enables more accurate epitope prediction. Immunity 2017;46(2):315–26.

98. Abelin JG, Harjanto D, Malloy M, et al. Defining HLA-II ligand processing and binding rules with mass spectrometry enhances cancer epitope prediction. Immunity 2019;51(4):766–779 e17.

99. Hundal J, Kiwala S, McMichael J, et al. pVACtools: a computational toolkit to identify and visualize cancer neoantigens. Cancer Immunol Res 2020;8(3):409–20.

100. Wells DK, van Buuren MM, Dang KK, et al. Key parameters of tumor epitope immunogenicity revealed through a consortium approach improve neoantigen prediction. Cell 2020;183(3):818–834 e13.

101. Carvalho T. Personalized anti-cancer vaccine combining mRNA and immuno-therapy tested in melanoma trial. Nat Med 2023;29(10):2379–80.
102. Ott PA, Hu Z, Keskin DB, et al. An immunogenic personal neoantigen vaccine for patients with melanoma. Nature 2017;547(7662):217–21.
103. Oliveira G, Stromhaug K, Klaeger S, et al. Phenotype, specificity and avidity of antitumour CD8(+) T cells in melanoma. Nature 2021;596(7870):119–25.
104. Oliveira G, Stromhaug K, Cieri N, et al. Landscape of helper and regulatory anti-tumour CD4(+) T cells in melanoma. Nature 2022;605(7910):532–8.
105. Sahin U, Derhovanessian E, Miller M, et al. Personalized RNA mutanome vac-cines mobilize poly-specific therapeutic immunity against cancer. Nature 2017;547(7662):222–6.
106. Dolgin E. Personalized cancer vaccines pass first major clinical test. Nat Rev Drug Discov 2023;22(8):607–9.
107. Burris HA, Patel MR, Cho DC, et al. A phase I multicenter study to assess the safety, tolerability, and immunogenicity of mRNA-4157 alone in patients with re-sected solid tumors and in combination with pembrolizumab in patients with un-resectable solid tumors. J Clin Oncol 2019;37(15_suppl):2523.
108. Weber JS, Carlino MS, Khattak A, et al. Individualised neoantigen therapy mRNA-4157 (V940) plus pembrolizumab versus pembrolizumab monotherapy in resected melanoma (KEYNOTE-942): a randomised, phase 2b study. Lancet 2024;403(10427):632–44.
109. Rojas LA, Sethna Z, Soares KC, et al. Personalized RNA neoantigen vaccines stimulate T cells in pancreatic cancer. Nature 2023;618(7963):144–50.
110. Verma V, Shrimali RK, Ahmad S, et al. PD-1 blockade in subprimed CD8 cells induces dysfunctional PD-1(+)CD38(hi) cells and anti-PD-1 resistance. Nat Im-munol 2019;20(9):1231–43.
111. Patel SP, Othus M, Chen Y, et al. Neoadjuvant-adjuvant or adjuvant-only pem-brolizumab in advanced melanoma. N Engl J Med 2023;388(9):813–23.
112. Liu S, Iorgulescu JB, Li S, et al. Spatial maps of T cell receptors and transcrip-tomes reveal distinct immune niches and interactions in the adaptive immune response. Immunity 2022;55(10):1940–1952 e5.
113. Sellars MC, Wu CJ, Fritsch EF. Cancer vaccines: building a bridge over troubled waters. Cell 2022;185(15):2770–88.
114. McLane LM, Abdel-Hakeem MS, Wherry EJ. CD8 T cell exhaustion during chronic viral infection and cancer. Annu Rev Immunol 2019;37:457–95.
115. Daniel B, Yost KE, Hsiung S, et al. Divergent clonal differentiation trajectories of T cell exhaustion. Nat Immunol 2022;23(11):1614–27.
116. Giles JR, Ngiow SF, Manne S, et al. Shared and distinct biological circuits in effector, memory and exhausted CD8(+) T cells revealed by temporal single-cell transcriptomics and epigenetics. Nat Immunol 2022;23(11):1600–13.

Microbiome and Immunotherapy for Melanoma
Are We Ready for Clinical Application?

Antony Haddad, MD[a], Ashley M. Holder, MD[a],*

KEYWORDS

- Microbiome • Immunotherapy • Melanoma • Fecal microbial transplant

KEY POINTS

- The understanding of the role of microbiome on patients receiving immune checkpoint blockade is increasing.
- The current evidence neither permits clinical management of patients based on information collected through gut microbiome sampling nor clearly delineates how to modulate the microbiome most effectively to impact the response to immunotherapy.
- High-fiber diet is associated with an increased response to immune checkpoint blockade, increased overall survival, and decreased immune-related adverse events in patients with metastatic melanoma.
- Antibiotics likely modulate the gut microbiome in an unfavorable manner for patients who are going to or are currently receiving immune checkpoint blockade.
- Over-the-counter probiotics are not necessarily beneficial for patients with melanoma receiving immunotherapy.

INTRODUCTION

The gut microbiome has been associated with healthy and disease states, and studies of the gut microbiome have begun to demystify many pathophysiologic states.[1] In cutaneous malignancies, and specifically melanoma, the gut microbiome has been associated with the development and progression of the disease.[2] Notably, the gut microbiome profile of healthy individuals is different from that of patients with melanoma. Likewise, the gut microbiome differs between patients with early-stage melanoma and patients with late-stage melanoma.[3] Immune checkpoint inhibitors are increasingly incorporated into the treatment of hematologic and solid metastatic

[a] Department of Surgical Oncology, The University of Texas MD Anderson Cancer Center, 1515 Holcombe Boulevard, Unit 1484, Houston, TX 77030, USA
* Corresponding author.
E-mail address: Amholder@mdanderson.org
Twitter: @Haddad_Antony (A.H.); @AshleyHolderMD (A.M.H.)

Hematol Oncol Clin N Am 38 (2024) 1061–1070
https://doi.org/10.1016/j.hoc.2024.05.010
0889-8588/24/© 2024 Elsevier Inc. All rights reserved.
hemonc.theclinics.com

malignancies, particularly melanoma.[4–6] The response of patients with melanoma to immunotherapy is dependent on many factors,[7] and the effect of the gut microbiome on this response has begun to be revealed.[7–9] In this review, we summarize the role of microbiome in the response (or lack thereof) of melanoma to immunotherapy, provide insights on the mediators of this interaction, and discuss interventions to alter the microbiome that will likely become the standard-of-care to improve response to immunotherapy for patients with melanoma.

IMPACT OF THE MICROBIOME ON IMMUNOTHERAPY FOR MELANOMA
Microbiome Landscape and Response to Immunotherapy

The effect of the gut microbiome on the responsiveness to immunotherapy was first demonstrated in mouse models with melanoma.[10,11] In the study by Sivan and colleagues, mice obtained from different facilities known to have different commensal microbiome composition had different melanoma growth rates. Interestingly, two alterations abolished the differences in melanoma growth rates: the first was cohousing the mice before implanting the tumors and the second was transferring the fecal material from mice with slow tumor growth rate to their counterparts with fast tumor growth. Furthermore, transferring fecal material from mice with controlled tumor growth rate led to better response and enhanced tumor control when combined with anti-programmed cell death protein 1 (anti-PD-1) immunotherapy. In-depth analysis of the abundance of different bacterial taxa among the two groups revealed that the Bifidobacterium was more abundant in the mice that demonstrated controlled tumor growth. Further experiments revealed that the inoculation of Bifidobacterium in preclinical melanoma models led to a slower melanoma growth rate. More importantly, the response to anti-PD-1 immunotherapy was superior in mouse models with melanoma inoculated with Bifidobacterium compared to those that were not.[11] In fact, inoculation of Bifidobacterium resulted in similar degree of tumor control as anti-PD-1 immunotherapy, and the combination of the two had a synergistic effect and nearly halted tumor growth.[11] Further studies in humans identified differences in the gut microbiome composition in patients with metastatic melanoma who respond compared to those who do not respond to immunotherapy. Responders to the anti-PD-1 immunotherapy had a more diverse gut microbiome in addition to higher abundance of Dorea formicigenerans, Faecalibacterium prausnitzii, Akkermansia muciniphila, Bifidobacterium longum, Collinsella aerofaciens, Enterococcus faecium, and bacteria from the Ruminococcaceae family.[8,12–15]

The role of the gut microbiome in the response of melanoma mouse models to anti-cytotoxic T-lymphocyte-associated protein 4 (anti-CTLA-4) seems different than its role in anti-PD-1 therapies. While the microbiome composition positively or negatively affects the response to anti-PD-1 therapy, the microbiome composition is essential for the efficacy of anti-CTLA-4 therapy. In fact, in germ-free mouse models with melanoma, treatment with anti-CTLA-4 therapy does not have any effect on tumor size. Absence of certain microbes results in a lack of response in mouse models receiving anti-CTLA-4 therapy. Recolonization of the germ-free mice with Burkholderia cepacia and different Bacteroides species, such as Bacteroides caccae, Bacteroides thetaiotaomicron, and Bacteroides fragilis, restored the therapeutic response of anti-CTLA-4 immune therapy.[10] Also, the microbiome profile of patients with melanoma demonstrating good response to anti-CTLA-4 therapy is distinct from that of patients with melanoma receiving anti-PD-1 therapy. For instance, patients with melanoma responding to anti-CTLA-4 therapy had a baseline microbiome with an abundance of Firmicutes.[16,17] Consistent with the studies using mouse models, distinct species of *Bacteroides*, such as, *B caccae* and *B thetaiotaomicron*, were associated with a better response to anti-CTLA-4 immunotherapy.[15] In addition, in patients with metastatic melanoma receiving combined anti-PD-1 and anti-CTLA-4 therapy, enrichment of *Faecalibacterium prausnitzii*, *B thetaiotaomicron*, and *Holdemania filiformis* was associated with improved response to therapy.[10,15]

The gut microbiome modulates not only the response to immunotherapy but also the associated toxicities (immune-related adverse events or irAEs). Toxicities related to immunotherapy can affect multiple organs and organs systems, with the most common irAE being immunotherapy-induced colitis.[16,17] The mechanism behind these irAEs is thought to be due to the loss of T-cell inhibition and decreased self-tolerance.[18,19] In patients receiving anti-CTLA-4 immunotherapy, abundance of *Faecalibacterium* and Firmicutes in pretreatment gut microbiota was associated with higher risk of colitis during or following treatment as compared to the higher relative abundance of *Bacteroides*, which was not associated with colitis.[16] Notably, the patients who had the greatest clinical benefit or response to anti-CTLA-4 immunotherapy were also those who were the most likely to develop colitis during or following treatment; the reverse was also true, in that patients with higher relative abundance of *Bacteroides* not only did not develop colitis but also did not have a favorable response to ipilimumab.[16] These findings were recapitulated in a study led by Dubin and colleagues[17] in which the presence of *Bacteroides intestinalis* was associated with decreased risk of irAEs in patients receiving anti-CTLA-4 and anti-PD-1 combination therapy.[20]

It is important to note that while some gut microbes are shown to be associated with a favorable response to immunotherapy, the mechanisms through which these microbes are contributing to response has not yet been well delineated.

Pathways and Metabolites Mediating the Effects of Microbiome on Immunotherapy Response

Enhancing T-cell function

The role of the microbiome in modulating the response to immunotherapy appears to be through the modulation of the tumor microenvironment (TME). The changes in TME resulting from immunotherapy are diverse and depends on multiple factors including the immunotherapeutic agent administered.[10,11] For instance, in mouse models with melanoma, anti-PD-1 immune therapy is mediated by an increase in CD8 cytotoxic T cells in TME that would target and kill tumor cells. In these mouse models, heat inactivation of administered *Bifidobacterium* and depletion of CD8 T cells led to abolishment of antitumor immunity.[11] The recruitment and activation of CD8 cytotoxic T cells occurs through multiple mechanisms, most notably through an increase in the activation of dendritic cells (**Fig. 1**).[11] Interestingly, microbiome-derived stimulator of interferon genes (STING) agonists induce type I interferon (IFN-I) production by intratumoral monocytes that, in turn, regulate macrophage polarization and induce dendritic cell activation.[21] Another pathway was described in preclinical models related to the activation of CD8 T cells by gavaging *Lactobacillus reuteri* that was shown to translocate to the TME. In these mice, CD8 T cells were directly activated through the acyl hydrocarbon receptor by *L reuteri*-derived indole-3-aldehyde (see **Fig. 1**).[22]

Microbiome-enhanced recruitment of CD4 T cells into the TME has also been shown to be associated with the efficacy of anti-PD-1 and anti-CTLA-4 immunotherapy in mouse models with melanoma.[10,13] In the study by Vetizou and colleagues, the role of CD4 T cells was clearly delineated. CD4 T cells isolated from mouse models with melanoma and patients with melanoma showed an increased Th1 phenotype. These cells were later transferred to germ-free mouse models with melanoma and were

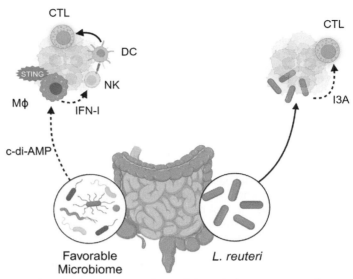

Fig. 1. Pathways by which the intestinal microbiome induce response of metastatic mela-noma to immune checkpoint blockage. On the left, activation of CTL occurs diectly by den-dritic cells (*solid arrow*). Microbiome-derived STING agonists (c-di-AMP, *dashed line*) induce intratumoral MΦ to produce IFN-I (*dashed line*) that subsequently activates DC though NK cells. On the right, activation of CTL occurs through stimulation of the acyl hydrocarbon re-ceptor by I3A (*dashed line*) produced by *Lactobacillus reuteri* that was shown to translocate to the TME (*solid line*). c-di-AMP, cyclic-di-adenosine monophosphate; CTL, cytotoxic T-lymphocyte; DC, dendritic cell; I3A, indole-3-aldehyde; IFN-1; type 1 interferon; MΦ, maco-phage; NK, natural killer cell; STING, stimulator of interferon genes.

capable of restoring the efficacy of anti-CTLA-4 immune therapy.[10] In addition, CD4 T cells are responsible for the increased responsiveness to anti-CTLA-4 immuno-therapy in metastatic melanoma patients with abundance of *Faecalibacterium*.[16] Not only do T cells differentiate into effector phenotypes of CD8 cytotoxic and CD4 Th1 cells but they can also differentiate into regulatory T cells. While differentiation into regulatory T cells is helpful in the treatment of autoimmune-related diseases,[23] their role in immunotherapy response is not favorable. For instance, increased abun-dance of intratumoral regulatory T cells is associated with a poor response in patients with solid tumors receiving anti-PD-1 therapy.[24]

Can the *Microbiome Profile Predict Response to Immunotherapy?*

The use of the microbiome profile for the prediction of response has been a topic of debate. Studies with metagenomic sequencing and metabolomics revealed several metabolites and bacterial species to be associated with response to immuno-therapy.[15] A meta-analysis of four cohorts with metagenomic sequencing introduced a classifier that was accurate in predicting responders to immunotherapy.[25] McCul-loch and colleagues developed a model that proved to be helpful in predicting response and irAEs in patients treated with anti-PD-1.[9] Despite these promising re-sults, studies have shown that the role of microbiome is heterogenous across cohorts and depends on the cohort studied.[9,26] Further investigations are needed to refine microbiome profiling before it can be implemented as a reliable, universal tool for the prediction of outcomes with immunotherapy.[9,26]

MODULATING THE GUT MICROBIOME FOR BETTER OUTCOMES WITH IMMUNOTHERAPY

Identification of bacteria and pathways associated with response or no response with immunotherapy is of utmost importance to power the clinical use of microbiome not only to predict and to improve the response to immunotherapy but also to potentially predict and prevent irAEs. In this section, we review the evidence for modification of the gut microbiome through dietary alterations and medication administration and ultimately the impact of modulation of gut microbiome on response to immunotherapy (**Fig. 2**).

Diet

What a patient eats has been shown to be associated with outcomes to immunotherapy in patients with cutaneous malignancies. For instance, high-fiber diet has been studied in mice, and somewhat surprisingly, it has been shown to trigger an improved response rate to immunotherapy by modulating the gut microbiome thus impacting microbe-produced metabolites and eventually altering TME to favor an anti-tumor response.[21] The beneficial effect of high-fiber diet on response to ICB was not present in germ-free mice. This finding further supports that the high-fiber diet exerts its beneficial effects through modulating the microbiome (see **Fig. 2**).[14] Obesity, well known to be associated with low-fiber diet, is paradoxically associated with improved progression-free and overall survival in patients with metastatic melanoma, especially in male patients receiving anti-PD-1 therapy.[27]

Probiotics

In preclinical models, commercially available probiotics and their impact on response to immune checkpoint blockade (ICB) were studied with different results depending on the bacterial constituents. For instance, commercially available probiotics with *Bifidobacterium longum* or *Lactobacillus rhamnosus* were shown to be associated with the worse outcomes after immunotherapy,[14] while the use of commercially available probiotics with a cocktail of *Bifidobacterium* was associated with improved tumor control

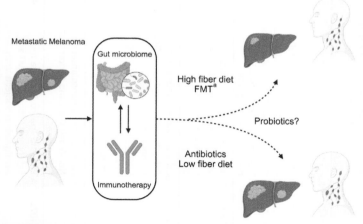

Fig. 2. The hypothesized interactions of lifestyle and medical practices with response of metastatic melanoma to immune checkpoint inhibitor through the microbiome. [a]Patient selection, donor profile, timing of FMT, and follow-up are essential for optimizing outcomes with FMT. FMT, fecal microbial transplant.

Table 1
Ongoing clinical trials for fecal microbial transplant and immunotherapy in patients with melanoma

Study Number	Title	N	Tumor Type	Immunotherapy	Microbiome
NCT0498841	Assessing the Tolerance and Clinical Benefit of feCal transplantation in patientS with melanoma (PICASSO)	60	Melanoma	Nivolumab (Anti-PD-1) Ipilimumab (Anti-CTLA-4)	MaaT013
NCT03341143	Fecal Microbiota Transplant in Melanoma Patients	18	Melanoma	Pembrolizumab (Anti-PD-1)	FMT from healthy donors
NCT03595683	Pembrolizumab and EDP1503 in Advanced Melanoma	8	Melanoma	Pembrolizumab (Anti-PD-1)	EDP1503
NCT05354102	A First-in-Human (FIH) Combination Treatment Study with a Single Dose Level of BMC 128	12	NSCLC, RCC, melanoma	Nivolumab (Anti-PD-1)	BMC128
NCT03637803	Live Biotherapeutic Product MRx0518 and Pembrolizumab Combination Study in Solid Tumors	132	NSCLC, RCC, bladder cancer, or melanoma	Pembrolizumab	MRx0518
NCT05273255	Fecal Microbiota Transplant in Patients with Malignancies Not Responding to Immune Checkpoint Inhibitor Therapy	30	Any malignancy	None	FMT from responders with solid tumors who had partial or complete response to ICI
NCT05251389	FMT to Convert Response to Immunotherapy	24	Melanoma	Anti-PD-1	FMT from donors undergoing ICI in either responders or non-responders
NCT04951583	Fecal Microbiota Transplantation Non-Small Cell Lung Cancer and Melanoma	70	NSCLC, melanoma	Pembrolizumab, Nivolumab (Anti-PD-1), Ipilimumab (Anti-CTLA-4)	FMT Capsules
NCT04521075	A Phase Ib Trial to Evaluate the Safety and Efficacy of FMT and Nivolumab in Subjects with Metastatic or Inoperable Melanoma, MSI-H, dMMR or NSCLC	42	Melanoma, MSI-H, dMMR, or NSCLC	Nivolumab (Anti-PD-1)	FMT Capsules

in melanoma mice models.[11] In patients with melanoma, commercially available probiotics were not associated with improved response to immunotherapy.[14]

Although probiotics are widely available, their use to achieve optimal results in patients and mouse models with melanoma is not yet established for many reasons (see **Fig. 2**). First, the ability of different probiotics to survive pH fluctuations in the gastrointestinal tract differs across products and their components, as do their ability to colonize the gastrointestinal tract.[28,29] Second, the colonization of probiotics in the diverse microbial system in humans remains a challenge,[30] and the implementation of antibiotics for gut conditioning followed by probiotics results in a less-diverse microbiome.[31] The inoculation of specific bacterial species may be necessary for an enhanced response in patients with melanoma.[14,32]

Furthermore, the combined effect of high-fiber diet and probiotics was studied in patients with metastatic melanoma, where patients who had high fiber intake but did not use probiotics had the best response to immunotherapy.[14]

Antibiotics

Antibiotics are known to alter the human microbiome, and this interaction in patients with cancer has been widely studied and well described.[1,33] Antibiotics modify the composition of the human microbiome by decreasing microbial diversity and causing population shifts that can persist up to twelve months.[34,35] The effect of antibiotics on response to immunotherapy was demonstrated in mouse models and assessed in patients. Administration of antibiotics to preclinical mice models of melanoma abolished the reduction in tumor growth rate after being treated with anti-PD-1 immunotherapy.[10] Similarly, administration of antibiotics prior to immunotherapy is associated with worse progression-free survival[36] and overall survival[37,38] in patients receiving immunotherapy for metastatic melanoma (see **Fig. 2**). Receipt of antibiotics prior to immunotherapy not only decreases its efficacy but also increases the risk of immune-mediated colitis.[39] Future observational studies with longitudinal microbiome analyses may uncover the relation among antibiotics, microbiome changes, and response to immunotherapy.

Fecal microbial transplant

The benefit of fecal microbial transplant (FMT) in health conditions such as *Clostridium difficile* colitis and the growing knowledge about the role of microbiome in the response to immunotherapy in patients with melanoma has fueled the investigation of the role of FMT in patients with melanoma receiving immunotherapy. Preclinical studies showed that mice receiving FMT from patients who had favorable response to immunotherapy ("Responder FMT") had reduced tumor growth and increased treatment efficacy compared to mice that received FMT from nonresponders.[8,12,13] Recently published pioneering clinical studies showed that responder FMT can overcome anti-PD-1 resistance in patients with PD-1 refractory melanoma (see **Fig. 2**).[40,41] The response was triggered by changes in immune cell recruitment and gene expression profiles in the TME.[40,41] Despite the promising results, several factors should be taken into consideration for optimizing outcomes with FMT including patient selection, donor profile, timing of FMT, and follow-up.[42,43] Several trials are underway to clearly establish the role of FMT in patients with melanoma and are summarized in **Table 1**.

SUMMARY

The role of the gut microbiome in the development, progression, and response of metastatic melanoma to immunotherapy is established. Multiple innovative studies have uncovered microbiome profiles that can serve as prognostic markers for immunotherapy response or can be modulated to augment response to immunotherapy.

Despite promising results observed regarding diagnostic and interventional aspects of the microbiome in patients with melanoma, the current applications in the clinical setting remain limited. These limitations result mainly from the heterogeneity of the microbiome profiles across different cohorts, which hinders our ability to derive universal conclusions about a suitable profile that would inform practice. On the other hand, the young nature of this field of research—the interaction between the microbiome and cancer—leaves many questions unanswered, especially the critical components for modulation and causality whether from the gut microbiome, its metabolites, or other factors yet to be identified. Nonetheless, the microbiome offers promising signals for changing clinical practice to benefit patients with melanoma through a highly scientific yet organic approach.

CLINICS CARE POINTS

- High-fiber diet is associated with increased response to ICB, increased overall survival, and decreased irAEs in patients with metastatic melanoma.
- Antibiotics likely modulate the gut microbiome in an unfavorable manner for patients who are going to or are currently receiving ICB for metastatic melanoma.
- Over-the-counter probiotics are not necessarily beneficial for patients with melanoma receiving immune therapy.

DISCLOSURE

The authors have nothing to disclose.

FUNDING

Dr Holder receives support from the American College of Surgeons Clowes Award, the Department of Defense Melanoma Academy Scholar Program, and the National Institutes of Health on grant R01CA289456.

REFERENCES

1. Routy B, Gopalakrishnan V, Daillere R, et al. The gut microbiota influences anti-cancer immunosurveillance and general health. Nat Rev Clin Oncol 2018;15(6): 382–96.
2. Khan MAW, Ologun G, Arora R, et al. Gut microbiome modulates response to cancer immunotherapy. Dig Dis Sci 2020;65(3):885–96.
3. Witt RG, Cass SH, Tran T, et al. Gut microbiome in patients with early-stage and late-stage melanoma. JAMA Dermatol 2023;159(10):1076–84.
4. Incorrect reference citations and figure labeling. JAMA 2016;315(22):2472.
5. Robert C, Thomas L, Bondarenko I, et al. Ipilimumab plus dacarbazine for previously untreated metastatic melanoma. N Engl J Med 2011;364(26):2517–26.
6. Topalian SL, Hodi FS, Brahmer JR, et al. Safety, activity, and immune correlates of anti-PD-1 antibody in cancer. N Engl J Med 2012;366(26):2443–54.
7. Pilard C, Ancion M, Delvenne P, et al. Cancer immunotherapy: it's time to better predict patients' response. Br J Cancer 2021;125(7):927–38.

8. Gopalakrishnan V, Spencer CN, Nezi L, et al. Gut microbiome modulates response to anti-PD-1 immunotherapy in melanoma patients. Science 2018;359(6371):97–103.

9. McCulloch JA, Davar D, Rodrigues RR, et al. Intestinal microbiota signatures of clinical response and immune-related adverse events in melanoma patients treated with anti-PD-1. Nat Med 2022;28(3):545–56.

10. Vetizou M, Pitt JM, Daillere R, et al. Anticancer immunotherapy by CTLA-4 blockade relies on the gut microbiota. Science 2015;350(6264):1079–84.

11. Sivan A, Corrales L, Hubert N, et al. Commensal Bifidobacterium promotes anti-tumor immunity and facilitates anti-PD-L1 efficacy. Science 2015;350(6264): 1084–9.

12. Matson V, Fessler J, Bao R, et al. The commensal microbiome is associated with anti-PD-1 efficacy in metastatic melanoma patients. Science 2018;359(6371): 104–8.

13. Routy B, Le Chatelier E, Derosa L, et al. Gut microbiome influences efficacy of PD-1-based immunotherapy against epithelial tumors. Science 2018;359(6371):91–7.

14. Spencer CN, McQuade JL, Gopalakrishnan V, et al. Dietary fiber and probiotics influence the gut microbiome and melanoma immunotherapy response. Science 2021;374(6575):1632–40.

15. Frankel AE, Coughlin LA, Kim J, et al. Metagenomic shotgun sequencing and unbiased metabolomic profiling identify specific human gut microbiota and metabolites associated with immune checkpoint therapy efficacy in melanoma patients. Neoplasia 2017;19(10):848–55.

16. Chaput N, Lepage P, Coutzac C, et al. Baseline gut microbiota predicts clinical response and colitis in metastatic melanoma patients treated with ipilimumab. Ann Oncol 2017;28(6):1368–79.

17. Dubin K, Callahan MK, Ren B, et al. Intestinal microbiome analyses identify melanoma patients at risk for checkpoint-blockade-induced colitis. Nat Commun 2016;7:10391.

18. Spain L, Diem S, Larkin J. Management of toxicities of immune checkpoint inhibitors. Cancer Treat Rev 2016;44:51–60.

19. Halsey T, Ologun G, Wargo J, et al. Uncovering the role of the gut microbiota in immune checkpoint blockade therapy: A mini-review. Semin Hematol 2020; 57(1):13–8.

20. Andrews MC, Duong CPM, Gopalakrishnan V, et al. Gut microbiota signatures are associated with toxicity to combined CTLA-4 and PD-1 blockade. Nat Med 2021; 27(8):1432–41.

21. Lam KC, Araya RE, Huang A, et al. Microbiota triggers STING-type I IFN-dependent monocyte reprogramming of the tumor microenvironment. Cell 2021;184(21): 5338–5356 e5321.

22. Bender MJ, McPherson AC, Phelps CM, et al. Dietary tryptophan metabolite released by intratumoral Lactobacillus reuteri facilitates immune checkpoint inhibitor treatment. Cell 2023;186(9):1846–1862 e1826.

23. Takahashi D, Hoshina N, Kabumoto Y, et al. Microbiota-derived butyrate limits the autoimmune response by promoting the differentiation of follicular regulatory T cells. EBioMedicine 2020;58:102913.

24. Kumagai S, Togashi Y, Kamada T, et al. The PD-1 expression balance between effector and regulatory T cells predicts the clinical efficacy of PD-1 blockade therapies. Nat Immunol 2020;21(11):1346–58.

25. Limeta A, Ji B, Levin M, et al. Meta-analysis of the gut microbiota in predicting response to cancer immunotherapy in metastatic melanoma. JCI Insight 2020; 5(23):e140940.

26. Lee KA, Thomas AM, Bolte LA, et al. Cross-cohort gut microbiome associations with immune checkpoint inhibitor response in advanced melanoma. Nat Med 2022;28(3):535–44.

27. McQuade JL, Daniel CR, Hess KR, et al. Association of body-mass index and outcomes in patients with metastatic melanoma treated with targeted therapy, immunotherapy, or chemotherapy: a retrospective, multicohort analysis. Lancet Oncol 2018;19(3):310–22.

28. Kristensen NB, Bryrup T, Allin KH, et al. Alterations in fecal microbiota composition by probiotic supplementation in healthy adults: a systematic review of randomized controlled trials. Genome Med 2016;8(1):52.

29. Sanders ME. Impact of probiotics on colonizing microbiota of the gut. J Clin Gastroenterol 2011;45(Suppl):S115–9.

30. Zmora N, Zilberman-Schapira G, Suez J, et al. Personalized gut mucosal colonization resistance to empiric probiotics is associated with unique host and microbiome features. Cell 2018;174(6):1388–1405 e1321.

31. Suez J, Zmora N, Zilberman-Schapira G, et al. Post-antibiotic gut mucosal microbiome reconstitution is impaired by probiotics and improved by autologous FMT. Cell 2018;174(6):1406–1423 e1416.

32. Tanoue T, Morita S, Plichta DR, et al. A defined commensal consortium elicits CD8 T cells and anti-cancer immunity. Nature 2019;565(7741):600–5.

33. Blaser MJ. Antibiotic use and its consequences for the normal microbiome. Science 2016;352(6285):544–5.

34. Palleja A, Mikkelsen KH, Forslund SK, et al. Recovery of gut microbiota of healthy adults following antibiotic exposure. Nat Microbiol 2018;3(11):1255–65.

35. Rashid MU, Zaura E, Buijs MJ, et al. Determining the long-term effect of antibiotic administration on the human normal intestinal microbiota using culture and pyrosequencing methods. Clin Infect Dis 2015;60(Suppl 2):S77–84.

36. Elkrief A, El Raichani L, Richard C, et al. Antibiotics are associated with decreased progression-free survival of advanced melanoma patients treated with immune checkpoint inhibitors. OncoImmunology 2019;8(4):e1568812.

37. Eng L, Sutradhar R, Niu Y, et al. Impact of antibiotic exposure before immune checkpoint inhibitor treatment on overall survival in older adults with cancer: a population-based study. J Clin Oncol 2023;41(17):3122–34.

38. Pinato DJ, Howlett S, Ottaviani D, et al. Association of prior antibiotic treatment with survival and response to immune checkpoint inhibitor therapy in patients with cancer. JAMA Oncol 2019;5(12):1774–8.

39. Mohiuddin JJ, Chu B, Facciabene A, et al. Association of antibiotic exposure with survival and toxicity in patients with melanoma receiving immunotherapy. J Natl Cancer Inst 2021;113(2):162–70.

40. Baruch EN, Youngster I, Ben-Betzalel G, et al. Fecal microbiota transplant promotes response in immunotherapy-refractory melanoma patients. Science 2021;371(6529):602–9.

41. Davar D, Dzutsev AK, McCulloch JA, et al. Fecal microbiota transplant overcomes resistance to anti-PD-1 therapy in melanoma patients. Science 2021;371(6529):595–602.

42. McQuade JL, Ologun GO, Arora R, et al. Gut microbiome modulation via fecal microbiota transplant to augment immunotherapy in patients with melanoma or other cancers. Curr Oncol Rep 2020;22(7):74.

43. McQuade JL, Daniel CR, Helmink BA, et al. Modulating the microbiome to improve therapeutic response in cancer. Lancet Oncol 2019;20(2):e77–91.

High-Risk Non-Melanoma Skin Cancers
Biological and Therapeutic Advances

Truelian Lee, BA[a,1], Tomonori Oka, MD, PhD[b,c,2],
Shadmehr Demehri, MD, PhD[a,b,c,*,3]

KEYWORDS

- High-risk non-melanoma skin cancer • Basal cell carcinoma
- Cutaneous squamous cell carcinoma • Merkel cell carcinoma • Ultraviolet radiation
- Cutaneous immunity

KEY POINTS

- Ultraviolet radiation is a main driver of non-melanoma skin cancers (NMSCs), emphasizing the importance of sun protection as the main primary prevention strategy.
- Mutations in the Hedgehog signaling pathway are a cardinal driver of basal cell carcinoma, with recent advances in therapeutics targeting this pathway.
- The epidermal growth factor receptor signaling pathway plays a crucial role in the development of cutaneous squamous cell carcinoma (cSCC), and there have been therapeutics developed targeting this pathway.
- Although knowledge about Merkel cell carcinoma (MCC) pathogenesis is limited, it has been associated with Merkel cell polyomavirus infection.
- cSCC and MCC are highly responsive to immunotherapy, which has become the primary treatment strategy for advanced disease.

INTRODUCTION

Non-melanoma skin cancers (NMSCs) are the most common cancer types. The global incidence of NMSCs increased 33% between 2007 and 2017, with 7.7 million new cases worldwide in 2017.[1] Studies predict that the incidence of NMSCs will continue

[a] Harvard Medical School, Boston, MA 02115, USA; [b] Center for Cancer Immunology, Center for Cancer Research, Massachusetts General Hospital, Boston, MA 02114, USA; [c] Department of Dermatology, Cutaneous Biology Research Center, Massachusetts General Hospital, Boston, MA 02114, USA
[1] Present address: 25 Shattuck Street, Boston MA 02115, USA.
[2] Present address: Building 149 13th Street, Room 3.215, Charlestown MA 02129, USA.
[3] Building 149 13th Street, Room 3.215, Charlestown MA 02129, USA.
* Corresponding author. Department of Dermatology, Cutaneous Biology Research Center, Massachusetts General Hospital, Boston, MA 02114.
E-mail address: sdemehri1@mgh.harvard.edu

Hematol Oncol Clin N Am 38 (2024) 1071–1085
https://doi.org/10.1016/j.hoc.2024.05.004
0889-8588/24/© 2024 Elsevier Inc. All rights reserved.

hemonc.theclinics.com

to increase for at least another decade.[1] Two major NMSCs are basal cell carcinoma (BCC) and cutaneous squamous cell carcinoma (cSCC). Together, BCC and cSCC are referred to as keratinocyte carcinomas, and their prevalence has increased over the past decades.[2] In addition, given underreporting of NMSCs in cancer registries, researchers have postulated that the mortality rate of NMSCs may be higher than that of melanoma.[3]

BCC is the most common NMSC, comprising of 70% of all NMSCs.[1] It is believed that BCC originates in hair follicle cells or the interfollicular epidermis.[4–6] There are multiple histopathologic subtypes of BCC, and many lesions contain multiple subtypes: nodular, superficial, infiltrative, micronodular, fibroepithelial, infundibulocystic, morpheaform, and basoquamous.[7] Nodular BCC is the most common subtype, seen in 50% to 80% of lesions, while superficial is the second most common at 10% to 30%.[7]

cSCC is the second most common NMSC, accounting for 25% of all NMSCs.[1] The histopathologic subtypes of cSCC extend from well-differentiated cSCC presenting as scaly erythematous nodules or plaques to poorly differentiated cSCC presenting as soft, ulcerated, or hemorrhagic lesions.[8]

Merkel cell carcinoma (MCC), another NMSC, is a rare neuroendocrine cancer believed to develop in the epidermis, potentially from dermal fibroblasts.[9] Common presentations of MCC include violaceous papulonodular lesions that grow rapidly.[9] MCC is characterized by high local recurrence rates, metastasis, and poor survival.[9]

There are several other NMSCs, which will not be discussed in this review. These include sebaceous carcinoma and other adnexal tumors, angiosarcoma, cutaneous B-cell lymphoma, cutaneous T-cell lymphoma, and dermatofibrosarcoma protuberans.

Characteristics of high-risk NMSCs include poor histologic differentiation, invasion into fat or deeper layers, perineural invasion, and development in high-risk anatomic locations.[10,11] This review will describe recent advances in the biological understanding of and therapeutic options for NMSCs.

BIOLOGICAL ADVANCES

Ultraviolet (UV) radiation is the main driver of NMSCs. Although DNA repair mechanisms such as nucleotide excision repair are evolved to fix pyrimidine dimers caused by UV, the accumulation of UV-induced mutations is readily detectable in an aging skin.[12] The clonal expansion of mutant keratinocytes leads to the formation of NMSCs. Silencing of the tumor suppressor gene *TP53* is found in 50% of patients with skin cancer.[13] However, a large array of UV-induced somatic mutations are found in NMSCs, which leads to tumor heterogeneity.

Basal Cell Carcinoma

Mutations in the Hedgehog signaling pathway are a cardinal driver of BCC.[14] Within the Hedgehog pathway, mutations in the transmembrane PTCH1 protein are the most common.[14] Mutations in the G-couple protein receptor smoothened (SMO) have also been implicated.[14] Some BCCs have also been reported to have a loss of function mutation in SUFU, which binds to the transcription factor Gli proteins.[14]

There have also been several other genetic pathways potentially implicated in BCC carcinogenesis. Research has suggested that variants in interleukin (IL)-6 are associated with a risk of BCC, and that overexpression of IL-6 can increase tumorigenic potency and growth.[15] Analysis of BCC tissue samples and genetic data have also brought forth stem cell differentiation regulator GREM1 and protein crosslinking gene TGM3 as candidate genes in the development of BCC.[16,17]

A recently conducted single-cell RNA sequencing analysis of human BCC reveals spatially heterogeneous cell populations with fibroblasts that promote inflammatory signaling pathways.[18] BCC overexpresses WNT5A, which regulates cancer cell metabolism, invasion, and metastasis.[18] Genes that code for heat shock protein are also upregulated, suggesting that BCC cells may use heat shock proteins to promote cell proliferation.[18]

Tumor microenvironment
The BCC microenvironment has been shown to help attenuate host immunity to the tumor. BCC tumors have reduced major histocompatibility complex (MHC)-I by down-regulating beta2-microglobulin, a component of MHC-I.[19–21] The BCC tumor microenvironment has been shown to be high in regulatory T cells and Th2 cytokines.[22] The BCC tumor microenvironment has also been suggested to promote pathogenesis and survival through the secretion of high levels of IL-17 and IL-22.[23] In addition, cancer-associated fibroblasts are abundant in BCC and secrete chemokines such as CXCL12 and CCL17, which are implicated in tumor progression and immunosuppression.[24] BCCs also upregulate several genes that form the extracellular matrix, including several cancer-associated fibroblast markers.[24] The expression of these genes promotes matrix remodeling.[24] The population of tumor-associated macrophages in BCC is enriched for the pro-tumorigenic M2 macrophages, which encourages tumor growth, invasion, and metastasis.[25] These macrophages can also act directly on BCC cancer cells to upregulate the expression of tumor-promoting genes.[25]

Cutaneous Squamous Cell Carcinoma
Several genetic mutations are implicated in cSCC carcinogenesis. Loss of expression in the NOTCH pathway, such as NOTCH1, disrupts its role in keratinocyte differentiation and has been associated with cSCC development.[12] Recent research has also shown the importance of epidermal growth factor receptor (EGFR) signaling on the Ras/Raf/Mek/Erk and PI3K/AKT/mTOR pathways.[26] Ras proteins, which influence cell proliferation, differentiation, and survival, have been theorized to promote epidermal invasion.[12] A meta-analysis of 105 tumors from 10 studies detected multiple tumors with mutations in the Ras/MAPK/PI3K pathways.[27] Studies with human tissue samples and murine models have also suggested that upregulating genes in the immune response, such as complement subunits C1r and C1s, can promote the growth of cSCC.[28]

Four tumor subpopulations are found in cSCC compared with matched normal samples analyzed with single-cell RNA-seq, spatial transcriptomics, and multiplex ion beam imaging.[29] Three of the subpopulations are analogous to subpopulations found in normal skin, expressing characteristic basal, cycling, and differentiating genes.[29] However, there is a fourth, tumor-specific subpopulation found in cSCC samples that is characterized by genes associated with cellular movement, extracellular matrix disassembly, and epithelial-mesenchymal transition markers.[29] These tumor-specific keratinocytes represented 2.7% to 13.8% of tumor cells and are situated within a fibrovascular niche at leading edges.[29] These findings suggest that a small population of keratinocytes drives the progression of cSCC.

Tumor microenvironment
Activated neutrophils and monocytes with immunosuppressive properties, also known as myeloid-derived suppressor cells, help cSCC avoid immune detection by limiting T cell localization to the tumor through the production of nitric oxide, which downregulates E-selectin on tumor vessels.[30,31] They also produce arginase and reactive oxygen species, both of which have also been shown to suppress T cell function.[30] The tumor

microenvironment in cSCC is believed to encourage tumor-associated macrophages to promote tumor growth.[32] They have been shown to increase the production of matrix metalloproteinases and lymphangiogenesis through the upregulation of vascular endothelial growth factor-C.[32] In addition, studies have shown that the population of Langerhans cells is decreased in cSCC lesions.[33] Dermal myeloid dendritic cells have also been shown to have a reduced ability to produce interferon-gamma and activate T cells, which is postulated to be due to increased levels of immunosuppressive cytokines.[34]

Merkel Cell Carcinoma

MCC can develop either through oncogenic events in the context of Merkel cell polyomavirus (MCPyV) infection, or through a nonviral pathway involving UV radiation and a high mutational burden.[35] Although it is unclear what cells MCC originates from, research suggests that MCPyV infects dermal fibroblasts, especially around the hair follicles based on cell culture and ex vivo models.[36] It is theorized that UV radiation upregulates Wnt signaling, which helps promote MCPyV infection.[36]

There has been extensive research elucidating the role of the immune system in curtailing MCC development.[35] Although MCC downregulates surface expression of MHC-I and upregulates T cell inhibitory signals, it is considered to be a highly immunogenic cancer.[35]

At a single-cell level, MCC shows several distinct tumor cell states.[37] Tumor cells also show plasticity, with some MCC tumors able to transition to a more "mesenchymal-like" state characterized by increased inflammation and correlated with favorable response to immune checkpoint inhibitors.[37] In contrast, a "well-differentiated neuroepithelial" state is associated with less active immune system in the tumor, as well as resistance to immune checkpoint inhibitors.[37]

Tumor microenvironment

Within the tumor microenvironment, a high level of $CD8^+$ T cell infiltration has been associated with favorable prognoses in patients with MCC.[38] In addition, increased numbers of regulatory T cells have been found in the tumor microenvironment, which promote tumor development and proliferation by secreting anti-inflammatory cytokines.[39] Another population of T cells that is enriched in MCC tumors is double negative T cells that express non-major histocompatibility complex antigen recognition, which allows them to regulate proinflammatory and antigen-driven responses.[40]

Over the past few years, several cellular and molecular pathways have been elucidated to play a role in the development of NMSCs (**Fig. 1**). An increased understanding of the biological underpinnings of NMSCs and their tumor microenvironment has led to the development of effective treatment strategies for NMSCs, including targeted therapy and immunotherapy.

THERAPEUTIC ADVANCES

Surgery is the first-line treatment for localized NMSCs. For higher risk NMSC, several strategies have been in development, including therapies that target specific molecular pathways in NMSC (**Fig. 2**).

Basal Cell Carcinoma

Although there is no formal staging system for BCC due to its rare metastasis, the National Comprehensive Cancer Network (NCCN) stratifies localized tumors into those at high versus low risk of recurrence.[41] One of the key factors in high-risk BCC is anatomic location.[42] Size, histologic subtype, and poorly demarcated borders also

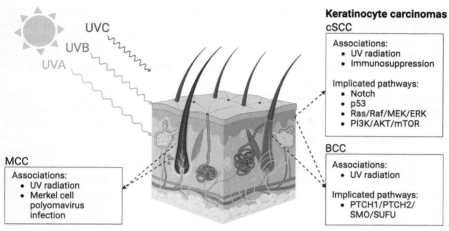

Fig. 1. Biological drivers of non-melanoma skin cancers (NMSCs). (Created with BioRender. com.)

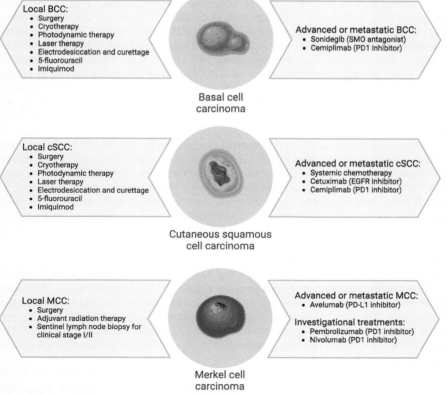

Fig. 2. Therapeutic approaches to NMSCs. (Created with BioRender.com.)

potentially have an impact depending on the risk associated with a particular anatomic location.[41] Treatments for low-risk BCC include standard excision, with the NCCN recommending 4 mm margins.[41] Other options also include cryotherapy, photodynamic therapy, laser therapy, electrodessication, curettage, topical 5-fluorouracil cream, and imiquimod cream.[43] Radiation therapy is indicated in patients where surgery is contraindicated or for unresectable tumors.[43]

Hedgehog pathway inhibitors, such as SHH inhibitors, SMO antagonists, and Gli inhibitors, have also been studied as promising treatments for BCC. Topical Hedgehog pathway inhibitors have been examined for primary BCC treatment and prevention, but they have not been shown to cure BCC on a histopathological level.[44] A trial of topical sonidegib was discontinued due to insufficient efficacy.[44] Patidegib, an analog to sonidegib, was studied in a phase II clinical trial applying it topically daily for 12 weeks in people who had untreated nodular BCCs to test for its efficacy on those tumors.[45] Compared to the control, patidegib led to more tumor reduction, and there were no serious adverse events noted.[45] Currently, patidegib is being investigated in a phase III clinical trial for BCC prevention in Gorlin syndrome patients.[46] Another investigational topical treatment for BCC is itraconazole, which is an anti-fungal agent that can inhibit SMO activity.[47] However, it is found not to significantly reduce BCC tumor size in a recent trial.[48]

Systemic formulations of Hedgehog inhibitors have been developed for BCC treatment, including SMO antagonists vismodegib and sonidegib. In ERIVANCE study, consisting of 63 patients with locally advanced BCC and 33 patients with metastatic BCC, vismodegib achieved a 42.9% objective response rate (ORR) with locally advanced BCC and 30.3% ORR with metastatic BCC.[49] However, the study showed that vismodegib also caused several side effects and adverse events. Serious adverse events were observed in 25% of the patients and associated with 7 deaths.[50] Adverse events included muscle spasms, dysgeusia, and weight loss.[49] Subsequent trials on vismodegib for BCC treatment, such as STEVIE and MIKIE, have arrived at similar safety profiles.[51] Sonidegib was approved by the U.S. Food and Drug Administration (FDA) in 2015 after the BOLT study.[51] This study showed that the drug at 200 mg achieved an ORR of 56% in locally advanced BCC and 8% in metastatic BCC, while having a better safety profile than vismodegib.[52,53]

There have also been a few immunotherapies approved for advanced NMSC, including immune checkpoint inhibitors (ICI).[54] Cemiplimab, a human IgG4 anti-PD-1 antibody, was approved by the FDA in 2021 for locally advanced and metastatic BCC.[54] The phase II EMPOWER-BCC 1 trial of cemiplimab treatment on 84 locally advanced BCC patients after first-line hedgehog inhibitor therapy showed an ORR of 31%, with 6% complete responses and 25% partial responses.[55] The most frequent adverse events were hypertension and colitis, which both occurred in 5% of the patients.[55]

Cutaneous Squamous Cell Carcinoma

The 2 main cSCC staging systems are the American Joint Committee on Cancer 9 (AJCC9) and Brigham and Women's Hospital systems.[56] These systems use TMN staging, in which T is based on tumor size, N lymph node involvement, and M the presence of metastases. The AJCC9 primarily uses tumor diameter to differentiate T1 and T2, and either tumor diameter, thickness, or invasion for T3, with T4 involving the bone.[56] The Brigham and Women's Hospital system factors in poorly differentiated histology and level of invasion.[56]

Treatment options for cSCC in situ include surgery, electrodessication and curettage, cryotherapy, laser therapy, topical 5-fluorouracil cream, topical imiquimod cream, and photodynamic therapy.[8] Recent research has also explored other options for cSCC in situ. A cohort study on the use of photodynamic therapy with aminolevulinic acid on facial cSCC in situ showed no pathologically residual tumor at 4 to 6 weeks after treatment.[57] Radiation therapy is indicated in patients where surgery is contraindicated or for unresectable tumors.[8]

Treatment for low-risk invasive cSCC consists of standard excision, with a recommended margin of 4 to 6 mm and a depth to the mid-adipose layer.[56] For cSCC of the scalp and face, and for higher risk cSCC, Mohs micrographic surgery is recommended.[58] Mohs surgery has been shown to lead to a lower recurrence rate than standard excision for cSCC of the ears, lips, and cSCC with perineural invasion.[58] Although research suggests that it is a safe and feasible staging technique, the role of sentinel lymph node biopsy in cSCC management remains uncertain.[59]

Systemic treatments for advanced cSCC include systemic chemotherapy, targeted therapy with EGFR inhibitors, and immunotherapy.[60] Systemic cytotoxic chemotherapy such as cisplatin and 5-fluorouracil was the main treatment for advanced cSCC prior to the advent of targeted therapy and immunotherapy.[61] EGFR inhibitors have been developed as a therapeutic option for advanced cSCC. A phase II study of cetuximab as a first-line monotherapy for 36 patients with unresectable cSCC achieved an disease control rate of 69%, with 3 serious adverse events consisting of infusion reactions or interstitial pneumopathy.[62] Another retrospective study in 58 patients with unresectable cSCC showed that first-line cetuximab achieved a 53% ORR, which was attributed to the population having less advanced disease with less lymph node involvement.[63] Cetuximab has also been explored as a second-line treatment after ICI therapy failure in locally advanced or metastatic cSCC, which is well-tolerated, with fast and durable responses in the patients treated successfully.[64]

Cemiplimab has been approved as a first-line treatment for locally advanced or metastatic cSCC.[65] The phase II EMPOWER-CSCC trial consisted of 193 patients with unresectable locally advanced or metastatic cSCC treated with cemiplimab.[66] Cemiplimab achieved a 46.1% ORR, with only 9% of the patients experiencing grade $\geq$3 immune-related adverse events and 10% discontinuing treatment.[66] The most common side effects were fatigue and diarrhea.[66] Another ICI therapy for advanced cSCC, pembrolizumab, was studied in the phase II KEYNOTE-629 trial, which consisted of 159 patients.[67] In this trial, pembrolizumab 200 mg had an ORR of 50% for patients with locally advanced cSCC and 35.2% for patients with recurrent or metastatic cSCC.[67] Common adverse events consisted of pruritus, fatigue, and asthenia, with 11.9% of the patients experiencing higher grade adverse events such as severe skin reactions.[67] Another phase II trial on 39 patients with unresectable cSCC showed an objective response rate of 41%, with 3 complete responses and 13 partial responses.[68] A total of 71% of patients experienced an adverse event, with common adverse events consisting of fatigue, diarrhea, and hypothyroidism.[68]

Although organ transplant recipients are at 100-fold increased risk of developing cSCC compared with the general population,[69] with re-transplanted patients at increased risk for more aggressive phenotypes,[70] ICI therapy may be counter indicated in this population due to increased risk of post-transplant complications and graft rejection.[71] In a systematic review of immunotherapy in patients with metastatic cancer and solid organ transplants, 37% experienced organ rejection and 14% died from it.[72] Thus, alternative therapeutic approaches are urgently needed to address cSCC in organ transplant recipients and other immunosuppressed patients.

Merkel Cell Carcinoma

MCC is classified with the AJCC/Union for International Cancer Control (UICC) 9 classification system, with head/neck lesions, tumor size equal or greater than 2 cm, chronic immunosuppression, pathologically positive lymph nodes, and lymphovascular invasion being the criteria that qualify MCC as high-risk.[73] Surgery is first-line treatment for MCC, with studies suggesting that adjuvant radiation therapy can be helpful.[73] Sentinel lymph node biopsy is recommended for clinical stage I/II MCC.[73]

ICI has also been investigated as a systemic treatment for virus-positive and virus-negative MCC, with the FDA having approved a PD-L1 inhibitor, avelumab, for metastatic MCC.[74] The phase 2 JAVELIN Merkel 200 trial showed a 31.8% ORR to avelumab in 88 patients who had metastatic MCC that previously failed chemotherapy.[75] A total of 5% of the patients experienced lymphopenia, aminotransferase increases, or other lab abnormalities.[75] When 39 patients who had never received any kind of treatment were studied, the ORR increased to 62.1%.[76] However, 71.8% of the patients experienced an adverse event, with 15.4% of the patients discontinuing the treatment because of it.[76] Other ICIs that are currently being studied for MCC include pembrolizumab and nivolumab, which have shown similar response rates and durability as avelumab.[77,78]

Although ICI therapy has proven effective in NMSC treatment, many high-risk patients, including immunosuppressed individuals, are not candidate for ICI therapy. Thus, novel strategies for NMSC prevention and treatment in high-risk patients remain an urgent unmet need.

FUTURE DIRECTIONS

Recent findings have suggested that cSCC is a highly immune-regulated disease, helping shift the framework of cSCC from a disease of immune suppression to a disease of immune dysregulation.[79] When organ transplant patients are compared to the general population, their risk of cSCC can be as high as 250-fold and their risk of BCC 10-fold.[80] Although research has shown that BCC is less immunogenic than cSCC, immune system suppression and dysregulation have been also found to play an important role in BCC development.[80] Understanding the role of immune cells and factors in these tumors can help efforts to identify novel immune pathways that can serve as targets for therapeutics, including immunoprevention (**Fig. 3**).[81]

Several ongoing trials are testing new treatment regimens for NMSC. Trials have also investigated immune checkpoint inhibitors in combination with other treatments. For instance, the CERPASS trial combines RP1, an intratumorally injected oncolytic virus, with cemiplimab.[82] In preliminary studies, this combination treatment achieved high response rates in patients with locally advanced cSCC and caused moderate side effects.[82] A combination of cemiplimab and pulsed dosing sonidegib treatment is being tested for patients with advanced BCC.[83]

Additional research has been done to optimize the delivery of medication into NMSC. Photodynamic therapy is often administered with 5-aminolaevulinic acid (5-AA) for superficial BCC, but a challenge is that 5-AA does not penetrate very deeply into the skin.[84] Administering 5-AA with nanoemulsion-based gel has been shown to induce a complete response in 23/31 patients after 3 months.[84] In addition, when ultradeformable liposomes were used to deliver vismodegib transdermally on ex vivo human skin samples, it achieved around 7 times increased penetration 1 hour after application compared to vismodegib in dimethyl sulfoxide.[85]

Strategies to prevent NMSCs have focused on UV protection as the cardinal primary prevention method. Individuals are counseled to protect their skin from UV exposure using sunscreen and protective clothing, avoidance of outdoor activities when the sun is the strongest (10:00 AM–3:00 PM), and avoidance of tanning beds. However, NMSC risk continues to increase despite the extensive campaign for UV protection around the world.

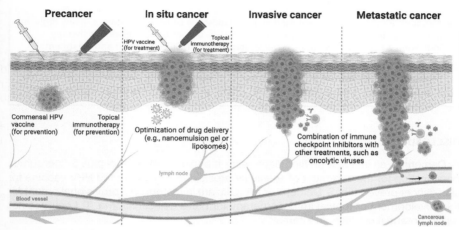

Fig. 3. Potential future directions in NMSC therapeutics. (Created with BioRender.com.)

A novel avenue for secondary NMSC prevention in immunocompetent and immuno-suppressed patients is topical immunotherapy, which could potentially prevent NMSCs without adverse systemic side effects.[81] In a recent randomized, double-blind clinical trial, 7% of the participants treated with topical calcipotriol (a low calcemic vitamin D analog) plus 5-fluorouracil combination therapy developed new cSCC compared to 28% in the Vaseline plus 5-fluorouracil group.[86,87]

Another future direction for NMSC prevention and early therapy takes advantage of skin virome-immune interactions to combat UV-induced carcinogenesis. Recent discoveries have revealed that T cell immunity to cutaneotropic human papillomaviruses (HPVs) cross-protects the skin from cancer development.[88] This fundamental concept can pave the way for the development of novel T cell-directed vaccines against commensal HPVs (eg, β- and γ-HPVs) that can help reduce the risk of NMSCs in immunosuppressed patients and older adults.

SUMMARY

High-risk NMSCs are characterized by poor histologic differentiation, invasion into fat or deeper layers, perineural invasion, and high-risk anatomic locations. Recent advances have suggested several different mutations that potentially drive NMSCs, with the Hedgehog pathway playing a major role in BCC and Notch and Ras playing a large role in cSCC. Given that research has highlighted the important role of immune system suppression or dysregulation in these tumors, multiple new therapies have been developed, such as targeted therapy, immune checkpoint inhibitors, and oncolytic viruses. Further elucidating the role of immune cells and factors in high-risk NMSCs can help identify novel immune pathways for NMSC prevention and early therapy.

CLINICS CARE POINTS

- An increased understanding of the genetic underpinnings of NMSCs and their tumor microenvironments has suggested several potential treatment strategies, including targeted therapy and immunotherapy.

- Although ICI therapy has revolutionized the landscape of NMSC treatment, many high-risk patients, including immunosuppressed individuals, do not benefit from this therapy, indicating a continued need for novel strategies for NMSC prevention and treatment.
- For primary NMSC prevention, individuals should be counseled to protect their skin from UV exposure through the use of sunscreen and protective clothing, avoidance of outdoor activities when the sun is the strongest (10:00 AM–3:00 PM), and avoidance of tanning beds.

DISCLOSURE

S. Demehri is an inventor on filed patents for the use of calcipotriol plus 5-fluorouracil combination for the treatment of actinic keratosis and T cell-directed HPV vaccine for skin cancer prevention. S. Demehri and T. Oka are inventors on a provisional patent for the development of topical immunotherapy for basal cell carcinoma. T. Lee does not report potential conflicts of interest.

REFERENCES

1. Ciuciulete AR, Stepan AE, Andreiana BC, et al. Non-melanoma skin cancer: statistical associations between clinical parameters. Curr Health Sci J 2022;48(1):110–5.
2. Urban K, Mehrmal S, Uppal P, et al. The global burden of skin cancer: A longitudinal analysis from the Global Burden of Disease Study, 1990-2017. JAAD Int 2021;2:98–108.
3. The ASCO Post Staff. Nonmelanoma skin cancers may have higher mortality rate than melanoma. 2023. Available at: https://ascopost.com/news/october-2023/nonmelanoma-skin-cancers-may-have-higher-mortality-rate-than-melanoma/. [Accessed 30 January 2024].
4. Donovan J. Review of the hair follicle origin hypothesis for basal cell carcinoma. Dermatol Surg 2009;35(9):1311–23.
5. Tan ST, Ghaznawie M, Heenan PJ, et al. Basal cell carcinoma arises from interfollicular layer of epidermis. JAMA Oncol 2018;2018:3098940.
6. Bansaccal N, Vieugue P, Sarate R, et al. The extracellular matrix dictates regional competence for tumour initiation. Nature 2023;623(7988):828–35.
7. Cameron MC, Lee E, Hibler BP, et al. Basal cell carcinoma: Epidemiology; pathophysiology; clinical and histological subtypes; and disease associations [published correction appears in J Am Acad Dermatol. 2021 Aug;85(2):535]. J Am Acad Dermatol 2019;80(2):303–17.
8. Fania L, Didona D, Di Pietro FR, et al. Cutaneous squamous cell carcinoma: from pathophysiology to novel therapeutic approaches. Biomedicines 2021;9(2):171.
9. Lewis DJ, Sobanko JF, Etzkorn JR, et al. Merkel Cell Carcinoma. Dermatol Clin 2023;41(1):101–15.
10. Burton KA, Ashack KA, Khachemoune A. Cutaneous squamous cell carcinoma: a review of high-risk and metastatic disease. Am J Clin Dermatol 2016;17(5):491–508.
11. Singh B, Dorelles A, Konnikov N, et al. Detection of high-risk histologic features and tumor upstaging of nonmelanoma skin cancers on debulk analysis: a quantitative systematic review. Dermatol Surg 2017;43(8):1003–11.
12. Zambrano-Román M, Padilla-Gutiérrez JR, Valle Y, et al. Non-Melanoma Skin Cancer: A Genetic Update and Future Perspectives. Cancers 2022;14(10):2371.
13. Giglia-Mari G, Sarasin A. TP53 mutations in human skin cancers. Hum Mutat 2003;21(3):217–28.

14. Pellegrini C, Maturo MG, Di Nardo L, et al. Understanding the molecular genetics of basal cell carcinoma. Int J Mol Sci 2017;18(11):2485.
15. Sternberg C, Gruber W, Eberl M, et al. Synergistic cross-talk of hedgehog and interleukin-6 signaling drives growth of basal cell carcinoma. Int J Cancer 2018; 143(11):2943–54.
16. Kim HS, Shin MS, Cheon MS, et al. GREM1 is expressed in the cancer-associated myofibroblasts of basal cell carcinomas. PLoS One 2017;12(3):e0174565.
17. Smirnov A, Anemona L, Montanaro M, et al. Transglutaminase 3 is expressed in basal cell carcinoma of the skin. Eur J Dermatol 2019;29(5):477–83.
18. Guerrero-Juarez CF, Lee GH, Liu Y, et al. Single-cell analysis of human basal cell carcinoma reveals novel regulators of tumor growth and the tumor microenvironment. Sci Adv 2022;8(23):eabm7981.
19. Hua LA, Kagen CN, Carpenter RJ, et al. HLA and beta 2-microglobulin expression in basal and squamous cell carcinomas of the skin. Int J Dermatol 1985; 24(10):660–3.
20. Cabrera T, Garrido V, Concha A, et al. HLA molecules in basal cell carcinoma of the skin. Immunobiology 1992;185(5):440–52.
21. Walter A, Barysch MJ, Behnke S, et al. Cancer-testis antigens and immunosurveillance in human cutaneous squamous cell and basal cell carcinomas. Clin Cancer Res 2010;16(14):3562–70.
22. Kaporis HG, Guttman-Yassky E, Lowes MA, et al. Human basal cell carcinoma is associated with Foxp3+ T cells in a Th2 dominant microenvironment. J Invest Dermatol 2007;127(10):2391–8.
23. Nardinocchi L, Sonego G, Passarelli F, et al. Interleukin-17 and interleukin-22 promote tumor progression in human nonmelanoma skin cancer. Eur J Immunol 2015;45(3):922–31.
24. Omland SH, Wettergren EE, Mollerup S, et al. Cancer associated fibroblasts (CAFs) are activated in cutaneous basal cell carcinoma and in the peritumoural skin [published correction appears in BMC Cancer. 2018 Jan 30;18(1):111]. BMC Cancer 2017;17(1):675.
25. Tjiu JW, Chen JS, Shun CT, et al. Tumor-associated macrophage-induced invasion and angiogenesis of human basal cell carcinoma cells by cyclooxygenase-2 induction [published correction appears in J Invest Dermatol. 2018 Feb;138(2):471]. J Invest Dermatol 2009;129(4):1016–25.
26. Di Nardo L, Pellegrini C, Di Stefani A, et al. Molecular genetics of cutaneous squamous cell carcinoma: perspective for treatment strategies. J Eur Acad Dermatol Venereol 2020;34(5):932–41.
27. Chang D, Shain AH. The landscape of driver mutations in cutaneous squamous cell carcinoma. NPJ Genom Med 2021;6(1):61.
28. Riihilä P, Viiklepp K, Nissinen L, et al. Tumour-cell-derived complement components C1r and C1s promote growth of cutaneous squamous cell carcinoma. Br J Dermatol 2020;182(3):658–70.
29. Ji AL, Rubin AJ, Thrane K, et al. Multimodal analysis of composition and spatial architecture in human squamous cell carcinoma [published correction appears in Cell. 2020 Sep 17;182(6):1661-1662]. Cell 2020;182(2):497–514.e22.
30. Gabrilovich DI, Nagaraj S. Myeloid-derived suppressor cells as regulators of the immune system. Nat Rev Immunol 2009;9(3):162–74.
31. Gehad AE, Lichtman MK, Schmults CD, et al. Nitric oxide-producing myeloid-derived suppressor cells inhibit vascular E-selectin expression in human squamous cell carcinomas. J Invest Dermatol 2012;132(11):2642–51.

32. Saeidi V, Doudican N, Carucci JA. Understanding the squamous cell carcinoma immune microenvironment. Front Immunol 2023;14:1084873.

33. Galan A, Ko CJ. Langerhans cells in squamous cell carcinoma vs. pseudoepitheliomatous hyperplasia of the skin. J Cutan Pathol 2007;34(12):950–2.

34. Bluth MJ, Zaba LC, Moussai D, et al. Myeloid dendritic cells from human cutaneous squamous cell carcinoma are poor stimulators of T-cell proliferation. J Invest Dermatol 2009;129(10):2451–62.

35. Samimi M, Kervarrec T, Touze A. Immunobiology of Merkel cell carcinoma. Curr Opin Oncol 2020;32(2):114–21.

36. Liu W, Yang R, Payne AS, et al. Identifying the target cells and mechanisms of merkel cell polyomavirus infection. Cell Host Microbe 2016;19(6):775–87.

37. Das BK, Kannan A, Velasco GJ, et al. Single-cell dissection of Merkel cell carcinoma heterogeneity unveils transcriptomic plasticity and therapeutic vulnerabilities. Cell Rep Med 2023;4(7):101101.

38. Paulson KG, Iyer JG, Tegeder AR, et al. Transcriptome-wide studies of Merkel cell carcinoma and validation of intratumoral CD8+ lymphocyte invasion as an independent predictor of survival. J Clin Oncol 2011;29(12):1539–46.

39. Dowlatshahi M, Huang V, Gehad AE, et al. Tumor-specific T cells in human Merkel cell carcinomas: a possible role for Tregs and T-cell exhaustion in reducing T-cell responses. J Invest Dermatol 2013;133(7):1879–89.

40. Liu Y, Zhang C. The role of human $\gamma\delta$ T cells in anti-tumor immunity and their potential for cancer immunotherapy. Cells 2020;9(5):1206.

41. Kim DP, Kus KJB, Ruiz E. Basal cell carcinoma review. Hematol Oncol Clin N Am 2019;33(1):13–24.

42. Batra RS, Kelley LC. Predictors of extensive subclinical spread in nonmelanoma skin cancer treated with Mohs micrographic surgery. Arch Dermatol 2002;138(8): 1043–51.

43. Cameron MC, Lee E, Hibler BP, et al. Basal cell carcinoma: Contemporary approaches to diagnosis, treatment, and prevention [published correction appears in J Am Acad Dermatol. 2019 Jul;81(1):310]. J Am Acad Dermatol 2019;80(2): 321–39.

44. Zhu H, Lewis DJ. Topical hedgehog inhibitors for basal cell carcinoma: how far away are we? Expet Opin Pharmacother 2022;23(6):739–40.

45. National Library of Medicine. Clinical trial of patidegib gel 2%, 4%, and Vehicle applied once or twice daily to decrease the GLI1 biomarker in sporadic nodular basal cell carcinomas (BCC). 2016. 2019. Available at: https://clinicaltrials.gov/study/NCT02828111. [Accessed 30 January 2024].

46. National Library of Medicine. Efficacy and Safety of Patidegib Gel 2% for Preventing Basal Cell Carcinomas on the Face of Adults With Gorlin Syndrome. 2023. Available at: https://clinicaltrials.gov/study/NCT06050122. [Accessed 30 January 2024].

47. Kim DJ, Kim J, Spaunhurst K, et al. Open-label, exploratory phase II trial of oral itraconazole for the treatment of basal cell carcinoma. J Clin Oncol 2014;32(8): 745–51.

48. Sohn GK, Kwon GP, Bailey-Healy I, et al. Topical itraconazole for the treatment of basal cell carcinoma in patients with basal cell nevus syndrome or high-frequency basal cell carcinomas: a phase 2, open-label, placebo-controlled trial. JAMA Dermatol 2019;155(9):1078–80.

49. Axelson M, Liu K, Jiang X, et al. U.S. Food and Drug Administration approval: vismodegib for recurrent, locally advanced, or metastatic basal cell carcinoma. Clin Cancer Res 2013;19(9):2289–93.

50. Sekulic A, Migden MR, Oro AE, et al. Efficacy and safety of vismodegib in advanced basal-cell carcinoma. N Engl J Med 2012;366(23):2171–9.
51. Chmiel P, Kłosińska M, Forma A, et al. Novel approaches in non-melanoma skin cancers-a focus on hedgehog pathway in basal cell carcinoma (BCC). Cells 2022;11(20):3210. Published 2022 Oct 13.
52. Lear JT, Migden MR, Lewis KD, et al. Long-term efficacy and safety of sonidegib in patients with locally advanced and metastatic basal cell carcinoma: 30-month analysis of the randomized phase 2 BOLT study. J Eur Acad Dermatol Venereol 2018;32(3):372–81.
53. Dummer R, Guminksi A, Gutzmer R, et al. Long-term efficacy and safety of sonidegib in patients with advanced basal cell carcinoma: 42-month analysis of the phase II randomized, double-blind BOLT study. Br J Dermatol 2020;182(6):1369–78.
54. U.S. Food and Drug Administration. FDA approves cemiplimab-rwlc for locally advanced and metastatic basal cell carcinoma. 2021. Available at: https://www.fda.gov/drugs/resources-information-approved-drugs/fda-approves-cemiplimab-rwlc-locally-advanced-and-metastatic-basal-cell-carcinoma. [Accessed 30 January 2024].
55. Stratigos AJ, Sekulic A, Peris K, et al. Cemiplimab in locally advanced basal cell carcinoma after hedgehog inhibitor therapy: an open-label, multi-centre, single-arm, phase 2 trial. Lancet Oncol 2021;22(6):848–57.
56. Guzman AK, Schmults CD, Ruiz ES. Squamous cell carcinoma: an update in staging, management, and postoperative surveillance strategies. Dermatol Clin 2023;41(1):1–11.
57. Nestor MS, Han H, Ceci FM, et al. Evaluating the safety and efficacy of aminolevulinic acid 20% topical solution activated by pulsed dye laser and blue light in the treatment of facial cutaneous squamous cell carcinoma in situ. J Cosmet Dermatol 2023;22(9):2471–5.
58. Kallini JR, Hamed N, Khachemoune A. Squamous cell carcinoma of the skin: epidemiology, classification, management, and novel trends. Int J Dermatol 2015;54(2):130–40.
59. Mooney CP, Martin RCW, Dirven R, et al. Sentinel Node Biopsy in 105 High-Risk Cutaneous SCCs of the Head and Neck: Results of a Multicenter Prospective Study. Ann Surg Oncol 2019;26(13):4481–8.
60. Fitzgerald K, Tsai KK. Systemic therapy for advanced cutaneous squamous cell carcinoma. Semin Cutan Med Surg 2019;38(1):E67–74.
61. Khansur T, Kennedy A. Cisplatin and 5-fluorouracil for advanced locoregional and metastatic squamous cell carcinoma of the skin. Cancer 1991;67(8):2030–2.
62. Maubec E, Petrow P, Scheer-Senyarich I, et al. Phase II study of cetuximab as first-line single-drug therapy in patients with unresectable squamous cell carcinoma of the skin. J Clin Oncol 2011;29(25):3419–26.
63. Montaudié H, Viotti J, Combemale P, et al. Cetuximab is efficient and safe in patients with advanced cutaneous squamous cell carcinoma: a retrospective, multi-centre study. Oncotarget 2020;11(4):378–85.
64. Marin-Acevedo JA, Withycombe BM, Kim Y, et al. Cetuximab for Immunotherapy-Refractory/Ineligible Cutaneous Squamous Cell Carcinoma. Cancers 2023;15(12):3180. Published 2023 Jun 14.
65. U.S. Food and Drug Administration. FDA approves cemiplimab-rwlc for metastatic or locally advanced cutaneous squamous cell carcinoma. 2019. Available at: https://www.fda.gov/drugs/drug-approvals-and-databases/fda-approves-cemiplimab-rwlc-metastatic-or-locally-advanced-cutaneous-squamous-cell-carcinoma. [Accessed 30 January 2024].

66. Rischin D, Khushalani NI, Schmults CD, et al. Integrated analysis of a phase 2 study of cemiplimab in advanced cutaneous squamous cell carcinoma: extended follow-up of outcomes and quality of life analysis. J Immunother Cancer 2021; 9(8):e002757.

67. Ascierto PA, Schadendorf D. Update in the treatment of non-melanoma skin cancers: the use of PD-1 inhibitors in basal cell carcinoma and cutaneous squamous-cell carcinoma. J Immunother Cancer 2022;10(12):e005082.

68. Maubec E, Boubaya M, Petrow P, et al. Phase II Study of Pembrolizumab As First-Line, Single-Drug Therapy for Patients With Unresectable Cutaneous Squamous Cell Carcinomas. J Clin Oncol 2020;38(26):3051–61.

69. Shope C, Andrews L, Atherton K, et al. Comparison of Patient and Provider Practices between Bone Marrow and Solid Organ Transplantation Programs for Patient Education on Increased Risk of Skin Cancer. Transplant Cell Ther 2023; 29(7):466.e1–7.

70. Ducroux E, Martin C, Bouwes Bavinck JN, et al. Risk of aggressive skin cancers after kidney retransplantation in patients with previous posttransplant cutaneous squamous cell carcinomas: a retrospective study of 53 cases. Transplantation 2017;101(4):e133–41.

71. Johnson DB, Sullivan RJ, Menzies AM. Immune checkpoint inhibitors in challenging populations. Cancer 2017;123(11):1904–11.

72. Fisher J, Zeitouni N, Fan W, et al. Immune checkpoint inhibitor therapy in solid organ transplant recipients: A patient-centered systematic review. J Am Acad Dermatol 2020;82(6):1490–500.

73. Gauci ML, Aristei C, Becker JC, et al. Diagnosis and treatment of Merkel cell carcinoma: European consensus-based interdisciplinary guideline - Update 2022. Eur J Cancer 2022;171:203–31.

74. U.S. Food and Drug Administration. FDA approves first treatment for rare form of skin cancer. 2018. Available at: https://www.fda.gov/news-events/press-announcements/fda-approves-first-treatment-rare-form-skin-cancer. [Accessed 30 January 2024].

75. Kaufman HL, Russell J, Hamid O, et al. Avelumab in patients with chemotherapy-refractory metastatic Merkel cell carcinoma: a multicentre, single-group, open-label, phase 2 trial. Lancet Oncol 2016;17(10):1374–85.

76. D'Angelo SP, Russell J, Lebbé C, et al. Efficacy and Safety of First-line Avelumab Treatment in Patients With Stage IV Metastatic Merkel Cell Carcinoma: A Preplanned Interim Analysis of a Clinical Trial. JAMA Oncol 2018;4(9):e180077.

77. Nghiem P, Bhatia S, Lipson EJ, et al. Durable Tumor Regression and Overall Survival in Patients With Advanced Merkel Cell Carcinoma Receiving Pembrolizumab as First-Line Therapy. J Clin Oncol 2019;37(9):693–702.

78. Topalian SL, Bhatia S, Amin A, et al. Neoadjuvant Nivolumab for Patients With Resectable Merkel Cell Carcinoma in the CheckMate 358 Trial. J Clin Oncol 2020;38(22):2476–87.

79. Chang MS, Azin M, Demehri S. Cutaneous Squamous Cell Carcinoma: The Frontier of Cancer Immunoprevention. Annu Rev Pathol 2022;17:101–19.

80. Zilberg C, Lyons JG, Gupta R, et al. The Immune Microenvironment in Basal Cell Carcinoma. Ann Dermatol 2023;35(4):243–55.

81. Mortaja M, Demehri S. Skin cancer prevention - Recent advances and unmet challenges. Cancer Lett 2023;575:216406.

82. Middleton M, Aroldi F, Sacco J, et al. 422 An open-label, multicenter, phase 1/2 clinical trial of RP1, an enhanced potency oncolytic HSV, combined with nivolumab: updated results from the skin cancer cohorts. J Immunother Cancer 2020;8(Suppl 3): A257.

83. Boerlin A, Ramelyte E, Maul JT, et al. 1089TiP Efficacy and tolerability of anti-PD1 antibody in combination with pulsed hedgehog inhibitor in advanced basal cell carcinoma. Ann Oncol 2021;32.
84. Navarro-Triviño FJ, Ayén-Rodríguez Á, Llamas-Molina JM, et al. Treatment of superficial basal cell carcinoma with 7.8% 5-aminolaevulinic acid nanoemulsion-based gel (BF-200 ALA) and photodynamic therapy: Results in clinical practice in a tertiary hospital. Dermatol Ther 2021;34(1):e14558.
85. Calienni MN, Febres-Molina C, Llovera RE, et al. Nanoformulation for potential topical delivery of Vismodegib in skin cancer treatment. Int J Pharm 2019;565:108–22.
86. Rosenberg AR, Tabacchi M, Ngo KH, et al. Skin cancer precursor immunotherapy for squamous cell carcinoma prevention. JCI Insight 2019;4(6):e125476.
87. Cunningham TJ, Tabacchi M, Eliane JP, et al. Randomized trial of calcipotriol combined with 5-fluorouracil for skin cancer precursor immunotherapy. J Clin Invest 2017;127(1):106–16.
88. Strickley JD, Messerschmidt JL, Awad ME, et al. Immunity to commensal papillomaviruses protects against skin cancer. Nature 2019;575(7783):519–22.

Cutaneous T-cell Lymphoma

David M. Weiner, MD, MBE[a],*, Alain H. Rook, MD[b]

KEYWORDS

- Mycosis fungoides • Sezary syndrome • Cutaneous T-cell lymphoma
- Lymphomatoid papulosis • Primary cutaneous anaplastic large cell lymphoma

KEY POINTS

- Cutaneous T-cell lymphoma is a group of non-Hodgkin T-cell lymphomas that develop in and affect the skin but can potentially spread to other organs.
- The etiology of cutaneous T-cell lymphoma is unknown. However, a leading theory is that the condition could result from prolonged exposure to an antigen stimulus.
- Cutaneous T-cell lymphoma is a common cause of chronic recalcitrant skin rash and frequently resembles other dermatologic conditions.
- Patients are typically treated by a multidisciplinary team including dermatologists, oncologists, and pathologists. Although general guidelines to treatment have been developed, individual centers have their own preferred therapies.
- Treatment options include skin-directed therapies (eg, topical steroids and phototherapy) and systemic therapies (eg, extracorporeal photopheresis, interferons, and chemotherapy).

INTRODUCTION

Cutaneous T-cell lymphoma (CTCL) is a group of non-Hodgkin T-cell lymphomas that by definition develop in and affect the skin but can potentially spread to other organs. There are many subtypes of CTCL, each characterized by distinct disease biology and clinical manifestations. The World Health Organization-European Organization for Research and Treatment of Cancer (WHO-EORTC) provides a classification of cutaneous lymphomas based on clinical, pathologic, and molecular characteristics (**Table 1**).[1] CTCL is rare overall, comprising about 1% to 2% of all non-Hodgkin's lymphomas.[2,3] In the United States, the estimated incidence rate is about 0.6 to 0.9 per 100,000 person-years.[4] However, cutaneous lymphoma is a common cause of recalcitrant chronic skin rash, and it is therefore important for medical providers to be aware of this condition.

---

[a] Department of Dermatology, Johns Hopkins University School of Medicine, 601 North Caroline Street, 8th Floor, Baltimore, MD 21287, USA; [b] Department of Dermatology, Cutaneous Lymphoma Program, Perelman School of Medicine, University of Pennsylvania, 3400 Civic Center Boulevard, 1st Floor, Philadelphia, PA 19104, USA
* Corresponding author.
E-mail address: dweine13@jh.edu

Hematol Oncol Clin N Am 38 (2024) 1087–1110
https://doi.org/10.1016/j.hoc.2024.05.012
0889-8588/24/© 2024 Elsevier Inc. All rights reserved, including those for text and data mining, AI training, and similar technologies.

Mycosis fungoides (MF) is the most prevalent form of CTCL, accounting for about 40% of all cutaneous lymphomas, and it is named after the fungating tumors that can develop when the disease is advanced.[1,5] The typical presentation of MF is slowly progressive erythematous patches and plaques that can gradually progress to thickened plaques and tumors and/or erythroderma. Although uncommon, MF can potentially involve extracutaneous tissues such as the lymph nodes, blood, bone marrow, and visceral organs. There are several variants, and atypical presentations are common. Therefore, MF is well known among dermatologists as an important imitator of other conditions and is frequently on the differential diagnosis for a persistent skin rash.

Sezary syndrome (SS) is a rare distinct form of CTCL (~5%–10% of CTCL) defined by leukemic involvement by malignant T cells (Sezary cells), as well as erythroderma

Table 1
Relative frequency and prognosis of primary cutaneous lymphomas included in the 2018 update of the World Health Organization-European Organization for Research and Treatment of Cancer classification[1]

WHO-EORTC Classification 2018	Frequency, %*	5 y DSS, %*
CTCL		
MF	39	88
MF variants	—	—
Folliculotropic MF	5	75
Pagetoid reticulosis	<1	100
Granulomatous slack skin	<1	100
SS	2	36
ATLL	<1	NDA
Primary cutaneous CD30+ LPDs	—	—
C-ALCL	8	95
LyP	12	99
Subcutaneous panniculitis-like T-cell lymphoma	1	87
Extranodal NK/T-cell lymphoma, nasal type	<1	16
Chronic active EBV infection	<1	NDA
Primary cutaneous peripheral T-cell lymphoma, rare subtypes	—	—
Primary cutaneous γ/δ T-cell lymphoma	<1	11
CD8+ AECTCL (provisional)	<1	31
Primary cutaneous CD4+ small/medium T-cell lymphoproliferative disorder (provisional)	6	100
Primary cutaneous acral CD8+ T-cell lymphoma (provisional)	<1	100
Primary cutaneous peripheral T-cell lymphoma, NOS	2	15
CBCL		
PCMZL	9	99
PCFCL	12	95
PCDLBLC, LT	4	56
EBV+ mucocutaneous ulcer (provisional)	<1	100
Intravascular large B-cell lymphoma	<1	72

Abbreviations: NDA, no data available

and lymphadenopathy.[1] The condition is named after Albert Sezary, a French dermatologist who first described erythroderma with "cellules monstrueues" in 1938.[6] SS generally has a more aggressive clinical course compared to MF; historical studies estimate a median survival of 3 to 4 years.[7,8] There is considerable overlap in the presentation and pathophysiology of MF and SS, and patients who initially present with MF can later meet the criteria for SS. Therefore, it is a topic of debate whether MF and SS are distinct disease entities versus a spectrum of disease.

CD30[+] lymphoproliferative disorders (CD30[+] LPDs) are a distinct subtype of CTCL defined by the expression of CD30[+] by the aberrant T cells. CD30[+] LPDs include lymphomatoid papulosis (LyP) and primary cutaneous anaplastic large cell lymphoma (pcALCL). CD30[+] LPDs are generally indolent and responsive to treatment but can be associated with comorbid systemic lymphoma.

The etiology of CTCL is unknown, and the disease likely occurs from multiple different pathways. A leading hypothesis is that CTCL can develop as a reaction to a chronic antigen stimulus, such as a viral, bacterial, or other environmental antigen.[9] A persistently stimulated genetically unstable T cell would acquire further mutations over time that eventually lead to self-sustained neoplastic growth. For example, patients with SS are usually highly colonized with *Staphylococcus aureus*, and antibiotic treatment can decrease clinical symptoms, supporting a link between this pathogen and tumor progression.[10] Associations with chemicals or pesticides have been suggested in epidemiologic studies but have not been definitively proven.[11,12]

CTCL preferentially affects the skin due to the skin-homing activity of the malignant T cells. In MF and SS, studies of the malignant T cells have revealed a mature memory CD4[+] helper T-cell phenotype.[13,14] Under normal conditions, memory T cells help the immune system respond efficiently to previously encountered pathogens.[15] In CTCL, an antigen-specific memory T cell becomes neoplastic and clonally expands.[14] The tumor microenvironment has an important role in the progression of MF and SS. In early MF, both neoplastic (CD4[+]/Th2) and reactive (CD8[+]/Th1) T cells are present in affected skin.[14] In advanced MF and SS, there is a predominance of malignant CD4[+] T cells, resulting in skewed Th2 cytokine expression, increasing immune suppression, and diminished antitumor immune response.[14]

This review serves as an introduction to CTCL, with a primary focus on the clinical presentation, diagnosis, immunopathogenesis, and management of the condition.

CLINICAL PRESENTATION AND DIAGNOSIS

CTCL frequently resembles other skin conditions, including psoriasis and atopic dermatitis, as well as benign LPDs, making the diagnosis challenging. Furthermore, some patients may present with overlapping features of multiple subtypes of CTCL. Therefore, the diagnosis of CTCL must be made carefully based on integration of clinical and pathologic findings as well as the patient's disease course over time.

In general, CTCL is diagnosed through a combination of clinical presentation, skin biopsy, peripheral flow cytometry, and molecular testing for T-cell clonality. Patients with more advanced disease on presentation may also have imaging and potentially a biopsy of lymph node and/or bone marrow to assess for spread of the disease to the lymph nodes or internal organs. Patients with possible CTCL are typically referred to specialty centers with specialized dermatologists, pathologists, and oncologists who conduct the diagnostic workup.

Patients' clinical and pathologic findings are always correlated to make an overall diagnosis that takes all data into context. Due to the variable presentation of CTCL and its tendency to mimic other conditions, multiple biopsies and follow-up assessments may be necessary over time to make a diagnosis. Algorithms based on expert experience have been proposed to aid in diagnosis of early MF but have not yet been validated.[16]

Clinical Presentation

On physical examination, patients are evaluated for the type, distribution, and extent of their skin lesions. For patients with MF or SS, a score termed the Modified Severity Weighted Assessment Tool is usually calculated to estimate the overall degree of skin involvement.[17] This tool determines a score based upon the percent body surface area affected, with plaques and tumors given a higher relative weight than patches. Palpation of peripheral lymph nodes should be performed to assess for lymphadenopathy, and an abdominal examination can be done to assess for hepatosplenomegaly.

Cutaneous manifestations can be variable and are stage-dependent. Patients with early-stage classic MF usually have erythematous patches or thin plaques that typically occur in sun-protected areas such as the trunk and proximal extremities (**Fig. 1**A–C). These lesions are typically slowly progressive and can remain stable in size and number for years to decades. Pruritus is variable. There may be a "cigarette paper" wrinkling appearance due to epidermal atrophy. Patients with more advanced MF can develop more extensive and thicker scaly plaques, fungating skin tumors that can ulcerate (see **Fig. 1**D, E), or erythroderma (patches/plaques involving >80% of body surface area; see **Fig. 1**G–J), often with lymphadenopathy and pruritus, as well as constitutional symptoms such as intermittent fever, drenching night sweats, and weight loss. Palpable lymph nodes on examination may be reactive in nature or may represent lymph node involvement by malignancy. Involvement of internal organs (eg, liver and spleen) is unusual and typically occurs in patients with tumor-stage or erythrodermic MF.[18]

MF can have variable clinical and histologic presentations, and there are many subtypes and atypical presentations (**Table 2**). The most common variants include folliculotropic and hypopigmented MF. Folliculotropic MF is a clinicopathologic variant defined by the presence of perifollicular and follicular infiltrates of atypical T cells on histology.[19] Folliculotropic MF usually presents with follicle-based patches or plaques, preferentially affecting the head and neck and other areas of hair growth, often with alopecia of affected areas.[19] Follicular plugging is quite characteristic (see **Fig. 1**F).[19] Hypopigmented MF is more easily clinically recognized in darkly pigmented individuals.[20] This variant is characterized by hypopigmented macules and patches rather than the more typical erythematous color.[20] Furthermore, the phenotype of hypopigmented MF is more often CD8+ rather than the usual CD4+ aberrant T cells on histology.[20] Less common variants include MF that is poikilodermatous, unilesional, palmoplantar, bullous, interstitial, syringotropic, pagetoid, or granulomatous.[21]

SS classically presents with a triad of erythroderma, lymphadenopathy, and leukemic involvement (see **Fig. 1**G–J). While patients with MF can develop erythroderma and may have some atypical lymphocytes in their blood, SS is defined by the presence of a particularly high burden of neoplastic T cells in the peripheral blood (see later sections on laboratory assessment and staging). Erythroderma can range from subtle and poorly defined (especially on initial presentation) to overt with widespread erythema and exfoliation of the skin (see **Fig. 1**). Other common skin changes in SS include palmoplantar keratoderma, ectropion, onychodystrophy, and alopecia. Leg edema can occur due to collection of fluid from skin inflammation. Uncommonly, infiltration of the facial skin can result in a "leonine facies" appearance. Pruritus is a common concern in SS and can be severe and debilitating.

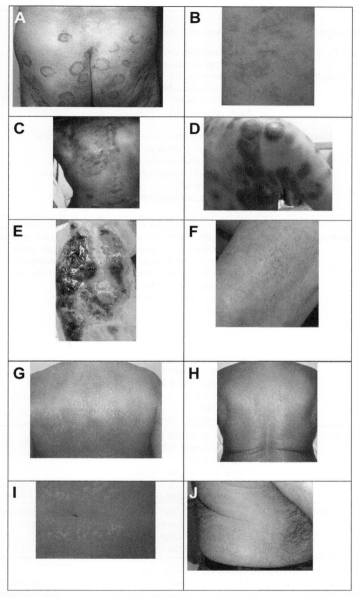

Fig. 1. MF and Sezary syndrome. (*A*) Patch stage MF. (*B*) Patch stage MF. (*C*) Plaque stage MF. (*D*) Tumor stage MF. (*E*) Tumor stage MF (ulcerated CD30⁺ tumor). (*F*) Folliculotropic MF (with follicular plugging). (*G*) Sezary syndrome (with erythroderma). (*H*) Sezary syndrome (with erythroderma). (*I*) Sezary syndrome (erythroderma with islands of sparing mimicking pityriasis rubra pilaris). (*J*) Sezary syndrome in Association with HTLV-1 infection.

LyP is a benign, nonaggressive CD30⁺ LPD characterized by recurrent, erythematous dome-shaped papules that can occur in crops on the trunk or limbs (**Fig. 2**A). The lesions of LyP are typically 1 to 2 cm in size and can be smooth, scaly, or necrotic. Larger nodules and ulcerations sometimes occur. The lesions usually spontaneously

Table 2
Clinicopathologic and phenotypic variants of mycosis fungoides

Clinical variants with "conventional" histopathological features	*Acanthosis nigricans-like MF* *Atopic dermatitis-like MF*[a] *Erythrodermic MF* *Hypopigmented MF* *Ichthyosiform MF* *Palmoplantar MF* *Papular MF* *Papuloerythroderma of Ofuji (subset of cases)* *Parapsoriasis ("large patch")* *Perioral dermatitis-like MF* *Pityriasis lichenoides-like MF (clinical variant)* *Psoriasiform MF* *Unilesional (solitary) MF* *Zosteriform MF*
Clinical variants with peculiar histopathological features	*Adnexotropic MF, including pilotropic (folliculotropic) MF (with or without follicular) and MF with eruptive infundibular cysts and comedones, and syringotropic MF*[b] *Anetodermic MF (MF with secondary anetoderma) (secondary anetoderma may be observed also in generalized follicular mucinosis)* *Bullous (vesiculobullous) MF* *Dyshidrotic MF* *Epidermal mucinosis in MF* *Granulomatous slack skin* *Hyperpigmented MF* *"Invisible" MF* *Pagetoid reticulosis (Woringer–Kolopp type)* *Poikilodermatous MF* *Purpuric MF* *Pustular MF* *Verrucous/hyperkeratotic MF*
Histopathological variants	*Annular lichenoid dermatitis of youth-like MF* *Granulomatous MF* *Interstitial MF* *Large cell transformation* *Pityriasis lichenoides-like MF (histopathological variant)* *Sclerosing MF (lichen sclerosus-like)*
Phenotypic variants[c]	*Cytotoxic MF (CD8+ and/or γ/δ+; rarely CD4+ with expression of cytotoxic proteins* *MF with T follicular helper phenotype* *MF with T-regulatory phenotype*

[a] Histopathologically characterized often by variable spongiotic changes.
[b] Pilotropic MF and syringotropic MF may be observed independently from one another, but in many instances of syringotropic MF, the hair follicles are involved as well, thus the term adnexotropic MF better reflects the clinicopathological features of this variant of the disease.
[c] A phenotypic switch may occur in sequential biopsies, and sometimes different phenotypic features are present in different biopsies taken on the same day.
From Skin Lymphoma: the Illustrated Guide by Lorenzo Cerroni)[85]

regress after a few weeks or months and often scar. However, the disease can wax and wane and may last for a patient's lifetime. Although LyP is a benign condition that is not life threatening, it can be associated with other lymphomas including MF/SS, Hodgkin's lymphoma, and anaplastic large cell lymphoma (ALCL) in up to 20%

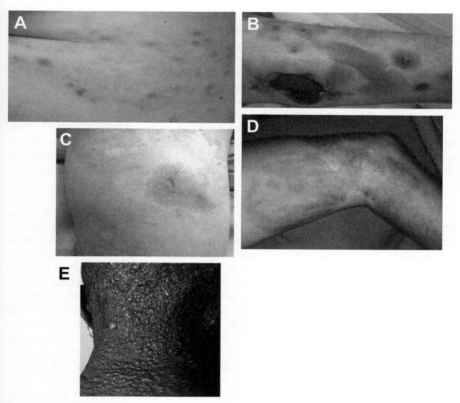

Fig. 2. Non-MF/SS subtypes of CTCL and related conditions. (*A*) Lymphomatoid papulosis (*B*) primary cutaneous gamma-delta T-cell lymphoma (*C*) subcutaneous panniculitis-like T-cell lymphoma (*D*) subcutaneous panniculitis-like T-cell lymphoma. (*E*) HTLV-1-associated adult T-cell leukemia/lymphoma. (Image Courtesy (a) Dr Peter Heald)

of patients.[22] In contrast to LyP, pcALCL typically presents as a single fast-growing large ulcerative nodule or tumor that usually does not regress (~20% chance of regression).[22] Multifocal pcALCL with multiple nodules sometimes occurs.[22] Of note, pcALCL is distinct from primary systemic ALCL, which can occasionally spread to the skin.

While MF/SS and CD30[+] LPDs are the most common subtypes of CTCL, it is important to rule out rare subtypes of CTCL as some are known to progress rapidly and portend a poor prognosis. Rare aggressive CTCL subtypes include primary cutaneous aggressive epidermotropic CD8[+] cytotoxic T-cell lymphoma (characterized by CD8 positivity and highly aggressive course) and primary cutaneous gamma-delta T-cell lymphoma (characterized by gamma-delta positivity and highly aggressive course; see **Fig. 2**B).[23,24] It is important to note that these are distinct subtypes of CTCL, and CD8 and gamma-delta positivity on their own do not always imply an aggressive course.[25] Subcutaneous panniculitis-like T-cell lymphoma is a rare alpha-beta T-cell lymphoma originating in the subcutis (see **Fig. 2**C, D).[26] Although SPTCL is usually positive for the cytotoxic markers CD8 and TIA-1, the condition is often indolent.[26] However, associated hemophagocytic syndrome can occur, which entails a poor prognosis.[26] SPTCL may not infrequently also manifest with autoimmune phenomena, including overlap with antinuclear antibody (ANA)-positive cutaneous or systemic lupus.[26] There are also rare distinct indolent subtypes of CTCL, such as primary cutaneous CD4+ small/medium T-cell lymphoproliferative disorder and primary cutaneous acral CD8+ T-cell lymphoma.[1] The former is not considered a true lymphoma.

Lastly, parapsoriasis is a controversial category of chronic dermatosis that may represent a precursor stage to MF.[27,28] Patients with a suggestive clinical presentation of small oval or digitiform macules may be diagnosed with small-plaque parapsoriasis, while patients with large erythematous scaly patches may be diagnosed with large-plaque parapsoriasis, which has a reported link to future development of MF.[28,29] Patients with parapsoriasis lack clear characteristic features of MF/SS on biopsy. Some experts do not consider parapsoriasis to be a distinct disease category but rather the early stages of evolving MF or other skin conditions (eg, nummular dermatitis).

Pathology

Skin biopsies are typically obtained from 2 or more different affected areas of skin. Skin biopsies can be assessed by immunohistochemical analysis for T-cell-associated antigens to help identify any atypical T-cell infiltrate in the skin, as well as by molecular tests of clonality such as T-cell receptor (TCR) polymerase chain reaction (PCR) analysis and high-throughput sequencing (HTS) of the T-cell receptor.

The standard immunohistochemistry used to evaluate for suspected MF and SS includes the T-cell markers CD2-CD5, CD7, CD8, and CD30.[30,31] In MF and SS, T cells are typically CD3 and CD4-positive, usually have decreased expression of CD7, and may have decreased CD2 and CD5.[30,31] However, hypopigmented MF is typically CD8+, and there are occasional CD8+ variants of classic MF/SS.[20,32] Expression of CD30 is most common in tumor-stage and large cell transformed MF/SS but can occur at any stage.[31,33]

The characteristic histologic appearance of MF/SS in skin biopsies is a superficial infiltrate of atypical lymphocytes with cerebriform nuclei (**Fig. 3**A, B).[31,34] Haloed lymphocytes, intraepidermal lymphocytes with clear space around the nuclei, are a common finding.[31,34] Pautrier microabscesses, intraepidermal clusters of atypical lymphocytes, are pathognomonic but have variable occurrence.[31,34]

Biopsies may be nonspecific in patients with patch-stage MF or thin plaques, with only subtle epidermotropism and nuclear atypia, and multiple biopsies may be required to confirm the diagnosis.[31,34] Characteristic histologic changes are typically present in biopsies of plaque lesions, although features suggestive of other diagnoses may also be present (eg, acanthosis and hyperparakeratosis may occur, suggesting psoriasis).[31,34] Biopsies of tumor-stage MF usually show dense infiltrates of atypical-appearing tumor cells in the dermis and epidermis.[31,34]

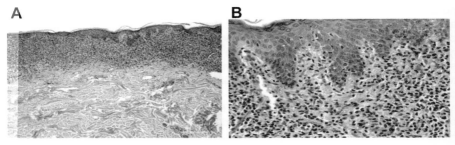

Fig. 3. Histopathology of CTCL demonstrating a lichenoid infiltrate and epidermotropism.

Skin biopsies obtained from individuals with SS are nondiagnostic in at least 50% of cases. Most often, a patchy papillary dermal lymphocytic infiltrate is observed, with epidermotropism being less common.[34,35] Thus, more than one biopsy is warranted to assist in making the diagnosis of SS. Moreover, patients with SS typically have a high burden of circulating malignant T cells, making blood flow cytometric analysis and/or performance of high-throughput sequencing on the blood mandatory. Those with erythrodermic CTCL without blood involvement should also have more than one skin biopsy to provide a higher level of certainty regarding the diagnosis.

Patients with plaques, tumors, or erythroderma may have large cell transformation (defined as large cells >4× the size of small lymphocytes in >25% of the lymphoid infiltrate), a pathologic finding associated with tumor formation and an inferior prognosis.[31,34] As described earlier, there are many clinical and pathologic variants of MF/SS, including folliculotropic MF, which is characterized by malignant cells around and within the hair follicles.[36,37]

By definition, CD30[+] LPDs are CD30[+] on immunohistochemistry. As MF and SS can also be CD30[+], clinicopathologic correlation is essential to make the correct diagnosis. The histologic findings of LyP are variable. In general, there is a dense infiltrate consisting of lymphocytes mixed with other immune cells.[22,31] There are several distinct histologic subtypes (A–F), some of which can resemble other types of CTCL and do not have prognostic significance.[22,31] Given the pathologic overlap with other conditions, LyP is diagnosed based on the characteristic clinical appearance and consistent histopathology. More than one subtype of LyP can occur in a single patient.[22,31] For pcALCL, at least 75% of the tumor cells must express CD30 in order to make the diagnosis.[22,31] There is typically a nodular dermal infiltrate of anaplastic large tumor cells with bizarre-appearing nuclei.[22,31] PcALCL is usually CD4[+] but can rarely be CD8[+]. PcALCL is usually negative for anaplastic lymphoma kinase-1 (ALK-1), in contrast to systemic ALCL.[22,31]

Molecular Testing

TCR gene rearrangement studies can help support a diagnosis of CTCL when taken into the context of the patient's clinical presentation and pathology findings. CTCL is characterized by clonal proliferation of T cells. Under normal circumstances, each T cell has a unique TCR sequence, allowing the immune system to recognize diverse pathogenic antigens. However, in CTCL, a T cell has undergone clonal expansion, resulting in a population of cells that share the same TCR sequence. Therefore, MF/SS and CD30[+] LPDs often have positive T-cell clonality, although the absence of detectable T-cell clonality does not necessarily refute the diagnosis of CTCL. PCR amplification of the TCR gamma chain gene is usually performed to evaluate for the presence of a clonal T-cell population in skin and blood samples.[38] If a sufficient percentage of cells with an identical TCR is present in a sample, this will manifest as a distinct peak during gel electrophoresis, in which PCR-amplified TCR regions are separated based on their base pair sizes. High-throughput sequencing of the TCR is a new alternative method for the assessment of T-cell clonality.[39,40] This technique can be used to determine the exact sequences of all TCR regions present in a sample, which can then be evaluated for a dominant clone. Both techniques, however, have limitations regarding diagnostic sensitivity and specificity for CTCL, as interpretation of these tests can be subjective, criteria for clonality can be variable, and T-cell clonality sometimes occurs in nonlymphomatous conditions.[38,39,41] Furthermore, benign TCR clones can sometimes occur in elderly patients and in patients with autoimmune inflammatory skin conditions.[42,43] Therefore, a single positive clone does not necessarily imply a diagnosis of CTCL. However, the presence of an identical T-cell clone in 2 or more biopsy specimens from distinct skin sites is more suggestive of CTCL in a patient with a compatible clinical presentation.[44]

Laboratory Testing

Routine laboratory studies include complete blood count (CBC), comprehensive metabolic panel (CMP), and lactate dehydrogenase (LDH). CBC and CMP are used to assess for lymphocytosis and eosinophilia and to monitor kidney and liver function, respectively. LDH is a tumor marker that is released by rapidly dividing lymphocytes. In most patients with MF and any patient with erythroderma, peripheral blood flow cytometry should be done to assess for blood involvement. Patients' blood is typically assessed for immunophenotypic abnormalities using a standard set of markers including CD3, CD4, CD8, CD7, and CD26.[45,46] CD25, CD30 and natural killer (NK) cell markers are also helpful.[45] Patients' blood can also be assessed for clonality by TCR or HTS, as well as by a novel technique involving analysis of T-cell receptor constant beta chain 1.[47] Malignant SS cells are clonal and usually CD4$^+$ and CD7$^-$ or CD26$^-$.[45] In addition to the characteristic clinical presentation of erythroderma and lymphadenopathy, the diagnosis of SS requires an absolute Sezary cell count of greater than 1000/μL in the peripheral blood, as well as traditionally a positive T-cell clone matching the skin.[48,49] Patients with MF may have small numbers of Sezary cells in the blood that do not reach the threshold for diagnosis of SS. Patients with LyP and pcALCL do not usually have detectable blood involvement from these conditions. Testing for human T-lymphotropic retroviruses 1 and 2 (HTLV-1 and 2), though less common in North America than in Japan, the Middle East, and the Caribbean, should be performed as these viruses may cause adult T-cell leukemia/lymphoma (ATLL), which can mimic MF and SS.[50]

Other Diagnostic Workup

Radiologic evaluation may include whole-body computed tomography (CT) or PET-CT. In general, imaging is recommended for any patient with SS or for patients with MF who have tumor stage disease, palpable lymphadenopathy, high-risk histologic features such as large-cell transformation, or abnormal hematologic laboratory findings.[51] Lymph node sampling is typically recommended for patients with suspicious lymph nodes that are large (>1.5 cm) and/or have increased standardized uptake value (>4.0) in a PET/CT scan.[51]

Criteria

Specific criteria have been developed to define MF/SS and aid in diagnosis.

Proposed criteria for early mycosis fungoides

The International Society for Cutaneous Lymphomas have proposed the following criteria to facilitate differentiation of early MF from other conditions (**Table 3**).[16] According to this algorithm, the diagnosis of early MF can be made if a total of 4 or more points is reached. However, these criteria have not been fully validated or adopted.

- Clinical criteria: Patient has persistent and/or progressive patches and plaques plus (2 points given if 2 of the following are present, 1 point is given if 1 of the following is present): lesions in a non-sun-exposed location, size/shape variation of lesions, and poikiloderma.
- Histopathologic criteria: Superficial lymphoid infiltrate present plus (2 points are given if both of the following are present, 1 point is given if only 1 of the following is present): epidermotropism without spongiosis and lymphoid atypia.

Table 3
Algorithm for diagnosis of early mycosis fungoides

Criteria	Scoring system
Clinical	
Basic	2 points for basic criteria and 2 additional criteria
Persistent and/or progressive patches/thin plaques	1 point for basic criteria and 1 additional criterion
Additional	
1. Non-sun-exposed location	
2. Size/shape variation	
3. Poikiloderma	
Histopathologic	
Basic	2 points for basic criteria and 2 additional criteria
Superficial lymphoid infiltrate	1 point for basic criteria and 1 additional criterion
Additional	
1. Epidermotropism without spongiosis	
2. Lymphoid atypia[a]	
Molecular biological	
1. Clonal TCR gene rearrangement	1 point for clonality
Immunopathologic	
1. <50% CD2[+], CD3[+], and/or CD5[+] T cells	1 point for 1 or more criteria
2. <10% CD7[+] T cells	
3. Epidermal/dermal discordance of CD2, CD3, CD5, or CD7[b]	

Abbreviations: MF, mycosis fungoides; TCR, T-cell receptor.
A total of 4 points is required for the diagnosis of MF based on any combination of points from the clinical, histopathologic, molecular biological, and immunopathologic criteria.
[a] Lymphoid atypia is defined as cells with enlarged hyperchromatic nuclei and irregular or cerebriform nuclear contours.
[b] T-cell antigen deficiency confined to the epidermis.
From: Pimpinelli et al., 2005.[16]

- Molecular biological criteria: If clonal TCR gene rearrangement is present, give 1 point.
- Immunopathologic criteria: Give 1 point if any of the following is present: less than 50% of the T cells express CD2, CD3, or CD5; less than 10% of the T cells express CD7; and there is discordance of the epidermal and dermal cells with regard to expression of CD2, CD3, CD5, or CD7.

Traditional criteria for Sezary syndrome

Traditionally, the diagnosis of SS requires fulfillment of all of the following criteria.[49] However, patients may present with some but not all of the following features (eg, missing a matching clonal TCR rearrangement in the blood and skin). These patients should be re-evaluated over time and may benefit from a similar treatment approach to classic SS.

- Erythroderma
- Skin biopsy diagnostic of MF/SS

○ *or* skin biopsy compatible with MF/SS plus (1) lymph node biopsy confirming MF/SS *or* (2) significant aberrant lymphocyte population in blood with TCR clone matching that in skin.
- Leukemic blood tumor burden: (1) B2 blood involvement defined by greater than 1000 cells by flow cytometry (in patients who are not lymphopenic) and (2) a clonal TCR rearrangement in blood that matches the skin.

Staging

Staging of CTCL is conducted by tumor, node, metastasis, blood (TNMB) classification **(Tables 4–6)**.[49] MF/SS have a separate staging system from other forms of CTCL. Skin involvement is staged based on the type and extent of lesions: T1 is patches or plaques less than 10% of the body surface area (BSA); T2 is patches or plaques greater than 10% BSA; T3 is the presence of at least one skin tumor; and T4 is erythroderma with greater than 80% BSA affected by patches, plaques, and/ or tumors.[49] Lymph node involvement is staged based on pathologic findings.[49] There are 2 main histopathologic grading systems: (1) the National Cancer Institute (NCI) system and (2) the Dutch system.[49,52,53] Per both systems, the presence of partial or complete effacement of nodal architecture constitutes high-grade involvement (NCI LN4 and Dutch grade 3/4), corresponding to an N3 stage by the TNMB staging system.[49,52,53] Patients with abnormal lymph nodes on examination or imaging that have not been biopsied are staged as "Nx."[49] Blood involvement is staged based on the number of circulating malignant cells.[49] The criteria for and staging of bone marrow involvement is not yet clear, but overt bone marrow involvement with a lymphomatous infiltrate has been shown to have negative prognostic significance.[54] An overall stage of IA-IVB can be determined based on patients' individual TNMB stages.

Advancing stage of MF/SS is associated with inferior prognosis, which is the purpose of the staging system. Patients with early MF, or patches and plaques less than 10%, have an excellent prognosis, with a disease-specific survival of 90% at 20 years.[55,56] However, there is an 18% risk of disease progression.[56] Those with T1 patch disease fare better than those with T1 with plaques.[57,58] Progression to tumor stage occurs in about 10% to 20% of patients with T2-stage MF.[57] Patients with advanced disease (IIB-IVB) have a poor prognosis, with a disease-specific survival of 20% to 50% at 5 years.[56] Large-cell transformation, lymph node effacement (corresponding to stage IVA2), and visceral involvement (corresponding to stage IVB) are important negative prognostic indicators indicative of advancing disease.[49,56] LyP is a benign condition with a disease-specific survival of 100% and is not life threatening unless associated with another lymphoma.[22] pcALCL has a good prognosis with a 5 year survival of greater than 90%, although prognosis is inferior in patients with multifocal pcALCL.[22]

Differential Diagnosis

The differential diagnosis is dependent on the exact clinical presentation, subtype, and stage of CTCL. Patch-stage classic MF frequently resembles benign inflammatory conditions such as atopic dermatitis, drug reactions, and psoriasis, which can also cause patches or lichenified-appearing plaques with reactive inflammation on histopathology. In these patients, a history of a chronic progressive and treatment-resistant skin rash raises the possibility of MF. Tumor-stage MF must be distinguished from other subtypes of CTCL (eg, ALCL, rare aggressive subtypes) and from cutaneous invasion by a systemic malignancy. In these patients, imaging and biopsy findings can help establish the diagnosis. Erythroderma can be caused by many conditions

Table 4
Tumor, node, metastasis, blood staging of mycosis fungoides and Sezary syndrome

Category		Description	
Skin (T)	T0[a]	Absence of Clinically Suspicious Lesions	
	T1	Patches, plaques, or papules <10% BSA	
			T1A Patch only lesions
			T1B Plaque/papule+/- patch lesions
	T2	Patches, plaques, or papules ≥10% BSA	
			T2A Patch only lesions
			T2B Plaque/papule+/- patch lesions
	T3	One or more tumors ≥1 cm diameter	
	T4	Confluence of erythema covering ≥80% BSA[b]	
Nodes (N)[c]	N0	No clinically abnormal lymph node (LN); no biopsy necessary	
	N1	Pathology Dutch grade 1 or NCI LN 0–2:	
			N1A clone negative or equivocal[d]
			N1B Pathology Dutch grade 1 or NCI LN 0–2: clone positive and identical to skin
	N2		N2A Dutch grade 2, NCI LN3: clone negative or equivocal
			N2B Dutch grade 2, NCI LN3: clone positive and identical to skin
	N3[c] (lymphoma)		N3A Dutch grade 3–4, NCI LN4: clone negative or equivocal
			N3B Dutch grade 3–4, NCI LN4: clone positive and identical to skin
	NX	Clinically abnormal peripheral or central lymph node but no pathologic determination of representative LN. Other surrogate means of determining involvement may be determined by Tri-Society consensus	
Viscera (M)	M0	No visceral involvement	
	M1a	BM only involvement	Clone positive and identical to skin
		Clone negative or indeterminate	
	M1b	Non-BM visceral involvement	Clone positive and identical to skin
		Clone negative or indeterminate	
	MX	Visceral involvement is neither confirmed nor refuted by available pathologic or imaging assessment	

(continued on next page)

Table 4
(continued)

Blood (B)[e]			
B_0	B_{0A}	Clone negative or equivocal	Absence of significant blood involvement
	B_{0B}	Clone positive and identical to skin	
B_1	B_{1A}	Clone negative or equivocal	Low blood tumor burden
	B_{1B}	Clone positive and identical to skin	
B_2	B_{2A}	Clone negative or equivocal	High blood tumor burden
	B_{2B}	Clone positive and identical to skin	
B_x	B_{xA}	Clone negative or equivocal	Unable to quantify blood involvement according to agreed upon guidelines
	B_{xB}	Clone positive and identical to skin	

Options for characterizing clonality further by designation as A (clone negative or equivocal) and B (clone positive and identical to skin) are presented. If a clone in LN or viscera is detected but different from that identified in the skin, another concurrent lymphoproliferative process should be considered.

[a] T_0 is used for clinical trials in order to track clearance of lesions in the skin compartment. No patient with primary cutaneous lymphoma (PCL) at time of diagnosis should be T_0.

[b] Patients with both erythroderma and tumors may be designated as T_4 (T_3).[7] The BSA of 80% is used to define erythroderma in MF/SS at study entry, but any decrease in BSA during the study does not affect the entry classification.

[c] Abnormal LNs are those now >1.5 cm longest diameter (LDi) according to the Lugano classification and confirmed by imaging. The pathologic findings of a representative abnormal LN may apply to all abnormal lymph nodes.

[d] Dutch system: grade 1, dermatopathic lymphadenopathy; grade 2, dermatopathic lymphadenopathy with an early involvement by MF (presence of cerebriform nuclei >7.5 um); grade 3, partial effacement of lymph node architecture; many atypical cerebriform mononuclear cells; and grade 4, complete effacement. NCI classification: LN0, no atypical lymphocytes; LN1, occasional and isolated atypical lymphocytes (not arranged in clusters); LN2, many atypical lymphocytes or in 3–6 cell clusters; LN3, aggregates of atypical lymphocytes, nodal architecture preserved; and LN4, partial/complete effacement of nodal architecture by atypical lymphocytes or frankly neoplastic cells.

[e] Blood staging for MF/SS is defined currently as B_0, <250/μL of CD4+/CD26− or CD4+/CD7− cells; B_1, does not meet criteria for B_0 or B_2; and B_2, ≥1000/μL of CD4+/CD26− or CD4+/CD7− cells or other aberrant population of lymphocytes identified by flow cytometry. It is expected that patients with high blood tumor burden (B_2) will have a clone in the blood that is identical to that in the skin. Nonidentical T-cell clones are often detected in peripheral blood with increasing age and are of unknown clinical significance.

From Olsen et al., 2022.[49]

Table 5
Overall staging of mycosis fungoides and Sezary syndrome

	T	N	M	B
IA	1	0	0	0,1
IB	2	0	0	0,1
II	1,2	1,2	0	0,1
IIB	3	0–2	0	0,1
III	4	0–2	0	0,1
IIIA	4	0–2	0	0
IIIB	4	0–2	0	1
IVA_1	1–4	0–2	0	2
IVA_2	1–4	3	0	0–2
IVB	1–4	0–3	1	0–2

including MF/SS, other systemic T-cell lymphomas/leukemias (eg, ATLL), atopic dermatitis, psoriasis, pityriasis rubra pilaris, and drug reactions. Skin biopsies, peripheral flow cytometry, and suggestive clinical features (eg, ectropion) can help clarify the etiology, although in some cases, it may be impossible clinically to distinguish MF/SS

Table 6
Immunotherapy options for cutaneous T-cell lymphoma: summary of mechanisms

Therapy	Mechanism
Established therapies	
IFN-α	Enhances cell-mediated cytotoxicity, decreases T_H2 production by tumor cells, and inhibits malignant T-cell proliferation
IFN-γ	Enhances cell-mediated cytotoxicity, decreases T_H2 production by tumor cells, enhances dendritic cell function, and inhibits malignant T-cell growth
Photopheresis	Apoptosis of tumor cells
Retinoids (RXRs)	Apoptosis of tumor cells, decreases T_H2 production by tumor cells, and inhibits CCR4 expression and skin trafficking
New and emerging therapies	
IL-12	Enhances cell-mediated cytotoxicity, activates IFN-γ production, decreases T_H2 production by tumor cells, and enhances dendritic cell function
TLR-agonists	TLR-7/9: activates IFN-α production; TLR-8: activates IL-12, tumor necrosis factor-α, and IFN-γ production
Targeting tumor antigens and checkpoint molecules	
Mogamulizumab	Antibody targeting of tumor cells via CCR4 and depletes $CCR4^+$ regulatory T cells
Anti–PD-1	Immune checkpoint inhibition
Anti-CD47	Antibody targeting of tumor cells via CD47 and enhances phagocytosis by macrophages
CAR-T	T cell targeting of tumor cells

Abbreviations: CAR-T, Chimeric antigen receptor T cells; CCR4, C-C chemokine receptor type 4; IFN, interferon; IL-12, interleukin-12; PD-1, programmed cell death protein 1; T_H2, T-helper 2; TLR, Toll-like receptor.
(*From* Weiner and colleagues, 2021[73])

from other causes of erythroderma. The differential diagnosis for LyP includes pcALCL, pityriasis lichenoides et varioliformis acuta, pityriasis lichenoides chronica, and reactive lymphoid hyperplasia from arthropod bites, scabies, medications, or infections. The differential diagnosis of pcALCL includes LyP, MF/SS, systemic ALCL with cutaneous involvement, and other systemic T-cell lymphomas with secondary cutaneous involvement (eg, ATLL).

Pathophysiology and Tumor Microenvironment

Mycosis fungoides/Sezary syndrome

While the etiology of MF/SS is unknown, a prevailing theory is that MF/SS can develop as a response to prolonged exposure to an antigen stimulus, resulting in persistent activation of a genetically unstable T cell that accumulates mutations favoring neoplastic growth.[9] Somatic copy number variations (eg, loss of part of chromosome 17 containing TP53) are the most common driving mutations found in MF/SS.[59,60] One potential antigen stimulus is S aureus, which may promote the proliferation of malignant T cells by binding to major histocompatibility complex class II molecules and TCRs.[10] Environmental stimuli such as chemicals and pesticides have also been suggested but not proven.[11,12] There are reports of CTCL clustering in certain regions and occurring in married couples, supporting the possibility of extrinsic disease triggers.[61,62] In general, CTCL is not hereditary, although there are rare reports of families with multiple cases of CTCL.[63]

A major focus of research has been to identify the "cell of origin," or the specific subtype of physiologic T cell that can transform into MF/SS. In general, both MF and SS likely arise from memory T cells, which comprise the majority of T cells in normal skin.[15] Both MF and SS usually express the skin-homing molecules C-C chemokine receptor type 4 (CCR4) and cutaneous lymphocyte antigen (CLA), consistent with the ability of the malignant cells to target and proliferate within the skin.[64] Based on analysis of classic T-cell markers, a prominent hypothesis is that MF arises from transformed skin-resident memory T cells, as studies have shown a CCR4$^+$/CLA$^+$/L-selectin$^-$/CCR7$^-$ expression pattern.[64] On the other hand, SS is believed to develop from central memory T cells based on a CCR4$^+$/CLA$^+$/L-selectin$^+$/CCR7$^+$ phenotype.[64] The biological function of these distinct cell types could explain the differing clinical behavior of MF and SS. Central memory T cells, which express the lymph node homing receptors L-selectin and CCR7, possess the ability to recirculate from the skin to the peripheral blood and lymph nodes, in keeping with the typical presentation of SS of erythroderma, blood involvement, and lymphadenopathy.[64] In contrast, tissue-resident memory T cells typically remain confined to the skin, which would explain the tendency for MF to remain limited to specific areas of the skin for extended periods.[64] However, this paradigm does not account for the plasticity in surface marker expression of the malignant T cells. While it is appealing to infer the cellular origin of MF/SS based on conventional T-cell classifications, single-cell RNA-sequencing studies have recently shown that MF/SS cells are highly heterogeneous and sometimes have features inconsistent with any known T-cell subtype.[65]

In MF/SS, neoplastic and inflammatory cells establish a microenvironment that drives disease progression. In general, early classic MF lesions contain few malignant T cells, whereas there are elevated CD8$^+$ T cells and a Th1 microenvironment.[14] As MF advances, the increased burden of CD4$^+$ malignant T cells promotes a shift toward a Th2 microenvironment, with a reduction in the number and function of CD8$^+$ T cells, NK cells, and dendritic cells, allowing for immune escape.[14] This Th2 skewing can permit tumor evasion and invasion and increase the risk of infection, a common cause of morbidity and mortality in patients with CTCL.[14] Other members of the tumor stroma such as cancer-associated fibroblasts, keratinocytes, dendritic cells, M2 type macrophages, and regulatory T cells are increasingly implicated in malignant T-cell expansion.[66,67] Key signaling pathways responsible for cell growth and immune responses (eg, Janus kinase/signal transducer and activator of transcription [JAK-STAT], nuclear factor kappa B [NF-κB], and mitogen-activated protein kinase [MAPK]) and immune checkpoint function (eg, T cell immunoreceptor with Ig and ITIM domains [TIGIT], CD47-signal regulatory protein α [SIRPα], and programmed cell death protein 1 [PD1]-programmed death-ligand 1 [PDL1]) also contribute to disease progression.[68,69]

Other subtypes

Less commonly, CD8[+] forms of MF/SS may occur, in which the neoplastic T cells are positive for CD8 and usually negative for CD4 (rather than dual positivity).[32,70] There appears to be a similar or even improved prognosis in patients with CD8[+] classic and hypopigmented MF.[32,70] However, clinical correlation is essential to rule out cutaneous aggressive epidermotropic CD8[+] cytotoxic T-cell lymphoma. The pathogenesis of CD8[+] MF/SS is not well-studied, and it is not understood how this subtype fits into the classic perspective of MF/SS as a Th2-driven process. In general, CD8[+] MF/SS responds well to the same treatments as classic MF/SS, although interferons should be avoided due to their ability to activate CD8[+] T cells. Hypopigmented MF is usually CD8[+]; hypopigmentation might occur due to cytotoxicity of CD8[+] T cells toward melanocytes, similar to vitiligo.[20] However, many cases of CD8[+] MF are not hypopigmented, and CD4[+] MF may also be hypopigmented. Therefore, a cytotoxic phenotype alone does not explain the hypopigmented presentation.

The pathogenesis of LyP and ALCL is largely unknown. However, it is likely that CD30 plays a role in the development of these conditions. CD30 is a member of the tumor necrosis factor superfamily that has a variety of physiologic functions such as activation of the NF-κB pathway, Th17 differentiation, and suppression of Th1-driven inflammation.[71] In addition to the CD30[+] LPDs, CD30 is often overexpressed in malignancies such as MF/SS, Hodgkin's lymphoma, diffuse large B-cell lymphoma, and embryonal carcinoma.[71] Binding of CD30 to its ligand appears to aid tumor cell apoptosis, potentially explaining the tendency of LyP and pcALCL to self-regress.[72]

Treatment

Skin-directed versus systemic therapy

Treatment options for MF/SS include skin-directed therapies and systemic therapies. Skin-directed therapies include topical steroids, imiquimod, carmustine (BCNU), mechlorethamine, phototherapy (narrow-band ultraviolet B [NB-UVB] or psoralen plus ultraviolet A [PUVA]), and local radiation. Systemic therapies include interferons, extracorporeal photopheresis (ECP), mogamulizumab, retinoids, methotrexate, pralatrexate, vorinostat, romidepsin, brentuximab, alemtuzumab, total-skin electron beam therapy, single-agent chemotherapy (gemcitabine, pegylated liposomal doxorubicin), combination chemotherapy (eg, cyclophosphamide, doxorubicin, vincristine and prednisolone [CHOP]), and allogeneic stem cell transplant.

Importance of immunotherapy

It is important to treat MF/SS with immune-preserving agents whenever possible (eg, retinoids, interferon, ECP, and topical chemotherapy) prior to the use of immunosuppressive systemic chemotherapy (see **Table 5**). As previously discussed, MF/SS is characterized by progressive immune impairment, and a major cause of mortality in MF/SS is systemic microbial infection.[14,73] Immunosuppression occurs in MF/SS due to tumor cell overexpression of Th2 cytokines that suppress the number and function of CD8[+] T cells, NK cells, and dendritic cells, as well as upregulation of immune checkpoint molecules (eg, PD1 and TIGIT).[14,73] Therefore, initial therapy should be directed at shifting immune function in favor of the Th1 or cytotoxic lymphocyte activity to help reinvigorate the host antitumor response.[14,73]

In general, immunotherapies help eradicate malignant T cells by causing apoptosis of malignant cells, enhancing the processing of apoptotic malignant cells, and augmenting the cytotoxic T-cell response.[14,73] Concurrent use of multiple immunotherapies with complementary mechanisms of action including interferon, ECP, oral retinoids, and monoclonal antibodies can help maximally boost these functions.[73,74] Agents such as interferon and toll-like receptor (TLR) agonists directly enhance cell-mediated cytotoxicity, while therapies such as bexarotene and ECP result in apoptosis of malignant T cells.[73] In addition, ECP induces monocytes to differentiate into dendritic cells that can process the apoptotic tumor cell antigens, while interferon-γ and TLR agonists can prime dendritic cells for interleukin-12 (IL-12) production.[73]

In contrast, chemotherapy weakens the host immune system, may impair the efficacy of future immunotherapy, and increases the risk of infection. However, it should be noted that certain patients with rapidly progressive symptoms limiting quality of life may require cytotoxic chemotherapy for more immediate disease control.

Treatment approach

In general, MF and SS are not curable conditions, and the majority of patients have a disease course spanning years to decades. The goal of treatment is, therefore, to control the disease in the long term rather than completely eradicate it. Due to the rarity of CTCL, there is limited clinical trial data to guide therapy. Based on the available data and the clinical experience of experts in the field, there are international guidelines (eg, National Comprehensive Cancer Network [NCCN], EORTC, and European Society for Medical Oncology [ESMO]) that recommend first-line treatment options for patients based on their disease subtype and stage.[51,75,76] However, there is no standard preferred therapy, and individual institutions have developed their own approach to treatment. In addition, patient-specific factors such as medical comorbidities, finances, the type and site of disease, and the pace of disease progression also influence treatment selection. Treatment may be monotherapy or a combination of immunomodulatory treatments. Skin-directed therapies should be used whenever possible, even among patients requiring systemic therapy. As most patients have indolent disease that waxes and wanes throughout their life, it is important to carefully upgrade treatment (eg, from skin-directed to systemic therapy) only when necessary and to downgrade whenever possible. For patients with advanced disease who do achieve remission, complete withdrawal of therapy may ultimately result in disease relapse. Thus, for those with complete remission during immunotherapy, it is recommended that they should be slowly tapered and perhaps maintained long term on low-dose interferon.

Early MF (patches or plaques <10% BSA) is typically treated with skin-directed therapies only, primarily topical steroids, topical chemotherapy, and/or phototherapy depending on the extent of skin involvement.[51,75,76] Thicker recalcitrant plaques can be treated by PUVA, local radiation or by addition of interferon or bexarotene.[51,75,76]

Patients with localized tumors are usually treated with local radiation or systemic therapy plus skin-directed therapy for any patch/plaque disease. Patients with MF with generalized tumors, erythroderma, or lymph node disease require systemic therapy in addition to skin-directed therapy. Options include bexarotene, interferon, total skin electron beam therapy, the CD30-specific immunotoxin brentuximab, methotrexate, single-agent chemotherapy, and ECP.[51,75,76] However, it is important to note that interferon should be avoided in CD8[+] MF/SS due to the ability of interferon to stimulate CD8[+] T cells. The first-line treatment of SS is ECP, either as monotherapy or in combination with bexarotene or interferon (IFN).[77] High-burden SS is often treated with mogamulizumab, a monoclonal antibody directed against CCR4 that is particularly effective in the blood.[74,78] Patients who have exhausted all standard treatment options are typically enrolled in clinical trials.

Allogeneic hematopoietic stem cell transplantation (HSCT) is a potentially curative approach for advanced MF and SS. Allo-HSCT is ideally performed in young otherwise healthy patients with aggressive MF/SS who have temporarily obtained disease remission.[79] There is a 50% rate of potentially life-threatening posttransplant graft versus host disease and a 50% rate of posttransplant disease relapse, although relapsed CTCL after transplant is often less aggressive.[80]

SS frequently results in pruritus that can be debilitating and affect quality of life. The cause of pruritus is multifactorial including imbalance of cytokines such as IL-31, infiltration of the skin by malignant cells, infection by S aureus, and disruption of the skin barrier resulting in transepidermal water loss.[48,81] In addition to targeted treatment of the disease, the initial management of pruritus includes the use of moisturizers, topical steroids, and antihistamines.[82] In patients with skin superinfection, antibiotics and bleach baths to reduce bacterial colonization may be helpful.[82] In patients with refractory pruritus, medications such as gabapentin, doxepin, and mirtazapine are useful.[82] Some patients with refractory pruritus may only experience improvement of their symptoms with chronic prednisone, although this should be limited to the lowest possible dose.

Management of CD30[+] LPDs depends on the extent of skin involvement. Among patients with solitary or localized LyP, the lesions can often be monitored without intervention due to their tendency to self-regress. If necessary, localized LyP can be treated with potent topical steroids or irradiated.[83] In patients with widespread LyP, low-dose methotrexate is an effective option.[83] While these treatments can facilitate healing of LyP lesions and potentially prevent new eruptions, they have not been proven to reduce the risk of developing an associated lymphoma.[84] However, this is a topic that requires further research. Solitary pcALCL can be treated by radiotherapy or steroid injection.[83] In widespread pcALCL, systemic treatment is recommended, typically with brentuximab or methotrexate.[83]

CLINICS CARE POINTS

- CTCL often presents with subtle or atypical symptoms that can overlap with other skin conditions. Diagnosis, therefore, requires careful correlation of clinical, pathologic, and laboratory findings and typically involves multiple biopsies and physical examinations over time.

- In general, MF and SS are not curable conditions, and the disease tends to wax and wane over years to decades. Therefore, the goal of treatment is to control the disease in the long term rather than achieve remission.

- It is important to treat MF and SS with immune-preserving agents whenever possible prior to the use of immunosuppressive systemic chemotherapy. MF and SS are characterized by progressive immune impairment, and initial therapy should be directed at reinvigorating the host antitumor response.

- Treatment options include skin-directed and systemic therapies. Based on the available data and the clinical experience of experts, there are international guidelines (eg, NCCN, EORTC, and ESMO) that recommend first-line treatment options for patients based on their disease subtype and stage. However, there is no standard preferred therapy, and individual institutions have developed their own approach to treatment.

DISCLOSURE

A.H. Rook is a consultant for TLR Biosciences and speaker for Mallinckrodt. D. M. Weiner has no disclosures.

REFERENCES

1. Willemze R, Cerroni L, Kempf W, et al. The 2018 update of the WHO-EORTC classification for primary cutaneous lymphomas. Blood 2019;133(16):1703–14.
2. Koh HK, Charif M, Weinstock MA. Epidemiology and clinical manifestations of cutaneous T-cell lymphoma. Hematol Oncol Clin N Am 1995;9(5):943–60.
3. Morton LM, Wang SS, Devesa SS, et al. Lymphoma incidence patterns by WHO subtype in the United States, 1992-2001. Blood 2006;107(1):265–76.
4. Dobos G, Pohrt A, Ram-Wolff C, et al. Epidemiology of cutaneous T-cell lymphomas: a systematic review and meta-analysis of 16,953 patients. Cancers 2020;12(10):2921.
5. Alibert, J.L. Description des maladies de la peau: observées à l'Hôpital Saint-Louis, et exposition des meilleures méthodes suivies pour leur traitement. Vol. 2. 1825: Wahlen.
6. Sézary A, Bouvrain Y. Erythrodermie avec présence de cellules monstrueuses dans le derme et le sang circulant. Bull Soc Fr Dermatol Syphiligr 1938;45: 254–60.
7. Kubica AW, Davis MDP, Weaver AL, et al. Sézary syndrome: a study of 176 patients at Mayo Clinic. J Am Acad Dermatol 2012;67(6):1189–99.
8. Kim YH, Liu HL, Mraz-Gernhard S, et al. Long-term outcome of 525 patients with mycosis fungoides and Sezary syndrome: clinical prognostic factors and risk for disease progression. Arch Dermatol 2003;139(7):857–66.
9. Girardi M, Heald PW, Wilson LD. The pathogenesis of mycosis fungoides. N Engl J Med 2004;350(19):1978–88.
10. Fujii K. Pathogenesis of cutaneous T cell lymphoma: Involvement of Staphylococcus aureus. J Dermatol (Tokyo) 2022;49(2):202–9.
11. Whittemore AS, Holly EA, Lee IM, et al. Mycosis fungoides in relation to environmental exposures and immune response: a case-control study. JNCI: J Natl Cancer Inst 1989;81(20):1560–7.
12. Tuyp E, Burgoyne A, Aitchison T, et al. A case-control study of possible causative factors in mycosis fungoides. Arch Dermatol 1987;123(2):196–200.
13. Berger CL, Warburton D, Raafat J, et al. Cutaneous T-cell lymphoma: neoplasm of T cells with helper activity. Blood 1979;53(4):642–51.
14. Kim EJ, Hess S, Richardson SK, et al. Immunopathogenesis and therapy of cutaneous T cell lymphoma. J Clin Invest 2005;115(4):798–812.
15. Kupper TS, Fuhlbrigge RC. Immune surveillance in the skin: mechanisms and clinical consequences. Nat Rev Immunol 2004;4(3):211–22.
16. Pimpinelli N, Olsen EA, Santucci M, et al. Defining early mycosis fungoides. J Am Acad Dermatol 2005;53(6):1053–63.

17. Hristov AC, Tejasvi T, Wilcox RA. Mycosis fungoides and Sézary syndrome: 2019 update on diagnosis, risk-stratification, and management. Am J Hematol 2019; 94(9):1027–41.
18. Zhuang TZ, McCook-Veal A, Switchenko J, et al. Characterizing outcomes in visceral cutaneous t-cell lymphoma: a single center retrospective study. Clin Lymphoma, Myeloma & Leukemia 2023;23(9):667–73.
19. Mitteldorf C, Stadler R, Sander CA, et al. Folliculotropic mycosis fungoides. JDDG J der Deutschen Dermatol Gesellschaft 2018;16(5):543–57.
20. Furlan FC, Sanches JA. Hypopigmented mycosis fungoides: a review of its clinical features and pathophysiology. An Bras Dermatol 2013;88:954–60.
21. Ahn CS, ALSayyah A, Sangüeza OP. Mycosis fungoides: an updated review of clinicopathologic variants. Am J Dermatopathol 2014;36(12):933–51.
22. Chen C, Gu YD, Geskin LJ. A review of primary cutaneous CD30+ lymphoproliferative disorders. Hematol/Oncol Clin 2019;33(1):121–34.
23. Toro JR, Liewehr DJ, Pabby N, et al. Gamma-delta T-cell phenotype is associated with significantly decreased survival in cutaneous T-cell lymphoma. Blood 2003; 101(9):3407–12.
24. Berti E, Tomasini D, Vermeer MH, et al. Primary cutaneous CD8-positive epidermotropic cytotoxic T cell lymphomas: A distinct clinicopathological entity with an aggressive clinical behavior. Am J Pathol 1999;155(2):483–92.
25. Endly DC, Weenig RH, Peters MS, et al. Indolent course of cutaneous gamma-delta T-cell lymphoma. J Cutan Pathol 2013;40(10):896–902.
26. Lin EC, Liao JB, Fang YH, et al. The pathophysiology and current treatments for the subcutaneous panniculitis-like T cell lymphoma: An updated review. Asia Pac J Clin Oncol 2023;19(1):27–34.
27. Brocq L. Les parapsoriasis. Ann Dermatol Syphiligr 1902;3:433–68.
28. Chairatchaneeboon M, Thanomkitti K, Kim EJ. Parapsoriasis—a diagnosis with an identity crisis: a narrative review. Dermatol Ther 2022;12(5):1091–102.
29. Väkevä L, Sarna S, Vaalasti A, et al. A retrospective study of the probability of the evolution of parapsoriasis en plaques into mycosis fungoides. Acta Derm Venereol 2005;85(4):318–23.
30. Zhang Y, Wang Y, Yu R, et al. Molecular markers of early-stage mycosis fungoides. J Invest Dermatol 2012;132(6):1698–706.
31. Junkins-Hopkins JM. Cutaneous Lymphomas. In: Handbook of practical immunohistochemistry: frequently asked questions. Cham, Switzerland: Springer; 2022. p. 833–96.
32. Martinez-Escala ME, Kantor RW, Cices A, et al. CD8+ mycosis fungoides: a low-grade lymphoproliferative disorder. J Am Acad Dermatol 2017;77(3):489–96.
33. Kampa F, Mitteldorf C. A review of CD30 expression in cutaneous neoplasms. J Cutan Pathol 2021;48(4):495–510.
34. Kempf W, Mitteldorf C. Pathologic Diagnosis of Cutaneous Lymphomas. Dermatol Clin 2015;33(4):655–81.
35. Vonderheid EC. On the diagnosis of erythrodermic cutaneous T-cell lymphoma. J Cutan Pathol 2006;33:27–42.
36. Kazakov DV, Burg G, Kempf W. Clinicopathological spectrum of mycosis fungoides. J Eur Acad Dermatol Venereol 2004;18(4):397–415.
37. Van Doorn R, Scheffer E, Willemze R. Follicular mycosis fungoides, a distinct disease entity with or without associated follicular mucinosis: A clinicopathologic and follow-up study of 51 patients. Arch Dermatol 2002;138(2):191–8.

38. Moczko A, Dimitriou F, Kresbach H, et al. Sensitivity and specificity of T-cell receptor PCR BIOMED-2 clonality analysis for the diagnosis of cutaneous T-cell lymphoma. Eur J Dermatol 2020;30:12–5.

39. Rea B, Haun P, Emerson R, et al. Role of high-throughput sequencing in the diagnosis of cutaneous T-cell lymphoma. J Clin Pathol 2018;71(9):814–20.

40. Kirsch IR, Watanabe R, O'Malley JT, et al. TCR sequencing facilitates diagnosis and identifies mature T cells as the cell of origin in CTCL. Sci Transl Med 2015; 7(308):308ra158.

41. Zimmermann C, Boisson M, Ram-Wolff C, et al. Diagnostic performance of high-throughput sequencing of the T-cell receptor beta gene for the diagnosis of cutaneous T-cell lymphoma. Br J Dermatol 2021;185(3):679–80.

42. Posnett DN, Sinha R, Kabak S, et al. Clonal populations of T cells in normal elderly humans: the T cell equivalent to" benign monoclonal gammapathy". J Exp Med 1994;179(2):609–18.

43. Zelickson BD, Peters MS, Muller SA, et al. T-cell receptor gene rearrangement analysis: cutaneous T cell lymphoma, peripheral T cell lymphoma, and premalignant and benign cutaneous lymphoproliferative disorders. J Am Acad Dermatol 1991;25(5):787–96.

44. Thurber SE, Zhang B, Kim YH, et al. T-cell clonality analysis in biopsy specimens from two different skin sites shows high specificity in the diagnosis of patients with suggested mycosis fungoides. J Am Acad Dermatol 2007;57(5):782–90.

45. Vermeer MH, Nicolay JP, Scarisbrick JJ, et al. Flow cytometry for the assessment of blood tumour burden in cutaneous T-cell lymphoma: towards a standardized approach. Br J Dermatol 2022;187(1):21–8.

46. Scarisbrick JJ, Hodak E, Bagot M, et al. Blood classification and blood response criteria in mycosis fungoides and Sézary syndrome using flow cytometry: recommendations from the EORTC cutaneous lymphoma task force. Eur J Cancer 2018;93:47–56.

47. Horna P, Shi M, Jevremovic D, et al. Utility of TRBC1 expression in the diagnosis of peripheral blood involvement by cutaneous T-cell lymphoma. J Invest Dermatol 2021;141(4):821–9. e2.

48. Olsen EA, Rook AH, Zic J, et al. Sézary syndrome: immunopathogenesis, literature review of therapeutic options, and recommendations for therapy by the United States Cutaneous Lymphoma Consortium (USCLC). J Am Acad Dermatol 2011;64(2):352–404.

49. Olsen EA, Whittaker S, Willemze R, et al. Primary cutaneous lymphoma: recommendations for clinical trial design and staging update from the ISCL, USCLC, and EORTC. Blood, The Journal of the American Society of Hematology 2022; 140(5):419–37.

50. Mahieux R, Gessain A. Adult T-cell leukemia/lymphoma and HTLV-1. Current Hematologic Malignancy Reports 2007;2:257–64.

51. Primary Cutaneous Lymphomas. 2024, NCCN clinical practice guidelines in oncology.

52. Scheffer E, Meijer C, Van Vloten W. Dermatopathic lymphadenopathy and lymph node involvement in mycosis fungoides. Cancer 1980;45(1):137–48.

53. Sausville E, Worsham GF, Matthews MJ, et al. Histologic assessment of lymph nodes in mycosis fungoides/Sezary syndrome (cutaneous T-cell lymphoma): clinical correlations and prognostic import of a new classification system. Hum Pathol 1985;16(11):1098–109.

54. Graham SJ, Sharpe RW, Steinberg SM, et al. Prognostic implications of a bone marrow histopathologic classification system in mycosis fungoides and the Sézary syndrome. Cancer 1993;72(3):726–34.

55. Kim YH, Bishop K, Varghese A, et al. Prognostic factors in erythrodermic mycosis fungoides and the Sézary syndrome. Arch Dermatol 1995;131(9):1003–8.

56. Agar NS, Wedgeworth E, Crichton S, et al. Survival outcomes and prognostic factors in mycosis fungoides/Sézary syndrome: validation of the revised International Society for Cutaneous Lymphomas/European Organisation for Research and Treatment of Cancer staging proposal. J Clin Oncol 2010;28(31):4730–9.

57. Vollmer RT. A review of survival in mycosis fungoides. Am J Clin Pathol 2014; 141(5):706–11.

58. Talpur R, Singh L, Daulat S, et al. Long-term outcomes of 1,263 patients with mycosis fungoides and Sézary syndrome from 1982 to 2009. Clin Cancer Res 2012;18(18):5051–60.

59. Choi J, Goh G, Walradt T, et al. Genomic landscape of cutaneous T cell lymphoma. Nat Genet 2015;47(9):1011–9.

60. Stadler R, Hain C, Cieslak C, et al. Molecular pathogenesis of cutaneous lymphoma–Future directions. Exp Dermatol 2020;29(11):1062–8.

61. Ghazawi FM, Netchiporouk E, Rahme E, et al. Distribution and clustering of cutaneous T-cell lymphoma (CTCL) cases in Canada during 1992 to 2010. J Cutan Med Surg 2018;22(2):154–65.

62. Lozano A, Duvic M. Cutaneous T-cell lymphoma in non-blood-related family members: Report of an additional case. J Am Acad Dermatol 2007;56(3):521.

63. Hodak E, Klein T, Gabay B, et al. Familial mycosis fungoides: report of 6 kindreds and a study of the HLA system. J Am Acad Dermatol 2005;52(3):393–402.

64. Campbell JJ, Clark RA, Watanabe R, et al. Sezary syndrome and mycosis fungoides arise from distinct T-cell subsets: a biologic rationale for their distinct clinical behaviors. Blood, The Journal of the American Society of Hematology 2010; 116(5):767–71.

65. Buus TB, Willerslev-Olsen A, Fredholm S, et al. Single-cell heterogeneity in Sézary syndrome. Blood Advances 2018;2(16):2115–26.

66. Kalliara E, Belfrage E, Gullberg U, et al. Spatially Guided and Single Cell Tools to Map the Microenvironment in Cutaneous T-Cell Lymphoma. Cancers 2023;15(8): 2362.

67. Rendón-Serna N, Correa-Londoño LA, Velásquez-Lopera MM, et al. Cell signaling in cutaneous T-cell lymphoma microenvironment: promising targets for molecular-specific treatment. Int J Dermatol 2021;60(12):1462–80.

68. Xiao A, Akilov OE. Targeting the CD47-SIRPα Axis: Present Therapies and the Future for Cutaneous T-cell Lymphoma. Cells 2022;11(22):3591.

69. Durgin JS, Weiner DM, Wysocka M, et al. The immunopathogenesis and immunotherapy of cutaneous T cell lymphoma: Pathways and targets for immune restoration and tumor eradication. J Am Acad Dermatol 2021;84(3):587–95.

70. Jaque A, Mereniuk A, Walsh S, et al. Influence of the phenotype on mycosis fungoides prognosis, a retrospective cohort study of 160 patients. Int J Dermatol 2019;58(8):933–9.

71. Van der Weyden C, Pileri SA, Feldman AL, et al. Understanding CD30 biology and therapeutic targeting: a historical perspective providing insight into future directions. Blood Cancer J 2017;7(9):e603.

72. Mori M, Manuelli C, Pimpinelli N, et al. CD30-CD30 ligand interaction in primary cutaneous CD30+ T-cell lymphomas: a clue to the pathophysiology of clinical

regression. Blood, The Journal of the American Society of Hematology 1999;
94(9):3077–83.

73. Weiner DM, Durgin JS, Wysocka M, et al. The immunopathogenesis and immuno-therapy of cutaneous T cell lymphoma: Current and future approaches. J Am Acad Dermatol 2021;84(3):597–604.

74. Weiner DM, Rastogi S, Lewis DJ, et al. Mogamulizumab multimodality therapy with systemic retinoids, interferon, or extracorporeal photopheresis for advanced cutaneous t-cell lymphoma. Dermatol Ther 2023;2023.

75. Willemze R, Hodak E, Zinzani PL, et al. Primary cutaneous lymphomas: ESMO Clinical Practice Guidelines for diagnosis, treatment and follow-up. Ann Oncol 2018;29:iv30–40.

76. Latzka J, Assaf C, Bagot M, et al. EORTC consensus recommendations for the treatment of mycosis fungoides/Sézary syndrome–update 2023. Eur J Cancer 2023;195:113343.

77. Richardson SK, Lin JH, Vittorio CC, et al. High clinical response rate with multimo-dality immunomodulatory therapy for Sezary syndrome. Clinical Lymphoma and Myeloma 2006;7(3):226–32.

78. Kim YH, Bagot M, Pinter-Brown L, et al. Mogamulizumab versus vorinostat in pre-viously treated cutaneous T-cell lymphoma (MAVORIC): an international, open-label, randomised, controlled phase 3 trial. Lancet Oncol 2018;19(9):1192–204.

79. Schlaak M, Theurich S, Pickenhain J, et al. Allogeneic stem cell transplantation for advanced primary cutaneous T-cell lymphoma: a systematic review. Crit Rev Oncol Hematol 2013;85(1):21–31.

80. Weiner DM, Lewis DJ, Spaccarelli NG, et al. Management of relapsed cutaneous T-Cell lymphoma following allogeneic hematopoietic stem cell transplantation: Review with representative patient case. Dermatol Ther 2022;35(7):e15538.

81. Rook AH, Rook KA, Lewis DJ. Interleukin-31, a potent pruritus-inducing cytokine and its role in inflammatory disease and in the tumor microenvironment. Adv Exp Med Biol 2021;1290:111–27.

82. Ahern K, Gilmore ES, Poligone B. Pruritus in cutaneous T-cell lymphoma: a re-view. J Am Acad Dermatol 2012;67(4):760–8.

83. Hughey LC. Practical management of CD30+ lymphoproliferative disorders. Der-matol Clin 2015;33(4):819–33.

84. Kempf W, EORTC ISCL, Vermeer MH, et al. USCLC consensus recommendations for the treatment of primary cutaneous CD30-positive lymphoproliferative disor-ders: lymphomatoid papulosis and primary cutaneous anaplastic large-cell lym-phoma. Blood, The Journal of the American Society of Hematology 2011;118(15): 4024–35.

85. Cerroni L. Skin Lymphoma: The Illustrated Guide. 5th Edition. Hoboken, NJ: John Wiley & Sons; 2020.

Cutaneous B-Cell Lymphomas

Jennifer Villasenor-Park, MD, PhD[a,1], Jina Chung, MD[b,1],
Ellen J. Kim, MD[c,*]

KEYWORDS

- Cutaneous B-cell lymphoma • PCBCL • PCMZL • PCFCL • PCDLBCL-leg type
- IVLBCL • EBV[+] mucocutaneous ulcer

KEY POINTS

- Primary cutaneous marginal zone lymphoma (PCMZL) is an indolent B-cell lymphoma that has 2 subtypes: class-switched (immunoglobulin [Ig]G, IgA, or IgE[+]) and non–class-switched (IgM[+]). PCMZL has recently been reclassified as a chronic lymphoproliferative disorder according to the 2022 International Consensus Classification, although the World Health Organization continues to view it as an indolent lymphoma.
- Both PCMZL and primary cutaneous follicle center lymphoma are characterized by indolent behavior and excellent prognosis, and treatment options include low-dose radiation therapy, excision, intralesional steroids, and rituximab.
- Primary cutaneous diffuse large B-cell lymphoma, leg type (PCDLBCL, leg type) and intravascular large B-cell lymphoma require a more aggressive approach, often with rituximab plus multiagent chemotherapy. Radiation therapy is also frequently utilized for PCDLBCL, leg type.
- Epstein-Barr virus (EBV)-positive mucocutaneous ulcer is an indolent, EBV-associated lymphoproliferative disorder seen in the setting of immunodeficiency or age-related immunosenescence, which often resolves after cessation of immunosuppression.

INTRODUCTION

Primary cutaneous B-cell lymphomas (PCBCLs) represent a type of non-Hodgkin's lymphoma (NHL) of the skin without evidence of extracutaneous involvement at the

[a] Department of Dermatology, Perelman School of Medicine at the University of Pennsylvania, Perelman Center for Advanced Medicine, 3400 Civic Center Boulevard, Philadelphia, PA 19104, USA; [b] Department of Dermatology, Perelman School of Medicine at the University of Pennsylvania, 2 Maloney Building, 3600 Spruce Street, Philadelphia, PA 19104, USA; [c] Department of Dermatology, Perelman School of Medicine at the University of Pennsylvania, Perelman Center for Advanced Medicine, 3400 Civic Center Boulevard, Room 721, 7th floor, Philadelphia, PA 19104, USA
[1] Drs Villasenor-Park and Chung contributed equally to this study.
* Corresponding author.
E-mail address: ellen.kim@pennmedicine.upenn.edu

Hematol Oncol Clin N Am 38 (2024) 1111–1131
https://doi.org/10.1016/j.hoc.2024.05.017   hemonc.theclinics.com

time of diagnosis. They represent 25% to 35% of all primary cutaneous lymphomas.[1,2] In the 2018 classification system by the World Health Organization (WHO) and the European Organization for Research and Treatment of Cancer (EORTC), PCBCLs were categorized into 3 distinct entities: primary cutaneous marginal zone lymphoma (PCMZL), primary cutaneous follicle center lymphoma (PCFCL), and primary cutaneous diffuse large B-cell lymphoma, leg type (PCDLBCL, leg type).[3] Two additional subtypes were included: Epstein-Barr virus (EBV)[+] mucocutaneous ulcer (provisional) and the cutaneous variant of intravascular large B-cell lymphoma (IVLBCL; **Table 1**).

Herein, we provide a comprehensive review of the updated literature on these entities, including clinical presentation, histopathology, immunophenotype, molecular genetics, prognosis, and treatment.

PRIMARY CUTANEOUS MARGINAL ZONE LYMPHOMA
Clinical Presentation

PCMZL is an indolent B-cell lymphoma of the skin that comprises around 7% to 9% of all primary cutaneous lymphomas and approximately a third of PCBCLs.[3–6] While PCMZL was previously included in the category of extranodal marginal zone lymphomas of mucosa-associated lymphoid tissue (MALT), it is now recognized as a separate entity according to the 2022 WHO classification of Hematolymphoid Tumors (fifth edition) and the 2022 International Consensus Classification (ICC), due to its distinct clinicopathologic and molecular features.[7,8] The ICC now designates PCMZL as a lymphoproliferative disorder due to its indolent behavior, while the WHO continues to categorize PCMZL as an indolent lymphoma.[8]

PCMZL typically presents as solitary or multiple, pink to reddish-brown dermal papules, plaques, or nodules without significant surface changes, most commonly on the trunk and upper extremities (**Fig. 1**). Lesions are usually asymptomatic but may be slightly pruritic, and ulceration is uncommon. Median age of onset is around 39 to 55 years, with higher prevalence in male individuals than female individuals.[5,6,9–12] Cases have also been reported in children aged as young as 6 years, as well as adolescents.[13–16]

Histopathology

PCMZL can present as a nodular or diffuse dermal infiltrate of small to medium-sized lymphocytes in the dermis, sometimes extending into the subcutis. The epidermis is usually uninvolved, although rare cases with epidermotropism have been reported.[17] It can also present as a superficial and deep, perivascular and periadnexal lymphocytic infiltrate, sometimes mimicking an inflammatory dermatosis. The infiltrate is often composed of admixed B cells and reactive T cells, sometimes with a greater density of T cells, despite being a B-cell neoplasm. There are often admixed eosinophils and histiocytes, as well as variable numbers of plasma cells that are usually located at the periphery of the infiltrate. Sometimes, the infiltrate is composed almost exclusively of plasma cells (plasmacytic variant). Rare blastic variants with predominance of large, blastoid cells with high proliferation index have also been reported.[18]

Immunophenotype

The neoplastic B cells express B-cell markers such as CD20, CD79a, and PAX-5, are positive for BCL-2, and are negative for CD5 (which is aberrantly expressed in B-cell chronic lymphocytic leukemia and mantle cell lymphoma), CD10, and BCL-6. In the plasmacytic variant, B-cell markers are usually negative, but the neoplastic plasma cells are positive for CD38 and CD138 (plasma cell markers) and show monoclonal

Table 1
Primary cutaneous B-cell lymphomas

	PCMZL	PCFCL	PCDLBCL, Leg Type	IVLBCL, Cutaneous Variant	EBV-Positive Mucocutaneous Ulcer
Age	Fourth to fifth decade; can also involve children, adolescents	Sixth decade	Seventh decade	Sixth decade	Sixth to seventh decade
Male:Female	2:1	1.5:1	1:4	Female predominance	Slight female predominance
Site	Trunk, upper extremities	Head, neck, and trunk	Lower extremities (most common)	Trunk, lower extremities	Oropharyngeal, skin, and gastrointestinal
Immunophenotype	$CD20^+$; $CD79a^+$; $PAX-5^+$; $BCL-2^+$; $BCL-6^-$; $CD10^-$; $CD5^-$; light chain restriction; and $CD138^+$ in plasmacytic variant	$CD20^+$; $CD79a^+$; $PAX-5^+$; $Bcl-6^+$; $Bcl-2^{-(+)}$; $CD10^{-(+)}$; $CD5^-$; and $MUM-1^-$	$CD20^+$; $CD79a^+$; $PAX-5^+$; $BCL-2^+$; $MUM-1^+$; $FOX-P1^+$, $cMYC^{+/-}$, and $BCL-6^{+/-}$	$CD20^+$; $CD79a^+$; $PAX-5^+$; $BCL-2^+$; $MUM-1^+$, $cMYC^{+/-}$, and $BCL-6^{+/-}$	$PAX5^+$; CD20 and CD79 usually + but can be reduced; $CD30^+$, $MUM-1^+$, and EBER ISH^+
Treatment	RT, excision, topical or intralesional steroids, intralesional or systemic rituximab	RT, excision, topical or intralesional steroids, intralesional or systemic rituximab	Radiotherapy, rituximab + anthracycline-based chemotherapy (R-CHOP)	Rituximab + anthracycline-based chemotherapy (R-CHOP)	Cessation/reduction of immunosuppression
Clinical behavior	Indolent	Indolent	Aggressive	Aggressive; cutaneous-only variant may have better prognosis	Indolent

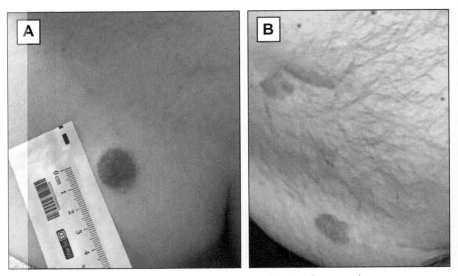

Fig. 1. PCMZL presenting as (A) solitary and (B) multifocal violaceous plaques.

expression of immunoglobulin light chains (kappa or lambda), which is a key diagnostic feature. A 10:1 ratio or greater is considered diagnostic of monoclonality. This can be detected by mRNA in situ hybridization, immunohistochemistry, or flow cytometry immunophenotyping, which are typically more sensitive than immunoglobulin heavy chain (IgH) gene rearrangement studies.[19]

Genetics

IgH gene rearrangement studies are positive for monoclonality in about 54% to 80% of cases.[20,21] Mutations in *FAS* are commonly found in PCMZL (>60%) but are uncommon in other extranodal marginal zone or MALT lymphomas, which distinguishes PCMZL from these entities.[22] Aberrant somatic hypermutation of protooncogenes such as *PAX5*, *RhoH/TTF*, *c-MYC*, and *PIM1* have been described in PCMZL, as well as preferential involvement of certain variable gene segments (V_H1-69 and V_H4-59).[23,24] Translocations involving t(11;18)(q21;q21) *API2/MALT1* and t(1;14)(p22;q32), detected in other MALT lymphomas, are usually absent in PCMZL.[25–29] Translocations of t(14;18)(q32;q21) involving *IGH/MALT1* and/or *IGH/BCL2*, and t(3;14)(p14.1;q32) *FOXP1/IGH*, which can be seen in a subset of MALT lymphomas, have rarely been described in PCMZL.[28,30,31]

There are 2 subtypes of PCMZL, based on IgH usage. The first subtype expresses class-switched immunoglobulins (most commonly IgG, less frequently IgA or IgE), are characterized by a T-helper type 2-like cytokine profile with a dense reactive T-cell infiltrate, and typically lack expression of CXCR3, which is thought to play an important role in the migration of B cells to MALT tissue.[32,33] This class-switched subtype comprises the vast majority of PCMZL cases (nearly 90% of cases). This subtype has also been reported to have variable rates of IgG4 expression (13%–39%) in the absence of a systemic IgG4-related disease, suggesting that this entity may lie on a spectrum with other chronic inflammatory disorders.[34–36] The class-switched subtype is sometimes preceded by cutaneous lymphoid hyperplasia, has lower rates of extracutaneous disease than the non–class-switched subtype, and it has been suggested that this subtype should be reclassified as a chronic clonal lymphoproliferative disorder.[32,35,36]

The second subtype, which comprises about 10% of PCMZL cases, is non–class-switched; these cases usually express IgM and display more MALT lymphoma-like features, such as expression of CXCR3 and IRTA1, and a Th1-like cytokine profile with a lower density of admixed reactive T cells.[32,35,37] MYD88 mutations have also been described in a small number of these non–class-switched IgM[+] cases; this mutation is more commonly found in lymphoplasmacytic lymphoma (>90% of cases), diffuse large B-cell lymphoma, splenic marginal zone lymphoma, and some extranodal MALT lymphomas.[38] This IgM[+] subtype is more commonly associated with extracutaneous involvement, and rare cases have also been associated with Borrelia burgdorferi infection.[32,39]

Staging and Prognosis

As with all cutaneous B-cell lymphomas (CBCLs), essential staging workup includes a complete history and physical examination, complete blood count (CBC) with differential, comprehensive metabolic panel (CMP), lactate dehydrogenase (LDH), and chest/abdominal/pelvic computed tomography (CT) with intravenous contrast or combined PET/CT scan to exclude a systemic lymphoma with secondary cutaneous involvement.[40] Tumors are staged according to the TNM classification system proposed by the International Society for Cutaneous Lymphomas and the EORTC, depending on the extent of skin, lymph node, and visceral involvement.[41] The use of PET-CT is somewhat controversial as marginal zone lymphoma often has low fluorodeoxyglcuose (FDG)-avidity, but some studies have suggested increased sensitivity for detection with PET-CT.[42] In the plasmacytic variant where the infiltrate is composed almost exclusively of plasma cells, serum protein electrophoresis or serum immunofixation studies may be considered.

Of note, while the 2022 ICC now classifies PCMZL as a lymphoproliferative disorder rather than a lymphoma, they do not specifically comment on whether staging workup is still indicated, and the 2023 National Comprehensive Cancer Network (NCCN) guidelines still recommend a staging workup including imaging studies. The ICC does mention that for IgM[+] non–class-switched cases, noncutaneous primary disease should be excluded, but immunoglobulin subtyping of PCMZL is not routinely performed in most pathology laboratories. Therefore, at this time, a staging workup is likely still necessary to exclude a systemic lymphoproliferative disorder. A bone marrow biopsy is usually not indicated for PCMZL unless there are unexplained hematologic abnormalities.

PCMZL is characterized by its indolent clinical course and excellent prognosis, with a 5 year disease-specific survival rate around 98% to 100%.[5,9] Cutaneous recurrences are common, seen in around half (44%–57%) of patients, and do not portend a worse prognosis; extracutaneous progression is rare (4%–8%).[5,9,10] The rates of recurrence are higher for patients presenting with multifocal or generalized disease than solitary lesions.[43]

Treatment

Solitary or locoregional lesions are usually treated with localized radiation therapy (RT), typically given at doses of 20 to 40 Gy.[40,44] RT is highly effective and can achieve complete remission in nearly 100% of cases, but relapses were frequent, in about half of cases.[44] There are also increasing reports of very low-dose RT (4–8 Gy) with excellent response, and no significant differences were seen in remission rates between standard-dose and very low-dose RT, with fewer toxicities observed with the very low-dose option.[45] Excision is reasonable for solitary lesions, but given the high risk of relapse, large disfiguring surgeries should be avoided. There are no significant differences in time to recurrence and recurrence risk among different treatment modalities.[43] For relapsed or multifocal disease, very low-dose palliative radiation (4 Gy), intralesional steroid injections, and watchful waiting are all reasonable options.[46,47] Rituximab is an option for treatment-refractory or generalized disease, but the risk–benefit ratio should be carefully considered, given that PCMZL is an indolent condition and eventual recurrences are frequent.[48–52] Chlorambucil has also rarely been utilized for disseminated lesions.[44,53] Other reported treatment modalities include intralesional rituximab, topical steroids, topical imiquimod, intralesional interferon-alpha, topical bexarotene, and topical nitrogen mustard.[52,54–59]

DNA evidence of *B burgdorferi* infection by polymerase chain reaction analysis has been documented in some cases of PCMZL from Europe (as well as in other types of CBCLs, including PCFCL and PCDLBCL, leg type), and there are rare reports of improvement after antibiotic therapy alone.[39,60–64] Other studies from North America, Asia, and other parts of Europe have failed to reproduce this link, however, suggesting that this association may only be significant in endemically infected areas, and there are also reports of *Borrelia*-positive cases that did not resolve with antibiotic therapy.[25,29,65–69] Antibiotic treatment with cephalosporins or tetracyclines may be considered in *Borrelia*-positive cases.

PRIMARY CUTANEOUS FOLLICLE CENTER LYMPHOMA
Clinical Presentation

PCFCL is the most common PCBCL and accounts for nearly 50% of all cases of PCBCL.[3] It is an extranodal, NHL that is distinct from follicular lymphoma and secondary cutaneous follicular lymphoma with a germinal center phenotype.[70] More commonly diagnosed in older individuals, with a median age of diagnosis of 51 years, and a slight predilection for male individuals (1.5:1), it can rarely occur in the pediatric population.[5,71,72]

PCFCL typically presents as nonulcerated erythematous or plum-colored papules, plaques, and tumors on the head, neck, upper extremities, and trunk. Most lesions are solitary, nonpruritic, and nontender with an intact epidermal surface, and progress slowly over months to years. Extracutaneous involvement is rare (<10%).[1,73] Other clinical presentations have been described including "reticulohistiocytoma of the dorsum" or "Crosti's lymphoma," which is a distinct clinical presentation of PCFCL

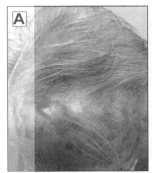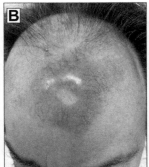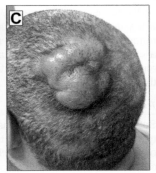

Fig. 2. Primary cutaneous follicle center cell lymphoma on the scalp presenting as red or pink patches (A), plaques (B), and exophytic tumor (C).

with plaques and tumors on the trunk with surrounding erythematous macules and papules.[74] On the scalp, PCFCL may present as seborrheic dermatitis like macular erythema (**Fig. 2**A, B), papules, erythematous nodules (**Fig. 2**C), noninflammatory sub-cutaneous nodules (mimicking benign pilar or epidermal inclusion cysts), or alopecia. Miliary or agminated lesions resembling rosacea or arthropod bites have also been described. However, it should be noted that there is not a specific clinical presentation that can reliably distinguish primary from secondary cutaneous follicular lymphoma.

Histopathology

Lesions of PCFCL typically demonstrate nodular or diffuse dermal and subcutaneous infiltrates; the epidermis is spared. The infiltrates are characterized by a predominance of centrocytes with admixed centroblasts and small lymphocytes, including reactive T cells. Three main growth patterns have been described: follicular, mixed follicular and diffuse, and diffuse. The neoplastic lymphoid follicles often have few-to-no tingible body macrophages (unlike reactive lymphoid follicles that typically have many), with a reduced or absent mantle zone.[75,76] In the diffuse type, there are dense nodular infiltrates of medium-to-large cells showing features of centrocytes and centroblasts, without clear lymphoid follicles. The presence of confluent sheets of immunoblasts should prompt consideration for diffuse large B-cell lymphoma, which can appear morphologically similar to PCFCL, diffuse type.

Immunophenotype

The neoplastic cells in PCFCL are positive for B-cell markers such as CD20, CD79a, and PAX-5 and are positive for BCL-6. Expression of CD10 is seen in fewer than 25% of cases and is more commonly associated with a follicular growth pattern. BCL-2 is typically negative in PCFCL. Expression of BCL-2 by immunohistochemistry (particularly if there is coexpression of CD10) and/or the presence of a t(14;18)(q32;q21) *IGH/BCL2* translocation by fluorescence in situ hybridization (FISH) should raise suspicion for a systemic follicular lymphoma with secondary cutaneous involvement. CD21+ follicular dendritic cell meshworks are easily identified in the follicular type but may be focal to absent in cases with a diffuse pattern. If present, they can help differentiate PCFCL, diffuse type, from diffuse large B-cell lymphoma (DLBCL). Negativity for BCL-2, MUM-1, and FOX-P1 can also help exclude PCDLBCL, leg type.[75]

Genetics

PCFCL often exhibits a monoclonal rearrangement of IgH genes. The gene expression profile of PCFCL is similar to germinal center-like large B-cell lymphomas with frequent amplification of the *REL* gene.[77,78] Unlike nodal follicular lymphoma, detection of the interchromosomal (14;18) translocation, which leads to overexpression of BCL-2, is uncommon in PCFCL and the incidence is reported to range from 0% to 30% to 40%.[74,79–81] Using targeted and whole exome next-generation sequencing techniques, PCFCL was also noted to have fewer chromatin-modifying gene mutations in characteristic genes including CREBBP or KMT2D compared to follicular lymphoma.[70,82] TNFRS14 loss-of-function mutations and copy number loss at chromosome 1p36, which are characteristic mutations in follicular lymphoma, are common in PCFCL and nodal follicular lymphoma.[70,82,83] Loss-of-function mutations in TNFRSF14 promote B-cell expansion.[84] Deletions of 9p21.3 involving *CDKN2A* and *CDKN2B* genes and *MYD88* mutations are rarely found in PCFCL and more common in PCDLBCL, leg type.[78,85]

Staging and Prognosis

Staging of PCFCL requires a complete physical examination and laboratory studies including a CBC with differential, CMP, and LDH. Radiographic imaging by CT scan of the chest, abdomen, and pelvis or combined PET/CT is important to exclude extracutaneous involvement given the relatively nonspecific clinical presentation of PCFCL, and other types of CBCL. Bone marrow biopsies typically are reserved for patients with unexplained cytopenias, or if there is concern for other subtypes such as PCDLBCL, leg type.[86]

PCFCL exhibits an indolent clinical course and excellent prognosis with 5 year and 10 year survival rates of approximately 95% and 85%, respectively.[4,5,9,80,87,88] Extracutaneous involvement is uncommon and can occur in 10% of patients.[5,9,89] Prognosis is not significantly affected by histologic type, extent of skin lesions, presence or absence of t(14;18) or BCL-2 expression. However, the presence of PCFCL lesions on the legs is associated with a poor prognosis; the reason for this is unclear, but it has been postulated that these cases may represent DLBCL, leg type with immunophenotypic aberrancies that led them to be miscategorized as PCFCL.[9,90,91]

Treatment

Consensus guidelines for the treatment of PCFCL are based on retrospective reviews and expert opinion. For solitary lesions, localized RT with intent to cure is the preferred treatment. The International Lymphoma Radiation Group and the NCCN guidelines recommend radiation at doses of 24 to 30 Gy with a margin of at least 1 to 1.5 cm, which results in excellent response rates.[86,92] Palliative treatment with low-dose radiation at doses between 4 and 8 Gy resulted in relatively high response rates of up to 70% to 90%.[9,93] Moreover, radiation treatment with doses between 4 and 12 Gy was shown to be equally effective as RT with 12 Gy or more.[94] Surgical excision may also be considered if it is minimally disfiguring given the high response rates; however, relapse rates of up to 40% have been reported.[44] Additional skin-directed treatments may be utilized in select patients including topical steroids, imiquimod, topical nitrogen mustard, bexarotene gel, or intralesional steroids.

For multifocal or refractory disease, intralesional or systemic treatment with rituximab have resulted in response rates of 80% to 90%.[44,50,51,95] However, relapses are common following treatment, with a median duration of response of approximately 40 months.[95] Noninferiority has been demonstrated with multiple-field radiotherapy compared to rituximab, and it is a reasonable treatment strategy in those with multifocal disease.[96]

PRIMARY CUTANEOUS DIFFUSE LARGE B-CELL LYMPHOMA, LEG TYPE
Clinical Presentation

PCDLBCL, leg type is rare and represents about 4% of all cutaneous lymphomas and 20% of primary CBCLs.[3,71] The median age of presentation is in the mid-to-late 70s and, predominantly occurs in women with a male-to-female ratio of 1.3 to 4.[9,97–99]

Erythematous or violaceous tumors or nodules presenting as solitary or grouped lesions on the lower extremities is the most common presentation (**Fig. 3**), although 10% to 15% can occur on other locations.[99,100] Other clinical presentations include ulcerated papules or nodules, confluent plaques and tumors, and lesions mimicking chronic venous ulcers.[75] Dissemination to extracutaneous sites is more common in PCDLBCL, leg type presenting on the lower legs and has reported to occur in about 33% of this population.[97]

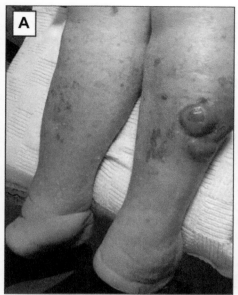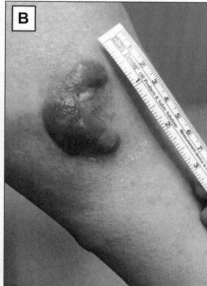

Fig. 3. PCDLBCL, leg type presenting as pink/red nodules with ulceration (*A, B*).

Histopathology

PCDLCBL, leg type is characterized by dense, diffuse infiltrates of large neoplastic B cells, composed of immunoblasts and centroblasts, often involving the entire dermis and extending into the subcutaneous fat. Ulceration is frequently present, and rarely the epidermis may be involved. Mitoses are readily identified, and reactive T-cell infiltrates are typically very focal.

Immunophenotype

The neoplastic cells in PCDLBCL, leg type express B-cell markers (CD20, CD79a, and PAX-5), and typically exhibit an activated B-cell phenotype with expression of BCL-2, IRF4/MUM1, and FOXP1, and variably express BCL-6.[77,97,101] Unlike PCFCL, CD21[+] follicular dendritic cell meshworks are typically absent in DLBCL. Double expression of BCL-2 and MYC is a negative prognostic indicator in nodal DLBCL, but its significance in primary cutaneous DLBCLs is unclear.[3,102–105]

Genetics

Neoplastic cells in PCDLBCL, leg type exhibit an activated B-cell phenotype and frequently show mutations in the nuclear factor kappa B (NF-κB) and B-cell signal transduction pathway.[106–108] The majority of cases exhibit gain-of-function mutations in *MYD88* (59%–77%) and *CD79 B* (~50%), which are important components in B-cell receptor signaling. Their presence may be disease-defining as they are notably absent in secondary cutaneous DLBCL and other CBCLs, particularly those with histologic similarities to PCDLBCL, leg type.[3,70] *MYD88* L265P mutations are associated with worse prognosis.[103] In about 30% of PCDLBCL, leg type cases, *MYD88* is in its wild-type form, and alternative mutations have been documented in pathways involving NF-κB signaling (*NFKBIE*), cell cycle (*CDKN1B* and *CCND3*), apoptosis (*CDKN2A*), and transcriptional regulation (*ASXL1*).[109,110] *MYC* rearrangements are seen in up to 32% of PCDLBCL, leg type cases and may be associated with worse prognosis.[103] Of note, there appears to be no correlation between MYC protein expression and the presence of *MYC* rearrangement on FISH.[103] Additional mutations thought to impair tumor-specific CD8$^+$ T-cell activation have also been noted in *HLA* genes and *CD58*.[110] Up to 25% of cases have copy number alternations and/or translocations in the *PDL1/L2* genes, resulting in impaired T-cell receptor signaling and increased T-cell exhaustion.[85,110,111]

Staging

Complete staging for all CBCLs includes a complete physical examination, CBC with differential, CMP, LDH, peripheral blood flow cytometry, and imaging by CT of the chest, abdomen, and pelvis or PET/CT. Secondary cutaneous DLBCL is more common than PCDLBCL, leg type and occurs in 7% to 10% of patients with systemic DLBCL. Therefore, imaging to rule out systemic involvement is important.[112,113] Bone marrow biopsy is essential for PCDLBCL, leg type, given its aggressive nature and requirement for systemic treatment.[86] In male patients with new cutaneous DLBCL, testicular ultrasound is helpful to rule out secondary cutaneous DLBCL.[114]

Prognosis

PCDLBCL, leg type usually exhibits an aggressive clinical course and is associated with poor prognosis with estimated 5 year survival rates between 41% and 66%.[9,97,99,115–117] The presence of multiple skin lesions at the time of diagnosis is associated with worse prognosis.[9,97] Five-year disease-specific survival for patients with single, localized, or generalized skin lesions was estimated to be 75%, 49%, and 0%, respectively, and 5 year overall survival of 70%, 27%, and 0%.[9,118] The presence of inactivating mutations of *CDKN2A* and *MYD88* L265P mutations are also associated with an unfavorable prognosis.[107,109]

Treatment

PCDLBCL, leg type requires a more aggressive approach with multiagent chemotherapy and radiation given its poor prognosis and high recurrence rates.[44] Treatment with anthracycline-based chemotherapy and rituximab is associated with favorable response rates. In a retrospective multicenter study, 12 patients treated with anthracycline-based chemotherapy and rituximab had a complete response (CR) rate of 92% compared to 62% in those treated with other modalities. A larger study involving 115 patients treated with multiagent chemotherapy and rituximab showed improved 3 year and 5 year survival rates of 80% and 74%, respectively, compared to those treated with less aggressive approaches.[97,115] Addition of radiation to Rituximab - Cyclophosphamide, Doxorubicin, Vincristine, Prednisone (R-CHOP) has been shown to result in improved progression-free survival.[119] Dose-limiting toxicities and high relapse rates preclude successful treatment with these regimens, and additional treatment strategies are needed. By exploiting known genetic mutations and identifying known altered pathways that are disease-defining in PCDLBCL and other CBCLs, the use of novel targeted therapies including Bruton tyrosine-kinase inhibitors (ibrutinib), BCL-2 inhibitors, and immune check-point inhibitors have been reported.[110,120–124]

INTRAVASCULAR LARGE B-CELL LYMPHOMA
Clinical Presentation

IVLBCL is a rare subtype of DLBCL included in the subset of CBCL, according to the 2022 WHO classification as well as the 2022 ICC.[7,8] Cutaneous involvement is present in about 40% of cases at presentation.[125,126] There are 3 primary variants of IVLBCL:

classic ("Western"), hemophagocytic syndrome-associated ("Asian"), and cutaneous. Clinical presentation can vary, but cutaneous findings range from indurated plaques, nodules, and telangiectasias, most frequently involving the trunk and lower extremities.[127] Median age of patients at diagnosis is around 60 to 70 years, with relatively equal prevalence in male and female individuals, although the cutaneous variant has been reported to occur in slightly younger patients (median age 59 years) and almost always in female individuals.[126,128] Neurologic symptoms are common in the classic variant, as well as other B-symptoms including fevers, night sweats, and weight loss.[129,130] The hemophagocytic syndrome-associated variant is mainly seen in Asian countries, has high rates of hemophagocytosis, and often presents with hepatosplenic and bone marrow involvement.[131] Cutaneous-only cases encompass about 25% of all cases, are usually seen in female individuals in Western countries, and are associated with a more favorable prognosis when compared to the classic variant (3 year overall survival 56% vs 22%).[125,126] In cases without apparent cutaneous involvement, IVLBCL may be diagnosed by random skin biopsy of healthy-appearing skin or sampling of cutaneous hemangiomas.[132–137]

Histopathology, Immunophenotype, and Genetics

IVLBCL is characterized by the proliferation of large B-cell immunoblasts confined within the blood vessels of the dermis and subcutaneous tissue. The neoplastic cells are positive for B-cell markers (CD20, CD79a, and PAX-5) and usually express BCL-2 and MUM-1, similar to PCDLBCL, leg type. There is also a high prevalence of *MYD88* and *CD79B* mutations in IVLBCL.[138] A t(14;18) translocation is usually absent in IVLBCL, suggesting a nongerminal center origin, but it has been detected in rare cases.[139,140] Structural aberrations in chromosomes 1, 6, and trisomy 18 have also been reported.[141]

Staging, Prognosis, and Treatment

Other than the cutaneous-only variant, IVLBCL is an aggressive disease and should be treated with rituximab and multiagent chemotherapy.[142] Some studies have also suggested a role for autologous peripheral blood stem cell transplantation, which may improve outcomes.[143,144]

EPSTEIN-BARR VIRUS-POSITIVE MUCOCUTANEOUS ULCER
Clinical Presentation

EBV-positive mucocutaneous ulcer (EBV-MCU) is a newly recognized clinicopathologic entity that usually presents in elderly or immunosuppressed patients. Causes of immunodeficiency include age-related immunosenescence, solid-organ or bone marrow transplant, human immunodeficiency virus/acquired immunodeficiency syndrome, and medications such as methotrexate (most common), cyclosporine, and azathioprine.[145–150] The median age is about 70 years and there is a slight female predominance, likely representing the increased prevalence of autoimmune diseases in women, for which immunosuppressives are commonly prescribed.[151] They often present as localized, sharply circumscribed ulcers involving the oropharyngeal mucosa (most common), skin, and gastrointestinal tract.[145] Cases are often triggered by local trauma.

Histopathology, Immunophenotype, and Genetics

EBV-MCU is characterized by an infiltrate of large B-cell immunoblasts and atypical cells with Hodgkin's and Reed-Sternberg-like morphology, which are often admixed with numerous reactive inflammatory cells. There is often tissue necrosis. The large cells are usually positive for PAX-5 (a B-cell marker) and CD30; expression of CD20 and CD79a may be reduced in about one-third of cases.[145] Expression of CD15 can be seen in about 40% of cases.[145] All cases are positive for EBER in situ hybridization, a marker for EBV. A monoclonal IgH rearrangement is found in a minority of cases (39%), and some cases may also display T-cell clonality.[145]

Staging, Prognosis, and Treatment

EBV-MCU follows an indolent clinical course, often displaying spontaneous remission after immunosuppression is reduced. This entity should be distinguished from other more aggressive EBV-associated lymphoproliferative disorders, such as EBV-positive DLBCL.

CLINICS CARE POINTS

- The indolent subtypes of PCBCL (PCMZL, PCFCL) have overall excellent prognosis, low risk of extracutaneous progression and are managed expectantly or with skin directed therapies in most cases.
- For PCMZL and PCFCL, cutaneous relapses are frequent (even after "curative" therapy of solitary lesions) and do not portent worse prognosis.
- Aggressive subtypes of PCBCL (PCDLBCL leg type, IVLBCL) require systemic therapy ± radiation.
- EBV-MCU has an indolent course and often responds to reduction of immunosuppression without additional therapy.

DISCLOSURE

The authors have nothing to disclose.

REFERENCES

1. Willemze R, Swerdlow S, Harris N, et al. Primary cutaneous follicle centre lymphoma. Classification of Tumours of Haematopoietic and Lymphoid Tissues 2008;227:228.
2. Olsen EA, Whittaker S, Willemze R, et al. Primary cutaneous lymphoma: recommendations for clinical trial design and staging update from the ISCL, USCLC, and EORTC. Blood 2022;140(5):419–37.
3. Willemze R, Cerroni L, Kempf W, et al. The 2018 update of the WHO-EORTC classification for primary cutaneous lymphomas. Blood 2019;133(16):1703–14.
4. Willemze R, Jaffe ES, Burg G, et al. WHO-EORTC classification for cutaneous lymphomas. Blood 2005;105(10):3768–85.
5. Zinzani PL, Quaglino P, Pimpinelli N, et al. Prognostic factors in primary cutaneous B-cell lymphoma: the Italian Study Group for Cutaneous Lymphomas. J Clin Oncol 2006;24(9):1376–82.
6. Bessell EM, Humber CE, O'Connor S, et al. Primary cutaneous B-cell lymphoma in Nottinghamshire U.K.: prognosis of subtypes defined in the WHO-EORTC classification. Br J Dermatol 2012;167(5):1118–23.
7. Alaggio R, Amador C, Anagnostopoulos I, et al. The 5th edition of the World Health Organization Classification of Haematolymphoid Tumours: Lymphoid Neoplasms. Leukemia 2022;36(7):1720–48.

8. Campo E, Jaffe ES, Cook JR, et al. The International Consensus Classification of Mature Lymphoid Neoplasms: a report from the Clinical Advisory Committee. Blood 2022;140(11):1229–53.

9. Senff NJ, Hoefnagel JJ, Jansen PM, et al. Reclassification of 300 primary cutaneous B-Cell lymphomas according to the new WHO-EORTC classification for cutaneous lymphomas: comparison with previous classifications and identification of prognostic markers. J Clin Oncol 2007;25(12):1581–7.

10. Servitje O, Muniesa C, Benavente Y, et al. Primary cutaneous marginal zone B-cell lymphoma: response to treatment and disease-free survival in a series of 137 patients. J Am Acad Dermatol 2013;69(3):357–65.

11. Golling P, Cozzio A, Dummer R, et al. Primary cutaneous B-cell lymphomas - clinicopathological, prognostic and therapeutic characterisation of 54 cases according to the WHO-EORTC classification and the ISCL/EORTC TNM classification system for primary cutaneous lymphomas other than mycosis fungoides and Sezary syndrome. Leuk Lymphoma 2008;49(6):1094–103.

12. Hoefnagel JJ, Vermeer MH, Jansen PM, et al. Primary cutaneous marginal zone b-cell lymphoma: clinical and therapeutic features in 50 cases. Arch Dermatol 2005;141(9):1139–45.

13. Amitay-Laish I, Tavallaee M, Kim J, et al. Paediatric primary cutaneous marginal zone B-cell lymphoma: does it differ from its adult counterpart? Br J Dermatol 2017;176(4):1010–20.

14. Torre-Castro J, Estrach T, Peñate Y, et al. Primary cutaneous lymphomas in children: A prospective study from the Spanish Academy of Dermatology and Venereology (AEDV) Primary Cutaneous Lymphoma Registry. Pediatr Dermatol 2021;38(6):1506–9.

15. Colmant C, Demers MA, Hatami A, et al. Pediatric cutaneous hematologic disorders: cutaneous lymphoma and leukemia cutis-experience of a tertiary-care pediatric institution and review of the literature. J Cutan Med Surg 2022;26(4): 349–60.

16. Bomze D, Sprecher E, Goldberg I, et al. Primary cutaneous b-cell lymphomas in children and adolescents: a SEER population-based study. Clin Lymphoma, Myeloma & Leukemia 2021;21(12):e1000–5.

17. Magro CM, Davis TL, Kurtzman DJB. Epidermotropic marginal zone lymphoma: An uncommon cutaneous B-cell lymphoma responsive to rituximab. JAAD Case Rep 2017;3(6):474–6.

18. Magro CM, Kalomeris T, Roberts A. Primary cutaneous blastic marginal zone lymphoma: a comprehensive clinical, light microscopic, phenotypic and cytogenetic appraisal. Ann Diagn Pathol 2023;63:152101.

19. Schafernak KT, Variakojis D, Goolsby CL, et al. Clonality assessment of cutaneous B-cell lymphoid proliferations: a comparison of flow cytometry immunophenotyping, molecular studies, and immunohistochemistry/in situ hybridization and review of the literature. Am J Dermatopathol 2014;36(10):781–95.

20. Lukowsky A, Marchwat M, Sterry W, et al. Evaluation of B-cell clonality in archival skin biopsy samples of cutaneous B-cell lymphoma by immunoglobulin heavy chain gene polymerase chain reaction. Leuk Lymphoma 2006;47(3):487–93.

21. Morales AV, Arber DA, Seo K, et al. Evaluation of B-cell clonality using the BIOMED-2 PCR method effectively distinguishes cutaneous B-cell lymphoma from benign lymphoid infiltrates. Am J Dermatopathol 2008;30(5):425–30.

22. Maurus K, Appenzeller S, Roth S, et al. Panel sequencing shows recurrent genetic FAS alterations in primary cutaneous marginal zone lymphoma. J Invest Dermatol 2018;138(7):1573–81.

23. Deutsch AJ, Frühwirth M, Aigelsreiter A, et al. Primary cutaneous marginal zone B-cell lymphomas are targeted by aberrant somatic hypermutation. J Invest Dermatol 2009;129(2):476–9.

24. Perez M, Pacchiarotti A, Frontani M, et al. Primary cutaneous B-cell lymphoma is associated with somatically hypermutated immunoglobulin variable genes and frequent use of VH1-69 and VH4-59 segments. Br J Dermatol 2010;162(3):611–8.

25. Li C, Inagaki H, Kuo TT, et al. Primary cutaneous marginal zone B-cell lymphoma: a molecular and clinicopathologic study of 24 asian cases. Am J Surg Pathol 2003;27(8):1061–9.

26. Gallardo F, Bellosillo B, Espinet B, et al. Aberrant nuclear BCL10 expression and lack of t(11;18)(q21;q21) in primary cutaneous marginal zone B-cell lymphoma. Hum Pathol 2006;37(7):867–73.

27. Streubel B, Lamprecht A, Dierlamm J, et al. T(14;18)(q32;q21) involving IGH and MALT1 is a frequent chromosomal aberration in MALT lymphoma. Blood 2003;101(6):2335–9.

28. Schreuder MI, Hoefnagel JJ, Jansen PM, et al. FISH analysis of MALT lymphoma-specific translocations and aneuploidy in primary cutaneous marginal zone lymphoma. J Pathol 2005;205(3):302–10.

29. Takino H, Li C, Hu S, et al. Primary cutaneous marginal zone B-cell lymphoma: a molecular and clinicopathological study of cases from Asia, Germany, and the United States. Mod Pathol 2008;21(12):1517–26.

30. Palmedo G, Hantschke M, Rütten A, et al. Primary cutaneous marginal zone B-cell lymphoma may exhibit both the t(14;18)(q32;q21) IGH/BCL2 and the t(14;18)(q32;q21) IGH/MALT1 translocation: an indicator for clonal transformation towards higher-grade B-cell lymphoma? Am J Dermatopathol 2007;29(3):231–6.

31. Streubel B, Vinatzer U, Lamprecht A, et al. T(3;14)(p14.1;q32) involving IGH and FOXP1 is a novel recurrent chromosomal aberration in MALT lymphoma. Leukemia 2005;19(4):652–8.

32. Edinger JT, Kant JA, Swerdlow SH. Cutaneous marginal zone lymphomas have distinctive features and include 2 subsets. Am J Surg Pathol 2010;34(12):1830–41.

33. van Maldegem F, van Dijk R, Wormhoudt TA, et al. The majority of cutaneous marginal zone B-cell lymphomas expresses class-switched immunoglobulins and develops in a T-helper type 2 inflammatory environment. Blood 2008;112(8):3355–61.

34. De Souza A, Ferry JA, Burghart DR, et al. IgG4 expression in primary cutaneous marginal zone lymphoma: a multicenter study. Appl Immunohistochem Mol Morphol 2018;26(7):462–7.

35. Carlsen ED, Swerdlow SH, Cook JR, et al. Class-switched primary cutaneous marginal zone lymphomas are frequently Igg4-positive and have features distinct from Igm-positive cases. Am J Surg Pathol 2019;43(10):1403–12.

36. Brenner I, Roth S, Puppe B, et al. Primary cutaneous marginal zone lymphomas with plasmacytic differentiation show frequent IgG4 expression. Mod Pathol 2013;26(12):1568–76.

37. Carlsen ED, Bhavsar S, Cook JR, et al. IRTA1 positivity helps identify a MALT-lymphoma-like subset of primary cutaneous marginal zone lymphomas, largely but not exclusively defined by IgM expression. J Cutan Pathol 2022;49(1):55–60.

38. Wobser M, Maurus K, Roth S, et al. Myeloid differentiation primary response 88 mutations in a distinct type of cutaneous marginal-zone lymphoma with a nonclass-switched immunoglobulin M immunophenotype. Br J Dermatol 2017; 177(2):564–6.
39. Roggero E, Zucca E, Mainetti C, et al. Eradication of Borrelia burgdorferi infection in primary marginal zone B-cell lymphoma of the skin. Hum Pathol 2000; 31(2):263–8.
40. National Comprehensive Cancer Network® (NCCN®) Clinical Practice Guidelines in Oncology. Primary Cutaneous Lymphomas. Version 1.2024 (December 21, 2023).
41. Kim YH, Willemze R, Pimpinelli N, et al. TNM classification system for primary cutaneous lymphomas other than mycosis fungoides and Sezary syndrome: a proposal of the International Society for Cutaneous Lymphomas (ISCL) and the Cutaneous Lymphoma Task Force of the European Organization of Research and Treatment of Cancer (EORTC). Blood 2007;110(2):479–84.
42. Carrillo-Cruz E, Marín-Oyaga VA, de la Cruz Vicente F, et al. Role of 18F-FDG-PET/CT in the management of marginal zone B cell lymphoma. Hematol Oncol 2015;33(4):151–8.
43. Haverkos B, Tyler K, Gru AA, et al. Primary cutaneous B-cell lymphoma: management and patterns of recurrence at the multimodality cutaneous lymphoma clinic of the Ohio State University. Oncol 2015;20(10):1161–6.
44. Senff NJ, Noordijk EM, Kim YH, et al. European Organization for Research and Treatment of Cancer and International Society for Cutaneous Lymphoma consensus recommendations for the management of cutaneous B-cell lymphomas. Blood 2008;112(5):1600–9.
45. Goyal A, Carter JB, Pashtan I, et al. Very low-dose versus standard dose radiation therapy for indolent primary cutaneous B-cell lymphomas: A retrospective study. J Am Acad Dermatol 2018;78(2):408–10.
46. Perry A, Vincent BJ, Parker SR. Intralesional corticosteroid therapy for primary cutaneous B-cell lymphoma. Br J Dermatol 2010;163(1):223–5.
47. Kollipara R, Hans A, Hall J, et al. A case report of primary cutaneous marginal zone lymphoma treated with intralesional steroids. Dermatol Online J 2015;21(8).
48. Heinzerling LM, Urbanek M, Funk JO, et al. Reduction of tumor burden and stabilization of disease by systemic therapy with anti-CD20 antibody (rituximab) in patients with primary cutaneous B-cell lymphoma. Cancer 2000;89(8):1835–44.
49. Gellrich S, Muche JM, Wilks A, et al. Systemic eight-cycle anti-CD20 monoclonal antibody (rituximab) therapy in primary cutaneous B-cell lymphomas–an applicational observation. Br J Dermatol 2005;153(1):167–73.
50. Morales AV, Advani R, Horwitz SM, et al. Indolent primary cutaneous B-cell lymphoma: experience using systemic rituximab. J Am Acad Dermatol 2008;59(6): 953–7.
51. Valencak J, Weihsengruber F, Rappersberger K, et al. Rituximab monotherapy for primary cutaneous B-cell lymphoma: response and follow-up in 16 patients. Ann Oncol 2009;20(2):326–30.
52. Kerl K, Prins C, Saurat JH, et al. Intralesional and intravenous treatment of cutaneous B-cell lymphomas with the monoclonal anti-CD20 antibody rituximab: report and follow-up of eight cases. Br J Dermatol 2006;155(6):1197–200.
53. Hoefnagel JJ, Vermeer MH, Jansen PM, et al. Primary cutaneous marginal zone B-cell lymphoma: clinical and therapeutic features in 50 cases. Arch Dermatol 2005;141(9):1139–45.

54. Heinzerling L, Dummer R, Kempf W, et al. Intralesional therapy with anti-CD20 monoclonal antibody rituximab in primary cutaneous B-cell lymphoma. Arch Dermatol 2000;136(3):374–8.

55. Kyrtsonis MC, Siakantaris MP, Kalpadakis C, et al. Favorable outcome of primary cutaneous marginal zone lymphoma treated with intralesional rituximab. Eur J Haematol 2006;77(4):300–3.

56. Trent JT, Romanelli P, Kerdel FA. Topical targretin and intralesional interferon alfa for cutaneous lymphoma of the scalp. Arch Dermatol 2002;138(11):1421–3.

57. Cozzio A, Kempf W, Schmid-Meyer R, et al. Intra-lesional low-dose interferon alpha2a therapy for primary cutaneous marginal zone B-cell lymphoma. Leuk Lymphoma 2006;47(5):865–9.

58. Bachmeyer C, Orlandini V, Aractingi S. Topical mechlorethamine and clobetasol in multifocal primary cutaneous marginal zone-B cell lymphoma. Br J Dermatol 2006;154(6):1207–9.

59. Coors EA, Schuler G, Von Den Driesch P. Topical imiquimod as treatment for different kinds of cutaneous lymphoma. Eur J Dermatol 2006;16(4):391–3.

60. Cerroni L, Zöchling N, Pütz B, et al. Infection by Borrelia burgdorferi and cutaneous B-cell lymphoma. J Cutan Pathol 1997;24(8):457–61.

61. Goodlad JR, Davidson MM, Hollowood K, et al. Primary cutaneous B-cell lymphoma and Borrelia burgdorferi infection in patients from the Highlands of Scotland. Am J Surg Pathol 2000;24(9):1279–85.

62. de la Fouchardiere A, Vandenesch F, Berger F. Borrelia-Associated Primary Cutaneous MALT Lymphoma in a Nonendemic Region. Am J Surg Pathol 2003;27(5).

63. Jothishankar B, Di Raimondo C, Mueller L, et al. Primary cutaneous marginal zone lymphoma treated with doxycycline in a pediatric patient. Pediatr Dermatol 2020;37(4):759–61.

64. Fühler M, Ottmann KW, Tronnier M. [Cutaneous marginal zone lymphoma (SALT) and infection with Borrelia burgdorferi]. Hautarzt 2010;61(2):145–7.

65. Ponzoni M, Ferreri AJ, Mappa S, et al. Prevalence of Borrelia burgdorferi infection in a series of 98 primary cutaneous lymphomas. Oncol 2011;16(11):1582–8.

66. Wood GS, Kamath NV, Guitart J, et al. Absence of Borrelia burgdorferi DNA in cutaneous B-cell lymphomas from the United States. J Cutan Pathol 2001;28(10):502–7.

67. Goteri G, Ranaldi R, Simonetti O, et al. Clinicopathological features of primary cutaneous B-cell lymphomas from an academic regional hospital in central Italy: no evidence of Borrelia burgdorferi association. Leuk Lymphoma 2007;48(11):2184–8.

68. Papadopoulou K, Falk TM, Metze D, et al. No evidence of Borrelia in cutaneous infiltrates of B-cell lymphomas with a highly sensitive, semi-nested real-time polymerase chain reaction targeting the 5S-23S intergenic spacer region. J Eur Acad Dermatol Venereol 2022;36(6):836–45.

69. Monari P, Farisoglio C, Calzavara Pinton PG. Borrelia burgdorferi-associated primary cutaneous marginal-zone B-cell lymphoma: a case report. Dermatology 2007;215(3):229–32.

70. Zhou XA, Yang J, Ringbloom KG, et al. Genomic landscape of cutaneous follicular lymphomas reveals 2 subgroups with clinically predictive molecular features. Blood Adv 2021;5(3):649–61.

71. Bradford PT, Devesa SS, Anderson WF, et al. Cutaneous lymphoma incidence patterns in the United States: a population-based study of 3884 cases. Blood 2009;113(21):5064–73.

72. Mirza I, Macpherson N, Paproski S, et al. Primary cutaneous follicular lymphoma: an assessment of clinical, histopathologic, immunophenotypic, and molecular features. J Clin Oncol 2002;20(3):647–55.

73. Bergman R, Kurtin PJ, Gibson LE, et al. Clinicopathologic, immunophenotypic, and molecular characterization of primary cutaneous follicular B-cell lymphoma. Arch Dermatol 2001;137(4):432–9.

74. Gulia A, Saggini A, Wiesner T, et al. Clinicopathologic features of early lesions of primary cutaneous follicle center lymphoma, diffuse type: implications for early diagnosis and treatment. J Am Acad Dermatol 2011;65(5):991–1000.

75. Cerroni L. Skin lymphoma : the illustrated guide. 5th edition. Hoboken (NJ): John Wiley & Sons; 2020.

76. Jaffe ES. Navigating the cutaneous B-cell lymphomas: avoiding the rocky shoals. Mod Pathol 2020;33(Suppl 1):96–106.

77. Hoefnagel JJ, Dijkman R, Basso K, et al. Distinct types of primary cutaneous large B-cell lymphoma identified by gene expression profiling. Blood 2005; 105(9):3671–8.

78. Dijkman R, Tensen CP, Jordanova ES, et al. Array-based comparative genomic hybridization analysis reveals recurrent chromosomal alterations and prognostic parameters in primary cutaneous large B-cell lymphoma. J Clin Oncol 2006; 24(2):296–305.

79. Harris NL, Jaffe ES, Stein H, et al. A revised European-American classification of lymphoid neoplasms: a proposal from the International Lymphoma Study Group. Blood 1994;84(5):1361–92.

80. Goodlad JR, Krajewski AS, Batstone PJ, et al. Primary cutaneous follicular lymphoma: a clinicopathologic and molecular study of 16 cases in support of a distinct entity. Am J Surg Pathol 2002;26(6):733–41.

81. Child FJ, Russell-Jones R, Woolford AJ, et al. Absence of the t(14;18) chromosomal translocation in primary cutaneous B-cell lymphoma. Br J Dermatol 2001; 144(4):735–44.

82. Barasch NJK, Liu YC, Ho J, et al. The molecular landscape and other distinctive features of primary cutaneous follicle center lymphoma. Hum Pathol 2020;106: 93–105.

83. Gángó A, Bátai B, Varga M, et al. Concomitant 1p36 deletion and TNFRSF14 mutations in primary cutaneous follicle center lymphoma frequently expressing high levels of EZH2 protein. Virchows Arch 2018;473(4):453–62.

84. Mintz MA, Felce JH, Chou MY, et al. The HVEM-BTLA Axis Restrains T Cell Help to Germinal Center B Cells and Functions as a Cell-Extrinsic Suppressor in Lymphomagenesis. Immunity 2019;51(2):310–323 e317.

85. Menguy S, Gros A, Pham-Ledard A, et al. MYD88 somatic mutation is a diagnostic criterior in primary cutaneous large b-cell lymphoma. J Invest Dermatol 2016;136:1741.

86. NCCN Guidelines for Primary Cutaneous B-cell Lymphomas. Available at: https://www.nccn.org/professionals/physician_gls/pdf/pcbcl.pdf. [Accessed 3 May 2024].

87. Abdul-Wahab A, Tang SY, Robson A, et al. Chromosomal anomalies in primary cutaneous follicle center cell lymphoma do not portend a poor prognosis. J Am Acad Dermatol 2014;70(6):1010–20.

88. Grange F, Bekkenk MW, Wechsler J, et al. Prognostic factors in primary cutaneous large B-cell lymphomas: a European multicenter study. J Clin Oncol 2001;19(16):3602–10.

89. Chan SA, Shah F, Chaganti S, et al. Primary cutaneous B-cell lymphoma: systemic spread is rare while cutaneous relapses and secondary malignancies are frequent. Br J Dermatol 2017;177(1):287–9.

90. Kodama K, Massone C, Chott A, et al. Primary cutaneous large B-cell lymphomas: clinicopathologic features, classification, and prognostic factors in a large series of patients. Blood 2005;106(7):2491–7.

91. Suárez AL, Pulitzer M, Horwitz S, et al. Primary cutaneous B-cell lymphomas: part I. Clinical features, diagnosis, and classification. J Am Acad Dermatol 2013;69(3):329, e321-313; quiz 341-322.

92. Specht L, Dabaja B, Illidge T, et al. Modern radiation therapy for primary cutaneous lymphomas: field and dose guidelines from the International Lymphoma Radiation Oncology Group. Int J Radiat Oncol Biol Phys 2015;92(1):32–9.

93. Neelis KJ, Schimmel EC, Vermeer MH, et al. Low-dose palliative radiotherapy for cutaneous B- and T-cell lymphomas. Int J Radiat Oncol Biol Phys 2009;74(1):154–8.

94. Akhtari M, Reddy JP, Pinnix CC, et al. Primary cutaneous B-cell lymphoma (non-leg type) has excellent outcomes even after very low dose radiation as single-modality therapy. Leuk Lymphoma 2016;57(1):34–8.

95. Brandenburg A, Humme D, Terhorst D, et al. Long-term outcome of intravenous therapy with rituximab in patients with primary cutaneous B-cell lymphomas. Br J Dermatol 2013;169(5):1126–32.

96. Vitiello P, Sica A, Ronchi A, et al. Primary cutaneous b-cell lymphomas: an update. Front Oncol 2020;10.

97. Grange F, Beylot-Barry M, Courville P, et al. Primary cutaneous diffuse large B-cell lymphoma, leg type: clinicopathologic features and prognostic analysis in 60 cases. Arch Dermatol 2007;143(9):1144–50.

98. Paulli M, Viglio A, Vivenza D, et al. Primary cutaneous large B-cell lymphoma of the leg: histogenetic analysis of a controversial clinicopathologic entity. Hum Pathol 2002;33(9):937–43.

99. Vermeer MH, Geelen FA, van Haselen CW, et al. Primary cutaneous large B-cell lymphomas of the legs. A distinct type of cutaneous B-cell lymphoma with an intermediate prognosis. Dutch Cutaneous Lymphoma Working Group. Arch Dermatol 1996;132(11):1304–8.

100. Hamilton SN, Wai ES, Tan K, et al. Treatment and outcomes in patients with primary cutaneous b-cell lymphoma: the BC cancer agency experience. Int J Radiat Oncol Biol Phys 2013;87(4):719–25.

101. Lucioni M, Berti E, Arcaini L, et al. Primary cutaneous B-cell lymphoma other than marginal zone: clinicopathologic analysis of 161 cases: Comparison with current classification and definition of prognostic markers. Cancer Med 2016;5(10):2740–55.

102. Lucioni M, Pescia C, Bonometti A, et al. Double expressor and double/triple hit status among primary cutaneous diffuse large B-cell lymphoma: a comparison between leg type and not otherwise specified subtypes. Hum Pathol 2021;111:1–9.

103. Schrader AMR, Jansen PM, Vermeer MH, et al. High incidence and clinical significance of MYC rearrangements in primary cutaneous diffuse large b-cell lymphoma, leg type. Am J Surg Pathol 2018;42(11):1488–94.

104. Kim YJ, Won CH, Chang SE, et al. MYC protein expression is associated with poor prognosis in cutaneous diffuse large B-cell lymphoma. Australas J Dermatol 2018;59(3):e240–2.

105. Menguy S, Frison E, Prochazkova-Carlotti M, et al. Double-hit or dual expression of MYC and BCL2 in primary cutaneous large B-cell lymphomas. Mod Pathol 2018;31(8):1332–42.
106. Mareschal S, Pham-Ledard A, Viailly PJ, et al. Identification of somatic mutations in primary cutaneous diffuse large b-cell lymphoma, leg type by massive parallel sequencing. J Invest Dermatol 2017;137(9):1984–94.
107. Pham-Ledard A, Beylot-Barry M, Barbe C, et al. High frequency and clinical prognostic value of MYD88 L265P mutation in primary cutaneous diffuse large B-cell lymphoma, leg-type. JAMA Dermatol 2014;150(11):1173–9.
108. Ducharme O, Beylot-Barry M, Pham-Ledard A, et al. Mutations of the b-cell receptor pathway confer chemoresistance in primary cutaneous diffuse large b-cell lymphoma leg type. J Invest Dermatol 2019;139(11):2334–2342 e2338.
109. Senff NJ, Zoutman WH, Vermeer MH, et al. Fine-mapping chromosomal loss at 9p21: correlation with prognosis in primary cutaneous diffuse large B-cell lymphoma, leg type. J Invest Dermatol 2009;129(5):1149–55.
110. Zhou XA, Louissaint A Jr, Wenzel A, et al. Genomic analyses identify recurrent alterations in immune evasion genes in diffuse large b-cell lymphoma, leg type. J Invest Dermatol 2018;138(11):2365–76.
111. Keir ME, Butte MJ, Freeman GJ, et al. PD-1 and its ligands in tolerance and immunity. Annu Rev Immunol 2008;26:677–704.
112. Morton LM, Wang SS, Devesa SS, et al. Lymphoma incidence patterns by WHO subtype in the United States, 1992-2001. Blood 2006;107(1):265–76.
113. Sterry W, Kruger GR, Steigleder GK. Skin involvement of malignant B-cell lymphomas. J Dermatol Surg Oncol 1984;10(4):276–7.
114. Muniesa C, Pujol RM, Estrach MT, et al. Primary cutaneous diffuse large B-cell lymphoma, leg type and secondary cutaneous involvement by testicular B-cell lymphoma share identical clinicopathological and immunophenotypical features. J Am Acad Dermatol 2012;66(4):650–4.
115. Grange F, Joly P, Barbe C, et al. Improvement of survival in patients with primary cutaneous diffuse large B-cell lymphoma, leg type, in France. JAMA Dermatol 2014;150(5):535–41.
116. Pandolfino TL, Siegel RS, Kuzel TM, et al. Primary cutaneous B-cell lymphoma: review and current concepts. J Clin Oncol 2000;18(10):2152–68.
117. Rijlaarsdam JU, Toonstra J, Meijer OW, et al. Treatment of primary cutaneous B-cell lymphomas of follicle center cell origin: a clinical follow-up study of 55 patients treated with radiotherapy or polychemotherapy. J Clin Oncol 1996;14(2):549–55.
118. Senff NJ, Willemze R. The applicability and prognostic value of the new TNM classification system for primary cutaneous lymphomas other than mycosis fungoides and Sezary syndrome: results on a large cohort of primary cutaneous B-cell lymphomas and comparison with the system used by the Dutch Cutaneous Lymphoma Group. Br J Dermatol 2007;157(6):1205–11.
119. Kraft RM, Ansell SM, Villasboas JC, et al. Outcomes in primary cutaneous diffuse large B-cell lymphoma, leg type. Hematol Oncol 2021;39(5):658–63.
120. Di Raimondo C, Abdulla FR, Zain J, et al. Rituximab, lenalidomide and pembrolizumab in refractory primary cutaneous diffuse large B-cell lymphoma, leg type. Br J Haematol 2019;187(3):e79–82.
121. Fox LC, Yannakou CK, Ryland G, et al. Molecular mechanisms of disease progression in primary cutaneous diffuse large b-cell lymphoma, leg type during ibrutinib therapy. Int J Mol Sci 2018;19(6).

122. Gupta E, Accurso J, Sluzevich J, et al. Excellent outcome of immunomodulation or bruton's tyrosine kinase inhibition in highly refractory primary cutaneous diffuse large b-cell lymphoma, leg type. Rare Tumors 2015;7(4):6067.

123. Walter HS, Trethewey CS, Ahearne MJ, et al. Successful treatment of primary cutaneous diffuse large b-cell lymphoma leg type with single-agent venetoclax. JCO Precis Oncol 2019;3:1–5.

124. Mitteldorf C, Berisha A, Pfaltz MC, et al. Tumor microenvironment and checkpoint molecules in primary cutaneous diffuse large b-cell lymphoma-new therapeutic targets. Am J Surg Pathol 2017;41(7):998–1004.

125. Röglin J, Böer A. Skin manifestations of intravascular lymphoma mimic inflammatory diseases of the skin. Br J Dermatol 2007;157(1):16–25.

126. Ferreri AJ, Campo E, Seymour JF, et al. Intravascular lymphoma: clinical presentation, natural history, management and prognostic factors in a series of 38 cases, with special emphasis on the 'cutaneous variant'. Br J Haematol 2004; 127(2):173–83.

127. Breakell T, Waibel H, Schliep S, et al. Intravascular large b-cell lymphoma: a review with a focus on the prognostic value of skin involvement. Curr Oncol 2022; 29(5):2909–19.

128. Murase T, Yamaguchi M, Suzuki R, et al. Intravascular large B-cell lymphoma (IVLBCL): a clinicopathologic study of 96 cases with special reference to the immunophenotypic heterogeneity of CD5. Blood 2007;109(2):478–85.

129. Fonkem E, Dayawansa S, Stroberg E, et al. Neurological presentations of intravascular lymphoma (IVL): meta-analysis of 654 patients. BMC Neurol 2016;16:9.

130. di Fonzo H, Contardo D, Carrozza D, et al. Intravascular large b cell lymphoma presenting as fever of unknown origin and diagnosed by random skin biopsies: a case report and literature review. Am J Case Rep 2017;18:482–6.

131. Ferreri AJ, Dognini GP, Campo E, et al. Variations in clinical presentation, frequency of hemophagocytosis and clinical behavior of intravascular lymphoma diagnosed in different geographical regions. Haematologica 2007;92(4):486–92.

132. Asada N, Odawara J, Kimura S-i, et al. Use of random skin biopsy for diagnosis of intravascular large b-cell lymphoma. Mayo Clin Proc 2007;82(12):1525–7.

133. Le EN, Gerstenblith MR, Gelber AC, et al. The use of blind skin biopsy in the diagnosis of intravascular B-cell lymphoma. J Am Acad Dermatol 2008;59(1): 148–51.

134. Matsue K, Abe Y, Kitadate A, et al. Sensitivity and specificity of incisional random skin biopsy for diagnosis of intravascular large B-cell lymphoma. Blood 2019;133(11):1257–9.

135. Rozenbaum D, Tung J, Xue Y, et al. Skin biopsy in the diagnosis of intravascular lymphoma: A retrospective diagnostic accuracy study. J Am Acad Dermatol 2021;85(3):665–70.

136. Sakurai T, Wakida K, Takahashi T, et al. Usefulness of senile hemangioma biopsy for diagnosis of intravascular large B-cell lymphoma: A report of two cases and a literature review. J Neurol Sci 2017;373:52–4.

137. MacGillivary ML, Purdy KS. Recommendations for an approach to random skin biopsy in the diagnosis of intravascular b-cell lymphoma. J Cutan Med Surg 2023;27(1):44–50.

138. Schrader AMR, Jansen PM, Willemze R, et al. High prevalence of MYD88 and CD79B mutations in intravascular large B-cell lymphoma. Blood 2018;131(18): 2086–9.

139. Kanda M, Suzumiya J, Ohshima K, et al. Analysis of the immunoglobulin heavy chain gene variable region of intravascular large B-cell lymphoma. Virchows Arch 2001;439(4):540–6.
140. Vieites B, Fraga M, Lopez-Presas E, et al. Detection of t(14;18) translocation in a case of intravascular large B-cell lymphoma: a germinal centre cell origin in a subset of these lymphomas? Histopathology 2005;46(4):466–8.
141. Tsukadaira A, Okubo Y, Ogasawara H, et al. Chromosomal aberrations in intravascular lymphomatosis. Am J Clin Oncol 2002;25(2).
142. Ferreri AJ, Dognini GP, Bairey O, et al. The addition of rituximab to anthracycline-based chemotherapy significantly improves outcome in 'Western' patients with intravascular large B-cell lymphoma. Br J Haematol 2008;143(2): 253–7.
143. Kato K, Mori T, Kim S-W, et al. Outcome of patients receiving consolidative autologous peripheral blood stem cell transplantation in the frontline treatment of intravascular large B-cell lymphoma: Adult Lymphoma Working Group of the Japan Society for Hematopoietic Cell Transplantation. Bone Marrow Transplant 2019;54(9):1515–7.
144. Meissner J, Finel H, Dietrich S, et al. Autologous hematopoietic stem cell transplantation for intravascular large B-cell lymphoma: the European Society for Blood and Marrow Transplantation experience. Bone Marrow Transplant 2017; 52(4):650–2.
145. Dojcinov SD, Venkataraman G, Raffeld M, et al. EBV positive mucocutaneous ulcer–a study of 26 cases associated with various sources of immunosuppression. Am J Surg Pathol 2010;34(3):405–17.
146. Magalhaes M, Ghorab Z, Morneault J, et al. Age-related Epstein–Barr virus-positive mucocutaneous ulcer: a case report. Clinical Case Reports 2015;3(7): 531–4.
147. Bunn B, van Heerden W. EBV-positive mucocutaneous ulcer of the oral cavity associated with HIV/AIDS. Oral Surg, Oral Med, Oral Pathol Oral Radiol 2015; 120(6):725–32.
148. Au WY, Loong F, Wan TSK, et al. Multi-focal EBV-mucocutaneous ulcer heralding late-onset T-cell immunodeficiency in a woman with lupus erythematosus. Int J Hematol 2011;94(5):501–2.
149. Hart M, Thakral B, Yohe S, et al. EBV-positive mucocutaneous ulcer in organ transplant recipients: a localized indolent posttransplant lymphoproliferative disorder. Am J Surg Pathol 2014;38(11).
150. Nelson AA, Harrington AM, Kroft S, et al. Presentation and management of post-allogeneic transplantation EBV-positive mucocutaneous ulcer. Bone Marrow Transplant 2016;51(2):300–2.
151. Ikeda T, Gion Y, Nishimura Y, et al. Epstein-Barr virus-positive mucocutaneous ulcer: a unique and curious disease entity. Int J Mol Sci 2021;22(3).

Merkel Cell Carcinoma

Jennifer Strong, BS, Patrick Hallaert, BS, Isaac Brownell, MD, PhD*

KEYWORDS

- Merkel cell carcinoma • Neuroendocrine • Skin cancer • Immunotherapy
- Merkel cell polyomavirus

KEY POINTS

- Merkel cell carcinoma (MCC) is associated with integrated Merkel cell polyomavirus and ultraviolet (UV) light exposure.
- Emerging biomarkers have prognostic value, can monitor treatment response, or screen for recurrence.
- MCC treatment includes surgical resection and radiation therapy for early-stage disease and immunotherapy for advanced disease.
- Clinical dilemmas in MCC treatment include optimal radiation therapy dosing, neoadjuvant versus adjuvant immunotherapy, optimal duration of immunotherapy, and second-line treatment options for disease refractory to anti-PD-(L)1 therapy.

INTRODUCTION

Merkel cell carcinoma (MCC) is a rare and aggressive neuroendocrine skin cancer driven by integrated Merkel cell polyomavirus (MCPyV) or UV signature mutations. MCC is associated with advanced age (>70 years), fair skin, male sex, and immunosuppression.[1,2] Here the authors review the characteristics and management of MCC.

EPIDEMIOLOGY

In the United States, MCC incidence is 0.7 per 100,000.[2] MCC incidence is higher in countries having more UV exposure, with Australia and New Zealand rates being 2.5 and 0.96 per 100,000 respectively.[3] Most MCC cases develop on UV-exposed skin with 42.6% of cases presenting on the head and neck, followed by 24.1%, 14.5%, and 9.4% of cases occurring on the upper limbs, lower limbs, and trunk. Fair skin is also a risk factor for MCC, with close to 90% of cases occurring in white patients.[4]

MCC is a disease of advanced age, with the median age of diagnosis being over 75 years old and less than 10% of patients presenting under the age of 50 years.[1,5] Male

Dermatology Branch, NIAMS, NIH, 10 Center Drive, 12N240C, Bethesda, MD 20892-1908, USA
* Corresponding author.
E-mail address: isaac.brownell@nih.gov

Hematol Oncol Clin N Am 38 (2024) 1133–1147
https://doi.org/10.1016/j.hoc.2024.05.013
0889-8588/24/Published by Elsevier Inc.

sex is also an MCC risk factor, as 63% of cases occur in men.[4] MCC risk is notably higher in immunosuppressed populations, yet most patients with MCC do not have a diagnosis of immunosuppression.[1,5]

PATHOGENESIS

MCC's name stems from its resemblance to Merkel cells, which are touch sensors in the basal epidermis. MCC probably does not arise from normal Merkel cells, but its precise cell of origin is currently unknown.[1,5] The majority of MCC cases in the United States are positive for MCPyV, a small double-stranded DNA polyomavirus. Episomal MCPyV skin infection is pervasive and asymptomatic. Commensal MCPyV infection is associated with low expression levels of viral oncogenes such as the large T antigen (LT) and small T antigen (ST). Virus-positive MCC (VP-MCC) occurs through clonal integration of MCPyV DNA into the host genome and a truncating mutation in LT. Integrated MCPyV is replication deficient but expresses high levels of ST and truncated LT, both of which are thought to be involved in VP-MCC transformation.[5]

Virus negative (VN)-MCC tumors are typically caused by chronic UV exposure as evidenced by a high tumor mutational burden and enrichment of somatic UV-signature mutations.[5] Although VP-MCC tumors lack enrichment of UV-signature mutations, they are nonetheless found at higher frequency on chronically sun exposed skin, suggesting an indirect role for UV in VP-MCC pathogenesis.[1,5]

DIAGNOSIS

MCC typically presents as a rapidly growing erythematous to violaceous skin nodule, although it may present in a skin-draining lymph node with no cutaneous primary.[5] Diagnosis requires histopathological evaluation of tissue biopsy by an experienced pathologist. Immunohistochemistry for neuroendocrine markers such as INSM1, chromogranin A, or synaptophysin is often used to support the diagnosis.[6,7] MCC typically stains with pan-cytokeratin and neurofilament antibodies, but the most commonly used MCC marker is cytokeratin 20 (CK20). A paranuclear dot-like staining pattern for CK20 or other intermediate filaments is highly supportive of an MCC diagnosis.[5,7]

STAGING

The American Joint Committee on Cancer staging system for MCC (8th edition) uses primary tumor size (2 cm threshold) and invasion to define Stages I and II. Stage III reflects nodal involvement or in-transit skin metastases. Stage IV requires distant metastasis with the most common sites being skin, nonregional lymph nodes, liver, bone, pancreas, and lung.[8] Because occult nodal disease is common in MCC, sentinel lymph node biopsy (SLNB) is recommended for most patients.[5] Recent literature also suggests that baseline imaging with fluorodeoxyglucose-PET/computed tomography (PET/CT) or CT should be considered before surgery. In a retrospective study involving 492 patients without clinical involvement of regional lymph nodes, 13.2% experienced an upstage in their MCC after baseline imaging. The same study reported that baseline imaging identified distant metastatic MCC in 10.8% of 92 patients with clinically involved regional nodes.[9] Another study of 23 patients similarly concluded that baseline PET/CT imaging led to a change in MCC staging in 39% of patients.[10] For MCC, PET/CT appears to be more sensitive than CT alone.[9] In addition to finding smaller lesions, PET/CT detects bone and bone marrow metastases missed by CT scans.[11]

PROGNOSIS

Tumor stage, advanced age, male sex, and virus status correlate with MCC prognosis. Approximate 5 year survival for stage I MCC is 62.8%, stage II is 34.8% to 54.6%, stage III is 26.8% to 40.3%, and stage IV is 13.5%.[1] However, more contemporary data suggest that prognosis has improved in recent years, likely due to the use of immunotherapy for advanced disease.[4] Men with MCC are approximately 50% more likely to die from their disease than women.[4] Similarly, advancing age is linked to increasingly lower survival.[3,4] Although VP-MCC is associated with better outcomes than VN-MCC,[12] clinical testing of tumors for MCPyV is not routinely performed.

Host immune status also impacts MCC outcomes. MCC is associated with earlier onset and poorer prognoses in immunosuppressed patient populations.[13] The importance of the immune response in MCC is further supported by the fact that heightened levels of intratumor and peritumoral CD8+ T cells, tumor-infiltrating MCPyV-specific T cells, and PD-(L)1 expression all correlate with more positive outcomes.[14–16]

An online MCC recurrence risk calculator that accounts for age, sex, tumor stage, primary site, immune status, and time since diagnosis is available at https://merkelcell. org/prognosis/recur/.[17]

DISCUSSION
Emerging Biomarkers of Merkel Cell Carcinoma Tumor Burden

Blood-based biomarker testing has the potential to predict prognosis, assess treatment response, and monitor for MCC recurrence while potentially sparing patients unnecessary imaging and biopsies. Both serology-based tests (eg, AMERK) and circulating tumor DNA (ctDNA) are particularly promising (**Table 1**). Optimally, a baseline assessment of one of these biomarkers would occur before treatment.

The AMERK test detects circulating antibodies against the MCPyV ST oncoprotein and is specific to VP-MCC. When detected, the titers correlate with tumor burden, falling after excision and rising in progressive disease, sometimes before clinical detection of recurrence.[18] In a study of 219 patients with MCC, 52% had positive AMERK titers. An increasing oncoprotein titer had a 66% positive predictive value for clinically evident recurrence whereas a decreasing titer had a negative predictive value of 97%. The UW MCC group, who developed AMERK, now routinely tests patients newly diagnosed with MCC with reassessment every 3 months for the first 3 to 4 years in those

Table 1
Comparison of emerging Merkel cell carcinoma peripheral blood biomarkers for surveillance

	AMERK[18,19]	Signatera (ctDNA)[20–22]
Assay	Serology for MCPyV ST antibodies	WGS + bespoke PCR
Positivity rate at diagnosis	~50%	90+%
Levels after treatment	Falls in 2–3 mo	Undetectable immediately
Effect of ICI	Possible impact	None
MCPyV requirement	+	None
Worse prognosis with	Negative test at diagnosis	Still + after treatment
Surveillance frequency	Every 3 mo	Every 3 mo
Recurrence detection	Rising titers	Rising levels

Abbreviations: ICI, immune checkpoint inhibitor; WGS, whole genome sequencing; PCR, polymerase chain reaction.

with positive baseline titers. Increasing titers prompt clinical and radiological evaluation.[19] Patients with undetectable AMERK titers at the time of diagnosis have higher risk of recurrence and may benefit from increased surveillance.[19] Given that immunotherapy can impact antibody production, it is possible that AMERK results may be altered in patients receiving immunotherapy. An additional serologic test of antibodies to MCPyV oncoprotein is under investigation in a large prospective MCC cohort in Europe (NCT04705389).

Quantifying ctDNA can also be used to assess recurrence risk, treatment response, and monitor for progression. MCC cells can release DNA as they die and ctDNA levels in the blood approximate real-time tumor burden, regardless of MCPyV status.[20] Signatera is the most widely used commercial ctDNA platform for MCC. It uses whole-genome sequencing of the tumor to identify patient-specific DNA sequence variants. Next, custom PCR primers are designed for targeted sequencing of multiple variants from the patient's blood.[20] In some patients serially assessed with Signatera, positive ctDNA results preceded a clinical diagnosis of recurrence, allowing for earlier therapeutic intervention. Additionally, among 75 patients with negative ctDNA tests during post-treatment surveillance, none experienced recurrence.[21,22] In contrast to the AMERK test, all patients with clinically evident MCC at diagnosis were found to have positive ctDNA testing.[22]

Treatment

The standard of care for locally advanced or metastatic MCC (mMCC) has changed significantly over time. Given MCC's rarity, randomized controlled trials are uncommon. As a result, patients with MCC benefit from evaluation by a multidisciplinary tumor board and consideration of clinical trials. We will highlight the current consensus on MCC treatment based on the NCCN and SITC guidelines with special attention to clinical dilemmas and areas actively assessed in current research (**Table 2**). A graphical summary of treatment guidelines is provided in **Fig. 1**.

Surgery

Per NCCN guidelines, surgical excision of the primary tumor is first-line therapy in MCC.[23,24] Around 1 to 2 cm surgical margins are recommended with narrower margins if adjuvant radiation therapy (RT) is performed.[23,24] Surgical excision may be performed by Mohs micrographic surgery (MMS) or wide local excision (WLE). In a retrospective study of 2359 patients with MCC in the SEER registry, there was no difference in MCC-specific survival between the MMS and WLE groups. However, patients undergoing MMS were less likely to receive an SLNB. Overall, patients in both the MMS and WLE groups who received an SLNB demonstrated improved survival.[25] This underscores the importance of performing SLNBs in conjunction with MMS. A benefit of WLE over MMS is that SLNB can be conducted concurrently.

Radiation Therapy

Prompt adjuvant radiation to the primary tumor site and, if involved, the regional lymph node basin is standard of care and reduces time to locoregional recurrence (LR) and improves disease-free survival (DFS) when compared to surgery alone.[23,24] The use of adjuvant RT is associated with an overall survival benefit in patients with stage I/II MCC (hazard ratio 0.783, $P<.02$).[26] However, if stage I tumors are resected with negative margins and the patient is deemed low risk (primary tumor <1 cm, no immunosuppression, not on the head and neck, and no lymphovascular invasion), foregoing adjuvant RT may be considered.[23,24] A recent retrospective study found no difference in LR in non-head and neck stage I MCC treated without RT.[27]

Table 2
Ongoing Merkel cell carcinoma

Intervention	Agent	Trial	EE
Adjuvant Immunotherapy			
Anti PD-L-1	Avelumab	ADAM (NCT03271372)	100
	Avelumab	I-MAT (NCT04291885)	132
Anti-PD-1 + RT/ anti-CTLA4	Nivolumab + RT/ipilimumab	NCT03798639	7
Neoadjuvant Immunotherapy			
Anti-PD-1	Pembrolizumab	STAMP (NCT03712605)	280
	Pembrolizumab	NCT05496036	15
Anti-PD-1 + VEGFR	Pembrolizumab + Lenvatinib	NCT04869137	26
Refractory to PD-(L)1 Inhibition			
Anti-PD1 + anti-LAG3 + anti-TIM3	Retifanlimab + Tuparstobart + Verzistobart	NCT06056895	20
Anti-PD-1 + RT	Avelumab ± CART	NCT04792073	18
	Pembrolizumab + PRRT	NCT05583708	18
ATRi	Tuvusertib ± Avelumab	MATRiX (NCT05947500)	50
MDM2i	Navtemadlin + Avelumab	NCT03787602	115
HDACi	Dominostat ± Avelumab	NCT04393753	19
First Line Systemic Therapy			
Anti-PD-1 + RT	Avelumab + PRRT/EBRT	NCT04261855	38
	Pembrolizumab ± SBRT	NCT03304639	9
Anti-PD-1 + platinum chemo	Pembrolizumab + cisplatin/ carboplatin and etoposide	NCT06086288	35
	Retifanlimab + platinum-etoposide	NCT05594290	36
Targeted Therapy			
DNA vaccine	ITI-3000	NCT05422781	6
Gene modified immune cells	aNK and ALT-803	NCT02465957	24
Surveillance Biomarkers			
Biomarkers	ctDNA + miR375	SUMMERTIME (NCT04705389)	150
Radiation Therapy			
RT vs surgery	Radical RT vs surgery	NCT05253144	64
RT	Hypofractionated RT	NCT05100095	

Abbreviations: aNK, activated NK-92 natural killer cells; CART, comprehensive ablative radiation therapy; EBRT, external beam radiation therapy; EE, estimated enrollment; PRRT, peptide receptor radionuclide therapy; RT; radiation therapy; SBRT, stereotactic body radiation.
Data from ClinicalTrials.gov.

The approach for RT in nodal disease is less well defined. Regional RT may be considered for clinically evident nodes, patients who are clinically node negative but at high risk for nodal disease, as a monotherapy for positive SLNB, or as adjuvant after lymph node dissection.[24]

In the United States, radiation monotherapy is typically reserved as palliative care in nonsurgical candidates.[24] In a systematic review of definitive RT for nonsurgical

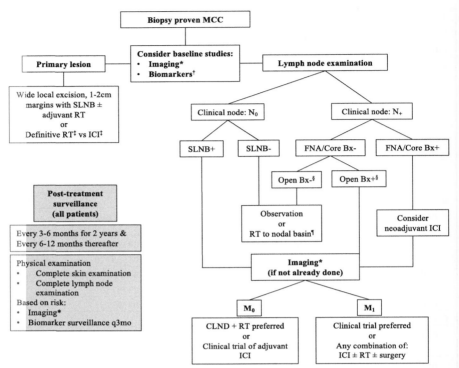

Fig. 1. MCC Treatment Algorithm. [a]PET/CT is preferred. [b]ctDNA[21,22] and AMERK[19] have demonstrated promising early results but are not yet recommended by treatment guidelines. [c]For patients ineligible for surgery. [d]If clinical suspicion remains high. [e]If high risk for false-negative SLNB. Bx, biopsy; CLND, complete lymph node dissection; FNA, fine needle aspiration; ICI, immune checkpoint inhibition; RT, radiation therapy; SLNB, sentinel lymph node biopsy.

candidates with macroscopic locoregional disease, 34.9% of patients were disease-free at final follow up.[28] MCC outcomes of definitive RT versus surgery are currently being assessed in patients without metastases beyond the regional lymph nodes (NCT05253144).

Data for RT dosing in MCC are limited and current recommendations are based on RT use in similar cancers. NCCN recommends conventionally fractionated adjuvant RT (50 Gy in 2 Gy doses) in cases with negative resection margins.[24] Single fraction (SF, 8 Gy) can be used in the palliative setting and may be an alternative to conventional dosing to decrease patient morbidity. In a retrospective study of patients with stage I/II MCC with at least one high-risk feature receiving adjuvant SF RT, no local reoccurrences were observed at a median follow up of 2.3 years.[29] The safety profile was favorable, with no side effects greater than grade 1 observed.[29] An additional hypofractionated, reduced dosing regimen using 10 fractions of 3.6 Gy is under investigation (NCT05100095).

Lymph Nodes

SLNB is recommended for all patients with MCC. Even if clinically node negative, patients still have a 30% risk of occult nodal disease.[23] In patients that are clinically node positive, a fine-needle aspiration or core biopsy is indicated. Patients with clinically enlarged nodes and negative biopsy results may still benefit from an excisional biopsy if at high risk for nodal disease. Patients with a positive FNA or core biopsy and no metastatic disease on imaging may receive a nodal dissection with or without RT.[24]

Immunotherapy

MCC is an immunogenic cancer, as demonstrated by an increased incidence in patients with immunosuppression and a dramatic response to immunotherapy.[13,30] PD-(L)1 immune checkpoint inhibitors (ICI) are recommended as a first-line (1L) treatment in locally advanced, recurrent or mMCC.[23,30] Avelumab, pembrolizumab, and retifanlimab are currently Food and Drug Administration (FDA) approved for MCC based on trial results detailed in **Table 3**. Nivolumab is not FDA approved for MCC but has been tested in clinical trials with positive results (**Table 3**). ICI immunotherapy has a similar safety profile in patients with MCC as in patients with melanoma and other solid cancers.[30]

Considerations for Selecting an Immunotherapy

The optimal first-line immunotherapy for MCC has not yet been determined as head-to-head trials are lacking. Heterogeneity in clinical trial designs limits drug comparisons. Of the landmark immunotherapy trials so far, objective response rate (ORR) ranges from 33% for second-line (2L) avelumab up to 100% for 1L nivolumab with ipilimumab (see **Table 3**). However, attempting to estimate response rates for these agents based on their small landmark studies is problematic as values often differ from real world use.

Avelumab was the first ICI approved for MCC and it also has the most real-world data reported. Prior to avelumab's FDA approval, a worldwide expanded access program allowed for the compassionate use of the drug outside of clinical trials. In a global cohort with 240 patients, real-world ORR (rwORR) was 46.7% and was consistent across 1L (n = 15) and 2L (n = 225) subgroups. In patients with a response, median duration of treatment was 7.9 months.[31] Several avelumab-treated cohorts in the United States have been studied with rwORR ranging between 53.57% and 75.3% in the 1L setting and between 35.0% and 64.7% in the 2L setting.[32–34] Overall, survival has also been reported in cohorts from England, Germany, Israel, and Japan, ranging from 13.3 to 52.0 months for patients with stage III and IV disease receiving 1L or 2L therapy.[35–38] No new safety signals arose in the real-world studies. These studies suggest a more favorable ORR for avelumab than was seen in the JAVELIN trial.

Significantly less real-world MCC data are available on other immunotherapies. Two cohort studies examine the ORR to anti-PD(L)-1 ICI overall. In 36 patients treated at the Moffit Cancer Center with various regimens of pembrolizumab, avelumab, nivolumab, or combination therapy, rwORR was 44%.[39] Notably, many patients received other systemic therapies prior to ICI. In 18 patients treated at 3 German clinical centers, 6 (33%) received nivolumab with a ORR of 43%, and 8 received pembrolizumab with a ORR of 29%.[40] In a case series of 7 patients receiving 1L pembrolizumab, ORR was 66.7%. At a median follow up of 16.5 months, 3 out of 4 responses were durable.[41] Moving forward, we hope to see real-world efficacy and safety data on larger cohorts of patients treated with pembrolizumab, retifanlimab, or nivolumab.

Besides ORR, there are many other factors to consider when choosing an ICI. In terms of safety, side effect profiles are similar across the ICI agents and consistent with what is expected for the PD-(L)1 inhibitor class. An exception is avelumab, which displays a higher incidence of low-grade infusion reactions, with 73.5% (n = 25) of

Table 3
Results of the landmark immunotherapy clinical trials for Merkel cell carcinoma

Trial	Overview	Participants (N)	ORR (%)	OS	Median DOR
JAVELIN A[55,56]	2L avelumab for advanced chemo refractory MCC	88	33.0	26.0% (5 y)	NR
JAVELIN B[42]	1L avelumab for treatment naïve mMCC	116	39.7	20.3 m (median)	18.2 m
KEYNOTE-017	1L pembrolizumab for advanced unresectable MCC	50	58.0[57]	59.4% (3 y)[58]	NR[59]
PODIUM-201[60,a]	1L retifanlimab for advanced/metastatic chemo naïve MCC	65	46.2	NR	NR
CheckMate 358[61]	1L nivolumab vs nivolumab + ipilimumab in recurrent or mMCC	68	60.0 N vs 58.1 N/I	80.7 m N vs 29.8 m N/I (median)	60.6 m N vs 25.9 m N/I
Kim et al,[48] 2022	Nivolumab + ipilimumab ± SBRT in advanced ICI naïve MCC	24	100 N/I vs 100 N/I + SBRT	NR	NE
	Nivolumab + ipilimumab ± SBRT in advanced MCC with previous ICI	26	42.0 N/I vs 21.0 N/I + SBRT	14.9 m vs 9.7 m (median)	15 m vs 5 m

Abbreviations: 1L, first line; 2L, second line; DOR, duration of response; ICI, immune checkpoint inhibitors; m, months; mMCC, metastatic Merkle cell carcinoma; N, nivolumab; N/I, nivolumab and ipilimumab; NE, not estimable; NR, not reached; ORR, objective response rate; OS, overall survival; SBRT, stereotactic body radiation therapy.

[a] Updated results on the full cohort of 101 patients were presented at the European Society for Medical Oncology Annual Meeting in 2023 and will be published shortly.

patients receiving 1L therapy experiencing reactions upon their first infusion.[42] Another difference between approved ICI drugs is dosing schedules. Avelumab is administered every 2 weeks, with pembrolizumab administered every 3 weeks and retifanlimab administered every 4 weeks.

Adjuvant and Neoadjuvant Immunotherapy

With the high therapeutic efficacy of ICIs in treating advanced MCC, there is considerable interest in the potential of neoadjuvant and adjuvant immunotherapy to reduce recurrence risk in patients with resectable disease. SITC guidelines recommend patients with resectable MCC at high risk for recurrence be enrolled in clinical trials of neoadjuvant or adjuvant immunotherapy.[30] Neoadjuvant immunotherapy is theorized to stimulate more robust antitumor T-cell responses due to more available tumor antigen, and it has the potential to decrease surgical morbidity by reducing tumor size before resection. On the other hand, surgical resection is delayed by neoadjuvant therapy, which may allow for disease progression to the point where surgery is no longer possible. Serious adverse events related to neoadjuvant therapy could potentially delay surgery even further.[43] Adjuvant therapy is thought to decrease disease recurrence by eliminating micrometastases after surgery and may counter the postoperative immunosuppressive environment.[44] Given the positive results of neoadjuvant and adjuvant ICI use in high-risk resectable melanoma,[45] it is reasonable to wonder whether a similar clinical benefit can be observed in MCC.

Nivolumab has been tested as a monotherapy for resectable MCC in both the neoadjuvant and adjuvant setting. In the CheckMate 358 trial, 36 patients with stage IIA to IV MCC received neoadjuvant nivolumab prior to surgery and 47.2% achieved a pathologic complete response.[46] Nivolumab was also tested in the adjuvant setting for completely resected MCC lesions of any stage. In 118 patients who received adjuvant nivolumab, interim data analysis demonstrated DFS rates of 85% at 12 months and 77% at 24 months, compared to 77% at 12 months and 73% at 24 months for in the observation group. Overall survival data were not mature, and the final survival analysis is pending.[47]

Further research on neoadjuvant or adjuvant ICI use in resectable MCC is needed before changes are made to clinical practice. Several ongoing prospective clinical trials address this question. Adjuvant nivolumab versus nivolumab with ipilimumab is under investigation for high risk or node positive MCC (NCT03798639). Adjuvant avelumab is being assessed in stage III (NCT03271372) and stage I to III MCC (NCT04291885). Pembrolizumab is under investigation in the adjuvant setting for patients with stage I to III MCC (NCT03712605) in the neoadjuvant–adjuvant setting alone (NCT05496036) and in combination with lenvatinib, a VEGR receptor inhibitor (NCT04869137). Neoadjuvant retifanlimab (NCT05594290) and cemiplimab (NCT04975152) are being tested as well.

Patients Refractory to PD-(L)1 Inhibition

Although immunotherapy is highly efficacious, almost half of patients with advanced MCC have tumors that are refractory to 1L anti-PD-(L)1 drugs. There are few effective therapeutic options for these patients, as switching from one anti-PD-(L)1 therapy to another is unlikely to be beneficial.[30] The addition of anti-CTLA-4 therapy to anti-PD-(L)1 therapy is a promising option. Kim and colleagues demonstrated an ORR of 31% in 26 patients with MCC and previous ICI who were treated with 2L nivolumab and ipilimumab, with no benefit from the addition of SBRT.[48] Additional retrospective studies have reported response rates of 31% and 50% to combination nivolumab and ipilimumab therapy for MCC refractory to prior anti-PD-(L)1 therapy.[49,50] Notably, patients had heterogenous treatment histories, with some having additional systemic therapies in between their initial anti-PD(L)1 treatment and the combination therapy.

Advancing effective treatments for anti-PD(L)1 resistant MCC is a key focus in current clinical trials. Active studies focus on the addition of new RT regimens (NCT04792073, NCT05583708), targeted therapies (NCT05947500, NCT03787602, NCT03787602), triplet immunotherapy (NCT06056895), and genetically modified immune cells (NCT03747484) (see **Table 2**).

When to Discontinue Immunotherapy

The optimal duration of ICI therapy for MCC remains unclear. Retrospective studies have investigated the duration of response after ICI discontinuation for reasons other than disease progression. Stege and colleagues demonstrated a 60% rate of relapse after ICI discontinuation in 20 patients with mMCC with a median ICI duration of 10 months.[51] In a more recent study by Weppler and colleagues of 40 patients with mMCC and a median ICI duration of 13.5 months, 35% of patients relapsed at a median follow up of 12.3 months.[52] Neither study demonstrated a relationship between duration of initial ICI and response durability. However, both studies noted a decreased risk of disease progression in those with a complete response.

Zijilker and colleagues recently published the first study with a uniform protocol for discontinuation of ICI in MCC. Sixty-five patients with mMCC were treated with avelumab for 1 year if complete response was observed on FDG-PET/CT or until unacceptable toxicity. Of the 25 patients with a complete response, only 2 (8%) relapsed.[53] In contrast, in the preceding retrospective Stege and colleagues and Weppler and colleagues studies, complete responders relapsed at a rate of 33% and 26% respectively.[51,52] However, these studies did not require PET/CT for confirmation of complete response and allowed multiple ICI agents. Another recent study investigated reducing ICI frequency to every 3 months after initial disease control for metastatic melanoma and MCC. Only 5 patients with MCC were included and 100% experienced a 36 month progression-free survival rate after reduced frequency dosing.[54]

Based on these studies, degree of response, rather than treatment duration, seems to be an important predictor of disease progression off ICI. In patients with PET/CT confirmed complete response, a year of ICI may be sufficient.[53] Alternative dosing regimens after complete or durable partial responses should be explored. As indefinite ICI is impractical and often unfeasible, larger studies investigating the optimal duration of ICI are required.

Chemotherapy

Historically, chemotherapies were the primary systemic treatments for advanced MCC. Chemotherapy demonstrated response rates comparable to those seen in immunotherapy. Yet responses were not durable, with a median duration of response ranging from 2 to 9 months.[24] As a result, chemotherapy is now reserved as a palliative treatment option or for patients who are ineligible for immunotherapy.[5]

CLINICS CARE POINTS

> - An MCC diagnosis is confirmed via histopathology, with CK20 immunostaining in a perinuclear dot pattern being most specific.
> - All eligible patients should receive an SLNB and most patients should receive PET/CT imaging in their initial staging workup.

- AMERK and ctDNA testing upon diagnosis can be tracked serially to assess tumor burden and monitor for recurrence.
- Locoregional MCC is typically treated with surgical resection and adjuvant RT. Immunotherapy is the mainstay of treatment for advanced disease.
- Multidisciplinary management and clinical trials are preferred for patients with MCC.

DISCLOSURE

The authors have nothing to disclose.

FUNDING

This work was supported by the National Institutes of Health (NIH) Intramural Research Program, National Institute of Arthritis and Musculoskeletal and Skin Diseases (NIAMS), grant ZIA AR041223 to IB. The opinions expressed in this article are those the authors and do not reflect the view of the National Institutes of Health, the Department of Health and Human Services, or the United States government.

REFERENCES

1. Becker JC, Stang A, DeCaprio JA, et al. Merkel cell carcinoma. Nat Rev Dis Primers 2017;3:17077.
2. Paulson KG, Park SY, Vandeven NA, et al. Merkel cell carcinoma: current US incidence and projected increases based on changing demographics. J Am Acad Dermatol 2018;78(3):457–63.e2.
3. Mohsen ST, Price EL, Chan AW, et al. Incidence, mortality, and survival of merkel cell carcinoma: a systematic review of population based-studies. Br J Dermatol 2023. https://doi.org/10.1093/bjd/ljad404.
4. Mohsin N, Martin MR, Reed DJ, et al. Differences in merkel cell carcinoma presentation and outcomes among racial and ethnic groups. JAMA Dermatol 2023;159(5): 536–40.
5. Harms PW, Harms KL, Moore PS, et al. The biology and treatment of Merkel cell carcinoma: current understanding and research priorities. Nat Rev Clin Oncol 2018;15(12):763–76.
6. Lilo MT, Chen Y, LeBlanc RE. INSM1 is more sensitive and interpretable than conventional immunohistochemical stains used to diagnose merkel cell carcinoma. Am J Surg Pathol 2018;42(11):1541–8.
7. Cassler NM, Merrill D, Bichakjian CK, et al. Merkel cell carcinoma therapeutic update. Curr Treat Options Oncol 2016;17(7):36.
8. Amin MB, Edge SB, Greene FL. In: Merkel Cell Carcinoma. In: AJCC Cancer Staging Manual. 8th edition. Cham, Switzerland: Springer International Publishing; 2017. p. 549–61.
9. Singh N, Alexander NA, Lachance K, et al. Clinical benefit of baseline imaging in Merkel cell carcinoma: Analysis of 584 patients. J Am Acad Dermatol 2021;84(2): 330–9.
10. George A, Girault S, Testard A, et al. The impact of (18)F-FDG-PET/CT on merkel cell carcinoma management: a retrospective study of 66 scans from a single institution. Nucl Med Commun 2014;35(3):282–90.
11. Hawryluk EB, O'Regan KN, Sheehy N, et al. Positron emission tomography/ computed tomography imaging in Merkel cell carcinoma: a study of 270 scans

in 97 patients at the Dana-Farber/Brigham and Women's Cancer Center. J Am Acad Dermatol 2013;68(4):592–9.

12. Harms KL, Zhao L, Johnson B, et al. Virus-positive merkel cell carcinoma is an independent prognostic group with distinct predictive biomarkers. Clin Cancer Res 2021;27(9):2494–504.

13. Ma JE, Brewer JD. Merkel cell carcinoma in immunosuppressed patients. Cancers (Basel) 2014;6(3):1328–50.

14. Paulson KG, Iyer JG, Simonson WT, et al. CD8+ lymphocyte intratumoral infiltration as a stage-independent predictor of Merkel cell carcinoma survival: a population-based study. Am J Clin Pathol 2014;142(4):452–8.

15. Miller NJ, Church CD, Dong L, et al. Tumor-infiltrating merkel cell polyomavirus-specific t cells are diverse and associated with improved patient survival. Cancer Immunol Res 2017;5(2):137–47.

16. Lipson EJ, Vincent JG, Loyo M, et al. PD-L1 expression in the Merkel cell carcinoma microenvironment: association with inflammation, Merkel cell polyomavirus and overall survival. Cancer Immunol Res 2013;1(1):54–63.

17. McEvoy AM, Hippe DS, Lachance K, et al. Merkel cell carcinoma recurrence risk estimation is improved by integrating factors beyond cancer stage: A multivariable model and web-based calculator. J Am Acad Dermatol 2024;90(3):569–76.

18. Paulson KG, Carter JJ, Johnson LG, et al. Antibodies to merkel cell polyomavirus T antigen oncoproteins reflect tumor burden in merkel cell carcinoma patients. Cancer Res 2010;70(21):8388–97.

19. Paulson KG, Lewis CW, Redman MW, et al. Viral oncoprotein antibodies as a marker for recurrence of Merkel cell carcinoma: A prospective validation study. Cancer 2017;123(8):1464–74.

20. Prakash V, Gao L, Park SJ. Evolving applications of circulating tumor DNA in merkel cell carcinoma. Cancers 2023;15(3). https://doi.org/10.3390/cancers15030609.

21. Park SJ, Kannan A, Harris JP, et al. Circulating tumor DNA as a predictive biomarker in Merkel cell carcinoma. J Am Acad Dermatol 2022;87(5):1209–11.

22. Akaike T, So N, Hippe DS, et al. The relationship between circulating tumor DNA with Merkel cell carcinoma tumor burden and detection of recurrence. J Clin Oncol 2022;40(16_suppl):9566.

23. Gauci M-L, Aristei C, Becker JC, et al. Diagnosis and treatment of Merkel cell carcinoma: European consensus-based interdisciplinary guideline – Update 2022. European Journal of Cancer 2022;171:203–31.

24. NCCN Guidelines Version 1.2023 Merkel Cell Carcinoma. National Comprehensive Cancer Network. Available at: https://www.nccn.org/docs/default-source/business-policy/nccn-referencing-guidance.pdf. Accessed September 4, 2023.

25. Moore KJ, Thakuria M, Ruiz ES. No difference in survival for primary cutaneous Merkel cell carcinoma after Mohs micrographic surgery and wide local excision. J Am Acad Dermatol 2023;89(2):254–60.

26. Wong WG, Stahl K, Olecki EJ, et al. Survival benefit of guideline-concordant postoperative radiation for local merkel cell carcinoma. J Surg Res 2021;266:168–79.

27. Bierma M, Goff PH, Hippe D, et al. Post-operative radiation therapy is indicated for "low-risk" pathologic stage I Merkel cell carcinoma of the head and neck region but not for other locations. Advances in Radiation Oncology 2023;101364. https://doi.org/10.1016/j.adro.2023.101364.

28. Gunaratne DA, Howle JR, Veness MJ. Definitive radiotherapy for Merkel cell carcinoma confers clinically meaningful in-field locoregional control: A review and analysis of the literature. J Am Acad Dermatol 2017;77(1):142–148 e1.

29. Goff PH, Huynh ET, Lachance K, et al. Efficacy of single-fraction postoperative radiotherapy in resected, early-stage merkel cell carcinoma with high-risk features. Int J Radiat Oncol Biol Phys 2023;117(2):e298.
30. Silk AW, Barker CA, Bhatia S, et al. Society for immunotherapy of cancer (SITC) clinical practice guideline on immunotherapy for the treatment of nonmelanoma skin cancer. J Immunother Cancer 2022;10(7). https://doi.org/10.1136/jitc-2021-004434.
31. Walker JW, Lebbe C, Grignani G, et al. Efficacy and safety of avelumab treatment in patients with metastatic Merkel cell carcinoma: experience from a global expanded access program. J Immunother Cancer 2020;8(1). https://doi.org/10.1136/jitc-2019-000313.
32. Bhatia S, Nghiem P, Veeranki SP, et al. Real-world clinical outcomes with avelumab in patients with Merkel cell carcinoma treated in the USA: a multicenter chart review study. J Immunother Cancer 2022;10(8). https://doi.org/10.1136/jitc-2022-004904.
33. Cowey CL, Liu FX, Kim R, et al. Real-world clinical outcomes with first-line avelumab in locally advanced/metastatic Merkel cell carcinoma in the USA: SPEAR-Merkel. Future Oncol 2021;17(18):2339–50.
34. Miller DM, Wright K, Silk AW, et al. A dual institution real-world study of avelumab for advanced Merkel cell carcinoma. J Clin Oncol 2023;41(16_suppl):e21514.
35. Knott C, Mahmoudpour S, Kearney M, et al. 1147P First-line treatment (tx) patterns and overall survival (OS) of patients (pts) with advanced Merkel cell carcinoma (aMCC) in England from 2013-2022: Results of a nationwide observational cohort study. Ann Oncol 2023;34:S686–7.
36. Becker JC, Mahmoudpour S, Schadendorf D, et al. 1145P Clinical characteristics and survival of patients with advanced Merkel cell carcinoma (MCC) treated with avelumab: Analysis of a prospective German MCC registry (MCC TRIM). Ann Oncol 2023;34:S685–6.
37. Averbuch I, Stoff R, Miodovnik M, et al. Avelumab for the treatment of locally advanced or metastatic Merkel cell carcinoma-A multicenter real-world experience in Israel. Cancer Med 2023;12(11):12065–70.
38. Yamazaki N, Kiyohara Y, Sato M, et al. 407P A post-marketing surveillance of the real-world safety and effectiveness of avelumab in patients with curatively unresectable Merkel cell carcinoma in Japan. Ann Oncol 2022;33:S1601–2.
39. Knepper TC, Montesion M, Russell JS, et al. The genomic landscape of merkel cell carcinoma and clinicogenomic biomarkers of response to immune checkpoint inhibitor therapy. Clin Cancer Res 2019;25(19):5961–71.
40. Spassova I, Ugurel S, Terheyden P, et al. Predominance of central memory t cells with high t-cell receptor repertoire diversity is associated with response to PD-1/PD-L1 inhibition in merkel cell carcinoma. Clin Cancer Res 2020;26(9):2257–67.
41. Bystrup Boyles T, Schødt M, Hendel HW, et al. Pembrolizumab as first line treatment of Merkel cell carcinoma patients - a case series of patients with various comorbidities. Acta Oncol 2020;59(7):793–6.
42. D'Angelo SP, Lebbé C, Mortier L, et al. First-line avelumab in a cohort of 116 patients with metastatic Merkel cell carcinoma (JAVELIN Merkel 200): primary and biomarker analyses of a phase II study. J Immunother Cancer 2021;9(7). https://doi.org/10.1136/jitc-2021-002646.
43. Lee AY, Brady MS. Neoadjuvant immunotherapy for melanoma. J Surg Oncol 2021;123(3):782–8.
44. Tang WF, Ye HY, Tang X, et al. Adjuvant immunotherapy in early-stage resectable non-small cell lung cancer: A new milestone. Front Oncol 2023;13:1063183.

45. Patel SP, Othus M, Chen Y, et al. Neoadjuvant-adjuvant or adjuvant-only pembro-lizumab in advanced melanoma. N Engl J Med 2023;388(9):813–23.

46. Topalian SL, Bhatia S, Amin A, et al. Neoadjuvant nivolumab for patients with resectable merkel cell carcinoma in the checkmate 358 trial. J Clin Oncol 2020; 38(22):2476–87.

47. Becker JC, Ugurel S, Leiter U, et al. Adjuvant immunotherapy with nivolumab versus observation in completely resected Merkel cell carcinoma (ADMEC-O): disease-free survival results from a randomised, open-label, phase 2 trial. Lancet 2023;402(10404):798–808.

48. Kim S, Wuthrick E, Blakaj D, et al. Combined nivolumab and ipilimumab with or without stereotactic body radiation therapy for advanced Merkel cell carcinoma: a randomised, open label, phase 2 trial. Lancet 2022;400(10357):1008–19.

49. Glutsch V, Schummer P, Kneitz H, et al. Ipilimumab plus nivolumab in avelumab-refractory Merkel cell carcinoma: a multicenter study of the prospective skin cancer registry ADOREG. J Immunother Cancer 2022;10(11). https://doi.org/10.1136/jitc-2022-005930.

50. LoPiccolo J, Schollenberger MD, Dakhil S, et al. Rescue therapy for patients with anti-PD-1-refractory Merkel cell carcinoma: a multicenter, retrospective case series. J Immunother Cancer 2019;7(1):170.

51. Stege HM, Haist M, Schultheis S, et al. Response durability after cessation of immune checkpoint inhibitors in patients with metastatic Merkel cell carcinoma: a retrospective multicenter DeCOG study. Cancer Immunol Immunother 2021; 70(11):3313–22.

52. Weppler AM, Da Meda L, Pires da Silva I, et al. Durability of response to immune checkpoint inhibitors in metastatic Merkel cell carcinoma after treatment cessation. Eur J Cancer 2023;183:109–18.

53. Zijlker LP, Levy S, Wolters W, et al. Avelumab treatment for patients with metastatic Merkel cell carcinoma can be safely stopped after 1 year and a PET/CT-confirmed complete response. Cancer 2023. https://doi.org/10.1002/cncr.35050.

54. Tachiki LML, Hippe DS, Williams Silva K, et al. Extended duration of treatment using reduced-frequency dosing of anti-PD-1 therapy in patients with advanced melanoma and Merkel cell carcinoma. Cancer Immunol Immunother 2023;72(11): 3839–50.

55. Kaufman HL, Russell JS, Hamid O, et al. Updated efficacy of avelumab in patients with previously treated metastatic Merkel cell carcinoma after ≥1 year of follow-up: JAVELIN Merkel 200, a phase 2 clinical trial. J Immunother Cancer 2018;6(1):7.

56. D'Angelo SP, Bhatia S, Brohl AS, et al. Avelumab in patients with previously treated metastatic Merkel cell carcinoma (JAVELIN Merkel 200): updated overall survival data after >5 years of follow-up. ESMO Open 2021;6(6):100290.

57. Nghiem PT, Bhatia S, Lipson EJ, et al. PD-1 blockade with pembrolizumab in advanced merkel-cell carcinoma. N Engl J Med 2016;374(26):2542–52.

58. Nghiem P, Bhatia S, Lipson EJ, et al. Three-year survival, correlates and salvage therapies in patients receiving first-line pembrolizumab for advanced Merkel cell carcinoma. J Immunother Cancer 2021;9(4). https://doi.org/10.1136/jitc-2021-002478.

59. Nghiem P, Bhatia S, Lipson EJ, et al. Durable tumor regression and overall survival in patients with advanced merkel cell carcinoma receiving pembrolizumab as first-line therapy. J Clin Oncol 2019;37(9):693–702.

60. Grignani G, Rutkowski P, Lebbe C, et al. A phase 2 study of retifanlimab in patients with advanced or metastatic merkel cell carcinoma (Mcc) (Pod1um-201). Journal for Immunotherapy of Cancer 2021;9:A574–5.
61. Bhatia S, Topalian SL, Sharfman WH, et al. Non-comparative, open-label, international, multicenter phase I/II study of nivolumab (NIVO) ± ipilimumab (IPI) in patients (pts) with recurrent/metastatic merkel cell carcinoma (MCC) (CheckMate 358). J Clin Oncol 2023;41(16_suppl):9506.

UNITED STATES POSTAL SERVICE® Statement of Ownership, Management, and Circulation
(All Periodicals Publications Except Requester Publications)

1. Publication Title	2. Publication Number	3. Filing Date
HEMATOLOGY/ONCOLOGY CLINICS OF NORTH AMERICA	002 – 473	9/18/2024

4. Issue Frequency	5. Number of Issues Published Annually	6. Annual Subscription Price
FEB, APR, JUN, AUG, OCT, DEC	6	$498.00

7. Complete Mailing Address of Known Office of Publication (Not printer) (Street, city, county, state, and ZIP+4®)

ELSEVIER INC.
230 Park Avenue, Suite 800
New York, NY 10169

Contact Person
Malathi Samayan

Telephone (Include area code)
91-44-4299-4507

8. Complete Mailing Address of Headquarters or General Business Office of Publisher (Not printer)

ELSEVIER INC.
230 Park Avenue, Suite 800
New York, NY 10169

9. Full Names and Complete Mailing Addresses of Publisher, Editor, and Managing Editor (Do not leave blank)

Publisher (Name and complete mailing address)

Dolores Meloni, ELSEVIER INC.
1600 JOHN F KENNEDY BLVD. SUITE 1600
PHILADELPHIA, PA 19103-2899

Editor (Name and complete mailing address)

STACY EASTMAN, ELSEVIER INC.
1600 JOHN F KENNEDY BLVD. SUITE 1600
PHILADELPHIA, PA 19103-2899

Managing Editor (Name and complete mailing address)

PATRICK MANLEY, ELSEVIER INC.
1600 JOHN F KENNEDY BLVD. SUITE 1600
PHILADELPHIA, PA 19103-2899

10. Owner (Do not leave blank. If the publication is owned by a corporation, give the name and address of the corporation immediately followed by the names and addresses of all stockholders owning or holding 1 percent or more of the total amount of stock. If not owned by a corporation, give the names and addresses of the individual owners. If owned by a partnership or other unincorporated firm, give its name and address as well as those of each individual owner. If the publication is published by a nonprofit organization, give its name and address.)

Full Name	Complete Mailing Address
WHOLLY OWNED SUBSIDIARY OF REED/ELSEVIER, US HOLDINGS	1600 JOHN F KENNEDY BLVD. SUITE 1600 PHILADELPHIA, PA 19103-2899

11. Known Bondholders, Mortgagees, and Other Security Holders Owning or Holding 1 Percent or More of Total Amount of Bonds, Mortgages, or Other Securities. If none, check box ▶ ☐ None

Full Name	Complete Mailing Address
N/A	

12. Tax Status (For completion by nonprofit organizations authorized to mail at nonprofit rates) (Check one)
The purpose, function, and nonprofit status of this organization and the exempt status for federal income tax purposes:
☒ Has Not Changed During Preceding 12 Months
☐ Has Changed During Preceding 12 Months (Publisher must submit explanation of change with this statement)

PS Form 3526, July 2014 [Page 1 of 4 (see instructions page 4)]   PSN: 7530-01-000-9931   PRIVACY NOTICE: See our privacy policy on www.usps.com.

13. Publication Title	14. Issue Date for Circulation Data Below
HEMATOLOGY/ONCOLOGY CLINICS OF NORTH AMERICA	AUGUST 2024

15. Extent and Nature of Circulation			Average No. Copies Each Issue During Preceding 12 Months	No. Copies of Single Issue Published Nearest to Filing Date
a. Total Number of Copies (Net press run)			109	92
b. Paid Circulation (By Mail and Outside the Mail)	(1)	Mailed Outside-County Paid Subscriptions Stated on PS Form 3541 (Include paid distribution above nominal rate, advertiser's proof copies, and exchange copies)	57	47
	(2)	Mailed In-County Paid Subscriptions Stated on PS Form 3541 (Include paid distribution above nominal rate, advertiser's proof copies, and exchange copies)	0	0
	(3)	Paid Distribution Outside the Mails Including Sales Through Dealers and Carriers, Street Vendors, Counter Sales, and Other Paid Distribution Outside USPS®	34	28
	(4)	Paid Distribution by Other Classes of Mail Through the USPS (e.g., First-Class Mail®)	7	6
c. Total Paid Distribution (Sum of 15b (1), (2), (3), and (4))		▶	98	81
d. Free or Nominal Rate Distribution (By Mail and Outside the Mail)	(1)	Free or Nominal Rate Outside-County Copies Included on PS Form 3541	9	10
	(2)	Free or Nominal Rate In-County Copies Included on PS Form 3541	0	0
	(3)	Free or Nominal Rate Copies Mailed at Other Classes Through the USPS (e.g., First-Class Mail)	0	0
	(4)	Free or Nominal Rate Distribution Outside the Mail (Carriers or other means)	1	1
e. Total Free or Nominal Rate Distribution (Sum of 15d (1), (2), (3) and (4))		▶	10	11
f. Total Distribution (Sum of 15c and 15e)		▶	109	92
g. Copies not Distributed (See Instructions to Publishers #4 (page 83))		▶	0	0
h. Total (Sum of 15f and g)		▶	109	92
i. Percent Paid (15c divided by 15f times 100)			90.63%	88.04%

* If you are claiming electronic copies, go to line 16 on page 3. If you are not claiming electronic copies, skip to line 17 on page 3.

16. Electronic Copy Circulation	Average No. Copies Each Issue During Preceding 12 Months	No. Copies of Single Issue Published Nearest to Filing Date
a. Paid Electronic Copies ▶		
b. Total Paid Print Copies (Line 15c) + Paid Electronic Copies (Line 16a) ▶		
c. Total Print Distribution (Line 15f) + Paid Electronic Copies (Line 16a) ▶		
d. Percent Paid (Both Print & Electronic Copies) (16b divided by 16c × 100) ▶		

☒ I certify that 50% of all my distributed copies (electronic and print) are paid above a nominal price.

17. Publication of Statement of Ownership
☒ If the publication is a general publication, publication of this statement is required. Will be printed
in the __OCTOBER 2024__ issue of this publication.   ☐ Publication not required.

18. Signature and Title of Editor, Publisher, Business Manager, or Owner	Date
Malathi Samayan - Distribution Controller *Malathi Samayan*	9/18/2024

I certify that all information furnished on this form is true and complete. I understand that anyone who furnishes false or misleading information on this form or who omits material or information requested on the form may be subject to criminal sanctions (including fines and imprisonment) and/or civil sanctions (including civil penalties).

PS Form 3526, July 2014 (Page 3 of 4)   PSN: 7530-01-000-9931   PRIVACY NOTICE: See our privacy policy on www.usps.com.

Moving?

Make sure your subscription moves with you!

To notify us of your new address, find your **Clinics Account Number** (located on your mailing label above your name), and contact customer service at:

Email: journalscustomerservice-usa@elsevier.com

800-654-2452 (subscribers in the U.S. & Canada)
314-447-8871 (subscribers outside of the U.S. & Canada)

Fax number: 314-447-8029

Elsevier Health Sciences Division
Subscription Customer Service
3251 Riverport Lane
Maryland Heights, MO 63043

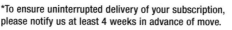

*To ensure uninterrupted delivery of your subscription, please notify us at least 4 weeks in advance of move.

ELSEVIER

Printed and bound by CPI Group (UK) Ltd, Croydon, CR0 4YY

08/05/2025

01864750-0004